A Special Issue of
Neuropsychological Rehabilitation

Cognitive Rehabilitation in Dementia

Edited by

Linda Clare
University College London, UK

and

Robert T. Woods
University of Wales, UK

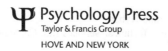

Psychology Press
Taylor & Francis Group

HOVE AND NEW YORK

First published in 2001 by Psychology Press Ltd
27 Church Road, Hove, East Sussex BN3 2FA

Simultaneously published in the USA and Canada
by Psychology Press
711 Third Avenue, New York, NY 10017

First issued in paperback 2015

Psychology Press is an imprint of the Taylor & Francis Group, an informa business

British Library Cataloguing in Publication Data
A catalogue record for this book is available from the British Library

ISBN 13: 978-1-138-87784-9 (pbk)
ISBN 13: 978-1-84169-912-7 (hbk)

ISSN 0960-2011

Cover design by Kate Hybert
Typeset by Quorum Technical Services Ltd, Cheltenham, UK

Contents*

---

* This book is also a special issue of the journal *Neuropsychological
Rehabilitation* which forms Issues 3 and 4 of Volume 11 (2001) and so begins
on page 193.

Editorial:
A role for cognitive rehabilitation in dementia care

Linda Clare

University College London, UK

Bob Woods

University of Wales, Bangor, UK

The importance of neuropsychological assesssment in establishing the diagnosis of dementia is widely acknowledged. In contrast, psychological aspects of intervention, including cognitive rehabilitation approaches, are all too often ignored within the framework of a largely medical approach to dementia (see, for example, Setting New Standards in the NHS Consensus Panel, 1997). It has been observed, however, that the psychological needs of the person with dementia are of paramount importance (British Psychological Society Professional Affairs Board, 1994).

In line with this view, researchers are starting to recognise the relevance of cognitive rehabilitation for people with dementia (e.g., Camp, 1998; Camp & Mattern, 1999). This special issue brings together a collection of papers by leading researchers in the dementia field that demonstrates the range and scope of the innovative research currently being undertaken in the area of cognitive rehabilitation, and reports new developments and recent findings.

Defining rehabilitation as "a process of active change" aimed at enabling people who are disabled by injury or disease to "achieve an optimal level of physical, psychological, and social function" (McLellan, 1991, p. 785) implies a focus on maximising functioning across a whole range of areas including physical health, psychological well-being, living skills, and social

Correspondence should be sent to Linda Clare, Sub-department of Clinical Health Psychology, University College London, Gower Street, London WC1E 6BT, UK (email: l.clare@ucl.ac.uk).

relationships. Such an approach is just as important for people with dementia and other progressive disorders as it is for people with non-progressive acquired brain injury. A firm theoretical basis for the application of rehabilitation approaches in dementia is provided by the development of alternatives to the medical model of dementia, such as the dialectical model of Kitwood (1997) and the social constructionist model of Sabat (Sabat, 1994; 1995; Sabat & Harré, 1992; Sabat, Wiggs, & Pinizzotto, 1984). These models clearly signal the need for a biopsychosocial approach to dementia care that aims to address the needs of people with dementia and their carers, taking into account the influence of biology, individual psychology, and social environment. Rehabilitation, in this context, provides a unifying core framework for conceptualising and developing interventions for people with dementia (Cohen & Eisdorfer, 1986).

The focus of rehabilitation will necessarily differ according to the needs of the individual and family, and according to the type and severity of dementia. By definition, however, dementia necessarily affects the cognitive domain. This means that cognitive rehabilitation, in the sense outlined by Wilson (1997), is particularly relevant:

"Any intervention strategy or technique which intends to enable clients or patients, and their families, to live with, manage, by-pass, reduce or come to terms with deficits. . ."

The aims of cognitive rehabilitation for the person with dementia include optimising functioning and well-being, minimising the risk of excess disability, and preventing the development of a "malignant social psychology" (Kitwood, 1997) within the person's family system and social environment. Compensatory models (e.g., Cottrell & Schulz, 1993; Hagberg, 1997; Woods & Britton, 1985) suggest that interventions should aim to enhance self-efficacy and coping skills, combat threats to self-esteem, and help the person make the best possible use of individual resources. These resources include the preserved capacity for a degree of learning and behavioural change, provided that appropriate support is available. However, the challenge of optimising function and well-being should not be underestimated in the context of disorders where progression of neuropathological damage is commonly the expectation. Rehabilitation approaches in this field have to be flexible and responsive to changes in the person's condition, and short-term effectiveness may be an adequate outcome. The advent of anti-dementia drugs by no means obviates the need for cognitive rehabilitation. The impact of pharmacological approaches for the forseeable future is likely to be partial and they will not be applicable in many cases; in addition there are possibilities of combined cognitive and pharmacological approaches to be explored.

As a newly developing area of research, cognitive rehabilitation requires the elaboration of theoretical and conceptual frameworks, the development of improved measures for assessment and outcome evaluation, the availability of effective rehabilitation methods, an understanding of the factors that influence the outcome of interventions, clear evidence of both effectiveness and the longer-term impact of gains, and a commitment to ensure that effective interventions are disseminated and implemented in standard clinical settings. While the main emphasis is on the development and evaluation of effective rehabilitation methods, the papers presented in this issue address each of these areas.

Issues of assessment and outcome evaluation are introduced with an opinion piece by Una Holden that argues strongly for a person-centred approach to assessment aimed at identifying individual strengths and needs. Janet Cockburn and Janet Keene explore ways of identifying preserved memory skills where memory impairments on standardised tests are severe, while Caroline Selai and colleagues present an innovative method for evaluating quality of life in dementia in which assessments are made in relation to areas identified as important by the individual.

The development and evaluation of rehabilitation methods is explored in a variety of ways. Stephanie Moore and colleagues describe a group programme incorporating the "novel event technique", Orazio Zanetti and colleagues focus on making use of preserved procedural memory, Sharon Arkin presents results from a multi-component elder rehabilitation programme, Mary and Margaret Quayhagen report new data from a family-based intervention, and Barbara Romero and Michael Wenz describe outcome data from a milieu programme based on self-maintenance therapy. Mike Bird advocates strongly for the use of cognitive rehabilitation techniques as a means of dealing with "problem" behaviours in residential care settings, while Aimee Spector and colleagues describe the implementation of an evidence-based cognitive stimulation programme in residential homes, and Laura Hoerster and colleagues report on the use of memory aids to enhance communication between residents and care staff. Relearning of semantic knowledge in fronto-temporal dementia, and implications for rehabilitation, are discussed by Kim Graham and colleagues.

Factors that influence the outcome of cognitive rehabilitation interventions are considered by Deborah Koltai and colleagues, who found that awareness of memory functioning was an important determinant of beneficial outcome for the participants in their memory group. Linda Clare and colleagues present evidence for long-term maintenance of treatment gains up to 3 years post-intervention. Finally, Cameron Camp highlights the challenge of ensuring that effective interventions are not only reported in the research literature, but also further developed for implementation in clinical settings, and considers how this essential goal may be achieved.

The evidence presented in this special issue strongly supports the relevance of cognitive rehabilitation approaches for people with dementia and their families, carers and supporters. As with any newly developing area of research, many questions remain to be answered, and there is a need to strengthen further the evidence base. We hope that this issue will encourage this process and serve as a stimulus for further research. Despite these limitations, the evidence currently available, the best of which is included here, suggests many avenues for the clinician wishing to enhance the care provided to people with dementia. We hope that this issue will encourage clinicians to make full use of this evidence and implement the ideas presented here in their own clinical settings within a person-centred approach to care that places the needs of the person with dementia firmly in the centre of the picture.

REFERENCES

British Psychological Society Professional Affairs Board (1994). *Psychological well-being for users of dementia services* (Division of Clinical Psychology Briefing Paper No. 2). Leicester, UK: British Psychological Society.

Camp, C.J. (1998). Memory interventions for normal and pathological older adults. In R. Schulz, G. Maddox, & M.P. Lawton (Eds.), *Annual review of gerontology and geriatrics, Vol 18: Interventions research with older adults*. New York: Springer.

Camp, C.J., & Mattern, J.M. (1999). Innovations in managing Alzheimer's disease. In D.E. Biegel & A. Blum (Eds.), *Innovations in practice and service delivery across the lifespan*. New York: Oxford University Press.

Cohen, D., & Eisdorfer, C. (1986). *The loss of self: A family resource for the care of Alzheimer's disease and related disorders*. New York: W. W. Norton.

Cottrell, V., & Schulz, R. (1993). The perspective of the patient with Alzheimer's disease: A neglected dimension of dementia research. *Gerontologist, 33*, 205–211.

Hagberg, B. (1997). The dementias in a psychodynamic perspective. In B.M.L. Miesen & G.M.M. Jones (Eds.), *Care-giving in dementia: Research and applications*, (Vol. 2). London: Routledge.

Kitwood, T. (1997). *Dementia reconsidered: The person comes first*. Buckingham: Open University Press.

McLellan, D.L. (1991). Functional recovery and the principles of disability medicine. In M. Swash & J. Oxbury (Eds.), *Clinical neurology*, (Vol. 1, pp. 768–790). London: Churchill Livingstone.

Sabat, S.R. (1994). Excess disability and malignant social psychology: A case study of Alzheimer's disease. *Journal of Community and Applied Social Psychology, 4*, 157–166.

Sabat, S. (1995). The Alzheimer's disease sufferer as a semiotic subject. *Philosophy, Psychiatry, and Psychology, 1*, 145–160.

Sabat, S.R., & Harré, R. (1992). The construction and deconstruction of self in Alzheimer's disease. *Ageing and Society, 12*, 443–461.

Sabat, S.B., Wiggs, C., & Pinizzotto, A. (1984). Alzheimer's disease: Clinical vs. observational studies of cognitive ability. *Journal of Clinical and Experimental Gerontology, 6*, 337–359.

Setting New Standards in the NHS Consensus Panel (1997). Setting new standards: The impact of Alzheimer's disease on the Health Service. *Health Service Journal, 11 Sept (Supplement)*.

Wilson, B.A. (1997). Cognitive rehabilitation: How it is and how it might be. *Journal of the International Neuropsychological Society, 3*, 487–496.

Woods, R.T., & Britton, P.G. (1985). *Clinical psychology with the elderly*. London: Croom Helm.

Crossing the i's and dotting the t's

Una Holden

Years ago I published an article in an American journal complaining that the use of test batteries was more appropriate for hens than people. Although such routine testing is no longer the norm there does appear to be a continued problem with providing appropriate assessment procedures for older people suffering from some form of cognitive or behavioural change.

The obvious first question here is why are tests required at all? There are various reasons which have been listed and recognised for many years, for instance, to establish a baseline or to identify changes in research programmes. However, if rehabilitation programmes are to be effective, it is absolutely essential to ascertain which abilities are retained in good working order, which are partially damaged, and which are severely impaired.

Over and over again errors in perception of a person's problems in functioning are demonstrated both in hospital and residential home as well as in a person's own home. Setting unrealistic goals only adds to the individual's stress and confusion. To treat someone with dysphasia as though he or she is a parrot and will eventually learn to copy through constant repetition, or to shout continually at a person with receptive dysphasia expecting that it will make him or her comprehend, will hardly prove to be successful as retraining programmes. Furthermore, misunderstandings can add emphasis to the assumption that a dementia is present. Not only those observing, but also the unfortunate patient him or herself, can be led to believe that serious degeneration is occurring. If a person presents with behavioural and cognitive changes it is no longer appropriate to conclude that "dementia" is the cause.

Unfortunately, despite tremendous progress in understanding the enormous number of conditions affecting brain function, the term "dementia" continues to be misused. Far too many staff and members of the public believe it to be a condition in its own right, see it as causing total damage to the brain, as

Correspondence should be sent to Una Holden-Cosgrove, Casa Ironmacannie, 0 12 Aiguaviva Parc, Vidreres, Girona 17411, Spain (email: cosgrove@girona.net).

irreversible, and as the explanation of every observed change in cognition or behaviour in people over the age of 65 years. Unfortunately, this persistent fallacy is held by older people themselves and frequently they react badly to self-perceptions of changes in ability, jumping to incorrect conclusions which can lead to depression and a pseudo-dementia state. In order to avoid errors, thorough investigations should be carried out, but this does not necessarily mean putting an individual in an examination situation. Although relevant testing is required, it should not be the initial step.

Good history taking can establish a person's previous social, educational, and occupational background. Careful observation of the person's behaviour and responses can prove invaluable. Challenging behaviour may be explained by watching, considering the possibilities of apraxia, agnosia, or neglect of one side. Does the person fight staff trying to feed, wash or dress him or her, does the person get lost, has he or she shown difficulty in recognising relatives, friends or even objects? What happens when the person is left alone to do things, is dressing suddenly done with ease? It is possible that a person may have, for example, an apraxia yet is capable of functioning normally apart from not being able to cope with being told what to do? Most human beings of any age are not too happy about being "told what to do"!

Have staff been trained to recognise or look for specific changes in ability or behaviour? Often there can be confusion over observed behaviour, and the person's difficulties may be seen as a conscious attempt to annoy or to seek attention instead of as clues to a more accurate interpretation. Staff and relatives may not appreciate that because a person sings but refuses to talk to them, he or she is not being deliberately rude—the fact that music and rhythm are located in another part of the brain is the real explanation.

Another situation when behaviour can be perceived as deliberate rudeness or offensive in some way can occur with frontal damage. Perseveration is a common indication of such damage and although it is usually demonstrated in the constant repetition of words or phrases and sometimes gestures, it can also appear in an unusual form. A person suddenly seems to ignore what is being said and continues to talk about a particular subject, so staff and relatives think that deafness, rudeness or boredom with the conversation are possible explanations. The person's attention has become focused on a subject and thought processes have got caught in a groove—the "stuck-needle syndrome" of frontal lobe damage. The only rehabilitation programme to minimise perseverations of this sort is one of sharp distraction—clapping hands, ringing bells or dropping something may provide the mental jerk that breaks the connection! Other forms of frontal damage such as poor sequencing and difficulties with using abstract thought need to be investigated with specific tests and simple retraining methods initiated. Day-to-day material such as shopping lists, order in dressing, in washing and making sense of mixed up picture stories are all useful tools.

Memory problems are cited as the start of a degenerative condition, but what form do these so-called memory lapses take? Does the teenager who forgets to pass on a message suffer from dementia? Does the person who climbs to the top of the stairs and wonders why he or she went up them, but recalls why after returning to the bottom, suffer from dementia? Memory lapses are common to everyone; those with heavy demands on recall are liable to forget some detail but are well within normal limits. The belief that memory error is a sign of deterioration is just an added stress which can precipitate misunderstandings of observed and perceived functions.

History taking and observation need also to be amplified by an awareness of the psychological and social situation of an individual. How do other people treat the person, what attitudes do they have, what social outlets are there, what are family relationships like? If the person is a patient on a ward, or a resident in a home, what knowledge do the staff have, what procedures are used, what attitudes and beliefs are current?

The first step in "diagnosis" is to ascertain if the problem is simply a matter of misconception, either by the patient, or the staff, or relatives. Why has a person's social behaviour deteriorated—is it because there has been no opportunity to employ social skills? Why does everyone think that a person is deteriorating—is it because the person has a high level of intelligence and has panicked because some errors in performance have arisen? Has the person been left alone for so long that depression has been the result and skills have not been employed and so have become rusty? Have the relatives or staff taken over and robbed the person of independence with the result that the unfortunate being has given up? All these are questions to be considered, along with a personal history. Rehabilitation takes on a different form when social and psychological influences are the root of the problem. Perhaps it is staff or relatives that require retraining! If the person has suffered a pseudo-dementia as a result of the social situation then therapy directed at restoring confidence and demonstrating retained abilities is required.

When a full history is available and no satisfactory explanation of changes has been found, more formal, relevant testing is appropriate. The emphasis must be placed on *relevant*. The person may be suffering from one of the many different degenerative conditions which damage part of the brain—from mere bruising of a small area to severe widespread damage. It is important, if at all possible, to identify the causal condition as well as identifying the functions and abilities affected, including the degree of impairment involved. The tests should cover not only basic intelligence, but should include useful neuro-psychological screening at levels commensurate with the person's basic level of ability. For instance if there is a problem with speech or language then tests will need to be modified or selected in order to obtain meaningful results. The rehabilitation programme and its goals should be planned to meet the needs of the individual as well as seeking ways to strengthen, retrain or compensate for the specific impairments identified.

Without taking all aspects and influences into consideration the result will be too many crossed i's and dotted t's.

FURTHER READING

Bender, M.P., & Cheston, R.I.L. (1997). Inhabitants of a Lost Kingdom: A model of the subjective experience of dementia. *Ageing & Society, 17*, 513–532.

Holden, U.P. (1984). Test batteries and elderly people. *Clinical Gerontologist, 32*, 48–52.

Holden, U.P. (1995). *Ageing, neuropsychology and the 'new' dementias*. London: Chapman and Hall.

Kitwood, T. (1997). *Dementia reconsidered*. Buckingham, UK: Open University.

Are changes in everyday memory over time in autopsy-confirmed Alzheimer's disease related to changes in reported behaviour?

Janet Cockburn

University of Reading, Reading, UK

Janet Keene

Warneford Hospital, Oxford, UK

Performance on an augmented version of the Rivermead Behavioural Memory Test (RBMT) was examined in 48 people with autopsy-confirmed Alzheimer's disease and compared with Mini Mental State Examination (MMSE) score and with ratings on a behavioural questionnaire. Highly significant correlations were found between RBMT and MMSE scores but there was little evidence of any systematic relationship between memory deficits and reported behavioural change. Longitudinal analyses of change over time were carried out on the scores of 22 participants who remained in the study for at least three years. Scores above zero were recorded for all but three RBMT items. Significant effects of reported change in two aspects of behaviour (losing one's way around the house; knowing the time of day) were identified on a number of memory test items. These results are interpreted as suggesting general rather than specific relationships between decline in cognition and behavioural change in Alzheimer's disease.

Correspondence should be sent to Janet Cockburn, Department of Psychology, University of Reading, Earley Gate, Reading, Berkshire, RG6 6AL, UK. Tel: 0118 931 8523, Fax: 0118 931 6715 (email: j.m.cockburn@reading.ac.uk).

This research was partly funded by grant no. G8516170 from the Medical Research Council of Great Britain.

The authors would like to thank Tony Hope for helpful advice and support and would like to acknowledge the contributions of Christopher Fairburn, Kathy Gedling and Sandra Cooper in setting up and carrying out the study; colleagues from OPTIMA (Oxford Project to Investigate Memory in Aging) for collaboration over post mortem data; Margaret Esiri and colleagues who carried out the post mortems; also the assistance of consultants, general practitioners, and community psychiatric nurses who helped to recruit participants, and the participants themselves and their carers without whom the study would not have been possible.

INTRODUCTION

Memory impairment is a common attribute of all dementias, often manifesting as marked difficulty in learning new information, although patterns of impaired and relatively preserved specific abilities vary across the dementia subtypes (Brandt & Rich, 1995). More specifically, there is evidence for a range of memory impairments among people with a clinical diagnosis of probable Alzheimer's disease (AD) that are not found in healthy older adults (Brandt & Rich, 1995). Patients are reported to show difficulty in encoding and acquiring new information as well as dysfunctional semantic memory but to demonstrate preservation of some types of implicit memory, such as perceptual priming and motor skill learning. Indication of the deficits usually begins with mild forgetfulness, a tendency to misplace objects, and forget familiar names. These are sometimes accompanied by compromised route-finding, and by word-finding difficulties, which may indicate either or both mnestic and language production problems. Memory for non-verbal material, such as faces, has been found to be severely impaired compared to that of healthy older adults (Wilson et al., 1982). Differences have even been reported in scores on delayed recall of a short word list and on confrontation naming between healthy controls and patients with mild probable AD, whose scores on the Mini Mental State Examination (MMSE; Folstein, Folstein, & McHugh, 1975) were borderline normal (Welsh et al., 1991, 1992).

Not only is it important to know whether or not a person has probable AD, but also understanding the relative speed of decline of different abilities makes an important contribution to improving management of the disease (Saxton, McGonigle, Swihart, & Boller, 1993). Few standard tests of memory allow for documentation of change in both verbal and non-verbal memory as the dementia progresses (Lezak, 1995). However, the Rivermead Behavioural Memory Test (RBMT; Wilson, Cockburn, & Baddeley, 1985), which was originally designed to detect memory problems that might interfere with rehabilitation of adults with acquired neurological damage (Wilson, Cockburn, Baddeley, & Hiorns, 1989), presents a different approach. It contains materials similar to those met in everyday life, has four parallel forms, thus facilitating longitudinal testing, and has norms for older people (Cockburn & Smith, 1989).

The variety of memory functions tapped by individual items in the RBMT suggest that it has scope for charting decline of different aspects of memory during progression of AD. The standard RBMT battery tests verbal and non-verbal recall and recognition as well as basic orientation. It includes immediate and delayed prose recall, immediate and delayed route recall, face and picture recognition, as well as tests of prospective memory. One of these, delayed recall of a message, has been found to be a sensitive discriminator between patients with minimal dementia and people without clinical signs of dementia who nevertheless score poorly on the MMSE (Huppert & Beardsall, 1993). However, the "prospective" nature of this particular task has subsequently been called into question (Maylor, 1995).

Despite the apparent advantages of the RBMT, score ranges of more frail community-dwelling older adults (Cockburn & Smith, 1989) indicate that floor level of performance on some, if not all, items might be reached at an early stage of the disease. Although the children's version of the RBMT (Wilson, Ivani-Chalian, & Aldrich, 1991) has been used successfully to assess memory problems in adults with Down's syndrome (Wilson & Ivani-Chalian, 1995) and may therefore have a score range more appropriate for people with AD, the nature of its material is, nevertheless, less appropriate for adults. The alternative, adopted in the study reported here, is to modify the original RBMT, retaining the existing materials but augmenting the scoring (see Methods section later).

In addition to memory impairments, a wide variety of behavioural changes have been noted in AD (Steele, Rovner, Chase, & Folstein, 1990), although the relationship between behavioural disturbance and severity of dementia is equivocal (Gilley et al., 1991; Hope et al., 1999). Nevertheless, understanding the nature and progression of behavioural change is of considerable clinical and practical importance because of the impact on carers and patient–carer relationships (Rabins, Mace, & Lucas, 1982). The findings reported in this paper form part of a large-scale longitudinal study, the main purpose of which was to describe the patterns of behavioural change observed in a sample of 100 adults with clinically defined dementia, who were living at home at the start of the study, and to examine relationships to other variables, such as age, clinical diagnosis, or dementia severity. Details of standardisation and validation of the behavioural questionnaire used are given in Hope and Fairburn (1992) and status of the sample at point of entry to the study are reported in Hope et al. (1997a; 1997b).

Previous papers have already reported on some aspects of behavioural change over the course of the disease. Hope et al. (1999) examined the sequence and pattern of 15 types of behaviour and psychiatric change. Their results indicate that there is not a systematic progression of change from normal to abnormal behaviour but, instead, wide individual variation, with changes occurring at almost any time in the course of the disease. There was no consistent change in behaviour in one direction with change in environment but entering a nursing home or hospital was found likely to produce some changes. For example, locked doors reduce the likelihood of wandering and getting lost. Nurses were also noted to differ in their tolerance of behaviour that might be rated "aggressive". McShane et al. (1998) examined occurrence of getting lost outside the home and found performance on the RBMT immediate route recall item on entry to the study discriminated significantly between people who did or did not get lost over the next two years.

We sought to answer the following questions in this paper:
1. Is there sufficient score distribution on all or some RBMT items to permit meaningful longitudinal analysis?
2. Do some RBMT items show faster deterioration than others?
3. What is the relationship between RBMT detailed score and MMSE score?
4. Is there a difference in RBMT scores between people who are or are not showing specific behavioural changes at the time of testing?

METHOD

Participants

At the beginning of the study, all 100 participants were living at home with a carer and had a clinical diagnosis of dementia that met DSM-IIIR criteria, following a full clinical examination, including CAMDEX, biochemical screen, full blood count, detailed review of past medical history, and computed tomography (CT) scan for most participants (Hope et al., 1997a). They were recruited through local general practitioners, community psychiatric nurses, and consultant old age psychiatrists. Clinical diagnosis of probable AD was made using NINCDS-ADRDA criteria (McKhann et al., 1984). Once included in the study, each participant was visited at four-monthly intervals until death and tested on the MMSE and RBMT. Results are reported here for the 48 people for whom there has to date been subsequent post mortem evidence of Alzheimer's disease and who had MMSE and RBMT scores at the first visit. Their mean age on entry to the study was 78.37 years (SD 6.26) and median time post-onset of dementia was five years. There were no significant differences on entry to the study in age, sex, time since onset of dementia, MMSE score, or overall detailed RBMT score between these 48 and the rest of the sample. Longitudinal analyses are reported for 22 people who remained in the study for at least three years. Again, there were no significant differences between these people and the rest of the sample. Fourteen of the 22 participants who were alive for at least three years continued to live at home during the course of the study period reported here.

Materials and methods

RBMT. The RBMT was administered according to instructions in the manual (Wilson et al., 1985). Additional scores were incorporated into each of the recognition items to give credit for correct naming of pictures when first presented for subsequent recognition and correct identification of the gender of the face in each photograph on initial presentation. A further addition of 10 questions to elicit cued recall after immediate and delayed story recall was also made. These, however, did not provide results significantly different from the free recall scores and have not been considered further in this paper.

Raw scores were recorded for each item (i.e., one point for every correct response, minus one point for false-positive responses in recognition items). Immediate and delayed message items were scored separately and knowing the correct date was scored with other orientation items to form a single orientation score. Thus 14 individual item scores plus an overall "detailed" score, formed from the sum of individual raw scores, were recorded at each four-monthly visit. Details are given in Appendix 1. Greater flexibility of scoring has been effected by using the raw scores for each item rather than the screening or standard profile scores of the standard RBMT, which require performance towards the upper end of the possible range for a score to be recorded.

MMSE.   The MMSE was administered at each visit and scored according to standard procedure.

Present Behaviour Examination.   The PBE (Hope & Fairburn, 1992) was administered. Each participant's main carer was interviewed at each four-monthly visit. The PBE is a semi-structured interview, with established validity and good test–retest and inter-rater reliability (Hope & Fairburn, 1992). It consists of 121 main questions and 66 "nested" questions in eight sections, and is designed to cover in detail the behaviour of the participant over the preceding four weeks. In order to minimise differences in scoring that might arise from a change in carer behavioural items were carefully defined, with ratings based on objective criteria. All interviews were carried out by one or other of two trained interviewers.

The majority of items were initially rated on a seven-point scale but this has been reduced to a three-point scale (change absent or no problem, mild change, severe change) for subsequent statistical analyses, with no loss of sensitivity. For the purposes of the present paper, a subset of six behaviours was selected on the basis of: (1) their relationship with psychiatric symptoms (Hope et al., 1999), (2) *a priori* likelihood of being related to memory test performance, and (3) presence of an adequate distribution across the three-point scale. These are listed in Appendix 2 together with their frequency of occurrence on entry to the study. There was no significant difference in distribution of ratings on these selected PBE variables between the 48 people with subsequent autopsy-confirmed AD and the rest of the sample.

RESULTS

Although data presented here are only for participants whose clinical diagnosis of probable AD has subsequently been confirmed at autopsy, equivalent analyses have been carried out for the whole sample of 100 people, of whom the majority ($n = 75$) had a clinical diagnosis of probable AD on entry to the study, and the pattern of results is substantially the same.

Score distribution on the RBMT

On entry to the study. The overall RBMT detailed score at the initial visit indicated a wide range of ability, from 0 (one person) to 65 (one person). The mean score was 31.17, SD 15.62, and the median 34.50. Table 1, however, indicates that already performance on some individual items was at or close to floor level. Only one individual scored above zero for the appointment item, and only three above zero for delayed story recall. Face gender identification, which has minimal memory content, showed best performance, followed by picture naming, for which semantic but not episodic memory is required, and then recognition memory items.

Analysis over time. Scores at each annual visit for the 22 participants who remained alive for at least three years were calculated (Table 2). Although this reduces overall numbers for analysis at earlier visits, it enables change over

TABLE 1
RBMT individual items: Median score, interquartile range and number scoring above zero on entry to the study ($N = 48$)

RBMT item	Median	Interquartile range	Number scoring above zero
Picture naming	9.00	7.25–10	47
Picture recognition	5.00	2.00–7.00	39
Face gender identification	5.00	4.00–5.00	44
Face recognition	2.00	1.00–4.00	38
Immediate route recall	2.00	0.00–3.00	34
Immediate message recall	1.50	0.00–2.00	31
Delayed route recall	0.00	0.00–2.00	22
Delayed message recall	0.00	0.00–1.00	18
Immediate story recall	0.00	0.00–1.00	19
Delayed story recall	0.00	0.00–0.00	3
Name recall	0.00	0.00–1.00	14
Orientation	3.50	1.00–6.00	43
Remembering a hidden belonging	0.00	0.00–1.00	16
Remembering an appointment	0.00	0.00–0.00	1

TABLE 2
Distribution of scores on MMSE and RBMT over 3 years
(22 patients alive and tested at all annual visits up to 10th visit)

Item	1st visit	1 year (4th visit)	2 years (7th visit)	3 years (10th visit)
	Mean (SD) Range	*Mean (SD) Range*	*Mean (SD) Range*	*Mean (SD) Range*
MMSE	14.86 (7.52) 0–26	10.77 (8.32) 0–25	8.09 (7.76) 0–26	4.77 (6.21) 0–13
RBMT				
Detailed	32.68 (16.99) 0–65	23.73 (16.67) 0–50	17.55 (15.55) 0–60	10.77 (11.56) 0–38
Picture naming	8.45 (2.87) 0–10	6.41 (3.87) 0–10	5.73 (4.28) 0–10	4.09 (4.32) 0–10
Picture recognition	4.77 (3.15) 0–10	3.45 (2.94) 0–10	2.05 (2.32) 0–7	1.09 (1.48) 0–4
Face gender identification	4.18 (1.74) 0–5	3.77 (2.14) 0–5	3.45 (2.04) 0–5	3.00 (2.37) 0–5
Face recognition	2.73 (1.75) 0–5	1.64 (1.53) 0–5	1.50 (1.82) 0–5	1.00 (1.57) 0–4
Immediate route	2.36 (1.73) 0–5	1.50 (1.82) 0–5	0.95 (1.36) 0–4	0.32 (0.78) 0–3
Immediate message	1.36 (1.18) 0–3	0.68 (1.09) 0–3	0.57 (0.93) 0–3	0.09 (0.29) 0–1
Delayed route	1.14 (1.32) 0–5	0.82 (1.10) 0–3	0.52 (1.12) 0–4	0.14 (0.47) 0–2
Delayed message	0.55 (0.91) 0–3	0.50 (0.86) 0–3	0.24 (0.70) 0–3	0.05 (0.21) 0–1
Immediate story recall	1.36 (2.04) 0–8	1.14 (1.78) 0–6	0.62 (1.77) 0–8	0.36 (0.85) 0–3
Delayed story recall	0.18 (0.85) 0–4	0.14 (0.64) 0–3	0.10 (0.44) 0–2	0.05 (0.21) 0–1
Name recall	0.41 (0.91) 0–3	0.32 (0.57) 0–2	0.10 (0.30) 0–1	——*
Orientation	3.73 (2.98) 0–9	2.36 (2.57) 0–8	1.41 (2.13) 0–8	0.50 (1.22) 0–5
Belonging recall	0.50 (0.86) 0–3	0.23 (0.75) 0–3	0.10 (0.30) 0–1	——*

* No patient scored above zero.

time to be shown without the potential distortion of lower scores at an earlier visit being due to people who died before the next assessment.

Rate of deterioration on RBMT items

The number of individuals who scored above zero at each visit over these three years was calculated. This is shown graphically in Figure 1. The appointment item, on which only one person scored at the initial visit and none thereafter, has been omitted.

Taken together, Table 2 and Figure 1 indicate that after three years there are only two other items on which no individual scored above zero (name recall, recall of a hidden belonging), although for a further two items (delayed story, delayed message) there was only one scoring individual. Rate of deterioration does vary between items. Immediate route and message items show the steepest drop in scoring participants over the first year, with little change for picture recognition and name recall and none for delayed message.

Relationship between RBMT and MMSE scores

Mean MMSE score on entry to the study was 14.25, SD 7.20, range 0–26, median 14, again suggesting a wide range of ability. The correlation between RBMT and MMSE scores at this time was $r = .89$, indicating a strong

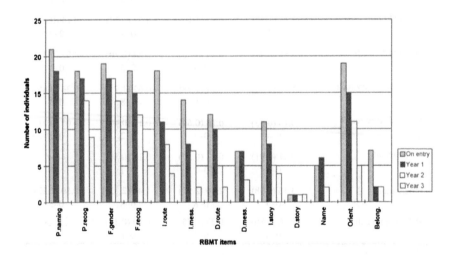

Figure 1.   Number of individuals tested over 3 years who scored above zero on RBMT items. Full names of the individual items are as given in Appendix 1.

relationship between overall memory test performance and general level of cognition. Over the three years covered here correlation coefficients between MMSE score and RBMT overall detailed score were robust, indicating that memory test performance was deteriorating at a similar rate to overall cognitive ability. For the 22 people tested over three years the annual correlation coefficients were: initial visit, $r = .92$; year 1, $r = .95$; year 2, $r = .93$; year 3, $r = .92$, all significant beyond the 0.1% level.

Relationship between RBMT scores and behavioural change

Behavioural change.   Changes in behaviour ratings on the six selected PBE variables are shown in Table 3. The relationship between memory test performance and reported behavioural disturbance was investigated by a series

TABLE 3

Change in distribution of categories on PBE variables over 3 years
(actual frequencies: 22 patients alive and tested at all annual visits up to 10th visit)

Variable	Category	Initial visit	1 year (4th visit)	2 years (7th visit)	3 years (10th visit)
Anxiety	Absent	16	15	15	17
	Mild	4	3	5	3
	Severe	2	4	2	1
Checking carer's	Absent	15	11	13	18
whereabouts	Mild	5	9	5	4
	Severe	2	2	4	0
Losing way around	No difficulty	13	11	4	4
home	Slight difficulty	5	4	7	2
	Great difficulty	3	6	8	14
	Immobile	1	1	3	2
Apparent sadness	Absent	11	9	10	13
	Mild	5	6	7	7
	Severe	6	7	5	2
Knowing time of day	Does know	15	11	6	3
	Does not know	4	7	13	19
	Diurnal rhythm disrupted	3	4	3	0
Verbal aggression	Absent	9	9	8	11
	Mild	6	8	8	4
	Severe	7	5	6	7

N.B. Where numbers do not add up to 22, information was not recorded for one or more patients at that visit.

of one-way ANOVAs with Bonferroni planned comparisons, using SPSS for Windows, version 6.1. We predicted that absence of behavioural change from premorbid state would be associated with higher RBMT scores than minor change which, in turn, would be associated with higher scores than marked change. Because of the number of comparisons only F values reaching the 1% significance level or better have been reported. Eight of the RBMT items (picture naming, picture recognition, face gender identification, face recognition, immediate route, immediate message, orientation, immediate story recall) were selected for analysis as having an adequate score range over three years of testing. Performance on each of these items, plus overall RBMT detailed score, according to rating on each of the six PBE variables was compared.

On entry to the study.   There were no overall significant differences in RBMT item scores at the initial visit according to rating on three of the PBE measures: checking carer's whereabouts; apparent sadness; knowing time of day; and only one significant individual planned comparison: people who did not check carer's whereabouts had significantly higher face gender identification scores than people who checked frequently. Two RBMT items, immediate route and immediate story, yielded significantly different scores according to anxiety ratings. For both items people rated as showing marked increase in anxiety levels scored significantly higher than people rated as showing no change from their premorbid behaviour, which may indicate knowledge in early dementia that something is wrong. There were three borderline significant differences for verbal aggression (face recognition, immediate route, immediate story recall), for all of which people displaying no change in aggressive behaviour from premorbid state scored significantly higher than people rated as showing marked change in aggressive behaviour. Change in behaviour on "losing one's way around the home" showed the strongest relationship with RBMT performance, producing three significant differences (for picture naming, face gender identification and overall detailed score) and one borderline with significant group differences on planned comparison (orientation) (Table 4). There is, nevertheless, little evidence of any consistent association between rated behavioural change and objective memory test performance on entry to the study.

Relationship over three years.   Analyses were carried out in the same manner for RBMT scores at the first visit of the 22 people remaining in the study for at least three years. Relationships with PBE variables were similar to those of the larger sample, although effects of anxiety and verbal aggression were no longer significant. Analyses were also carried out on RBMT scores of these 22 people at one, two and three years into the study (4th, 7th, and 10th

TABLE 4
Significant differences in RBMT items scores at initial visit according
to rating on PBE variable: Losing way around the home (N = 48)

RBMT item	F (2,43)	p	Planned comparison (mean score)
Picture naming	6.57	**	Not (9.31) > frequently (6.17)
Face gender identification	5.17	**	Not (4.65) > occasionally (4.64) > frequently (3.00)
Orientation	4.40	(**)	Not (4.73) > occasionally (2.57)
Detailed score total	5.12	**	Not (37.85) > occasionally (26.43), frequently (22.00)

** p < .01; (**) borderline significance (p < .02).

TABLE 5
Relationships over 3 years between RBMT scores and PBE variable:
Losing way around the home (N = 22)

	Initial visit F(2,18)	p	1 year F(2,18)	p	2 years F(2,16)	p	3 years F(2,17)	p
Picture naming	1.53	n.s.	5.69	**	3.58	n.s.	5.09	(**)
Picture recognition	0.18	n.s.	4.95	(**)	0.89	n.s.	7.91	**
Face gender	1.57	n.s.	10.71	**	3.60	n.s.	1.18	n.s.
Face recognition	0.23	n.s.	4.76	(**)	13.71	***	5.94	**
Orientation	1.58	n.s.	2.98	n.s.	15.58	***	4.51	(**)
Detailed score	1.02	n.s.	6.26	**	8.43	**	5.25	(**)

** = p < .01; *** = p < .001; (**) borderline significance (p < .02).
N.B. Only statistically significant effects are shown. In all comparisons people showing no sign of behavioural change score highest. Differences in degrees of freedom result from some individuals being immobile at one or more visits.

visits). Results of these analyses indicate more evidence of an association between memory test performance and reported behavioural change as RBMT scores declined and frequency of behavioural change increased. However, significant relationships were restricted to two of the PBE variables: losing one's way around the home and knowing the time of day. Sequential comparisons are shown in Tables 5 and 6. These indicate that some of the RBMT items show a consistent relationship over time with behavioural changes associated with spatial or temporal disorientation.

TABLE 6
Relationships over 3 years between RBMT scores and PBE variable: Knowing the time
of day (N = 22)

	Initial visit		1 year		2 years		3 years	
	F(2,19)	p	F(2,19)	p	F(2,19)	p	F(1,20)	p
Picture naming	2.29	n.s.	7.35	**	6.48	**	8.97	**
Picture recognition	3.76	(**)	6.52	**	5.51	**	4.64	(**)
Face gender identification	1.51	n.s.	7.49	**	5.32	(**)	2.67	n.s.
Face recognition	1.15	n.s.	6.48	**	3.61	(**)	4.56	(**)
Immediate route recall	1.95	n.s.	7.63	**	2.92	n.s.	19.57	***
Immediate message	0.59	n.s.	6.80	**	1.84	n.s.	2.53	n.s.
Immediate story recall	0.42	n.s.	4.15	(**)	2.62	n.s.	12.83	**
Orientation	3.24	n.s.	5.50	**	2.83	n.s.	6.60	(**)
Detailed score total	3.31	n.s.	15.45	***	6.37	**	10.92	**

** $p < .01$; *** $p < .001$; (**) borderline significance ($p < .02$).

NB. Only statistically significant effects are shown. In all comparisons people showing no sign of behavioural change score highest.

DISCUSSION

There were two broad aims of this paper: to examine response patterns over time to items of the RBMT as general cognitive ability deteriorated in a group of people with autopsy-confirmed Alzheimer's disease; and to explore the relationship between specific changes in behaviour and changes in memory test performance in the same group. Our results are, perhaps, easier to interpret with respect to the first aim than the second. There is evidence that three years into the study some people with profound cognitive impairment (bar one outlier scoring 23, MMSE scores ranged from 0 to 13, with a median of 1.00) are able to make correct responses to some items in tests of picture naming, picture recognition, face gender identification, face recognition, immediate route recall, immediate story recall, and orientation. That performance has dropped off almost completely for items testing delayed retrieval is not surprising. The one person who scored above zero at the 10th visit for delayed story recall was also the only person to score on the delayed message item and he was the individual with an MMSE score of 23. Nor is it, perhaps, surprising that participants continue to score highest on the two additional items—picture naming, face gender identification—neither of which requires episodic memory. Naming to confrontation, represented by the picture naming, has been shown to be sensitive to AD, with deficits reflecting a breakdown in semantic processes despite intact phonemic processes, in contrast to the disruptions of perceptual analysis found in patients with Huntington's disease (Hodges, Salmon, & Butters, 1991). The nature of the naming errors made by participants in our study was not routinely recorded and so we cannot analyse individual performance further. However, everyday speech output was rated as "normal" on the PBE at each visit over the three years for all the participants whose performances are reported here. Our results nevertheless indicate that preservation of access to the semantic representation of familiar everyday objects (picture naming) is substantially better preserved than episodic recognition memory for the same objects after a brief delay (picture recognition).

Taken as a whole, the results suggest that people with advanced AD may be more aware and responsive to what is going on around them than is sometimes assumed. We cannot, of course, entirely discount the possibility that some responses were a function of practice engendered by repeat testing every four months. However, routine use of each of the four parallel versions of the RBMT in turn meant, for example, that each set of pictures for naming and each route sequence would be presented once every 16 months. Therefore, we suggest that any benefits solely attributable to practice are likely to be extremely small.

In answer to our first question we conclude that there is a sufficient score distribution on at least some of the RBMT items to permit meaningful longitudinal analysis. Some of the RBMT items show faster deterioration than others (question 2), as shown in Figure 1, and the decline is in line with what has previously been reported about memory loss in dementia (Brandt & Rich, 1995). Most notably, performance on the prospective memory item of remembering an appointment was at floor level at the start of the study but scores on remembering a hidden belonging, name recall, and delayed story recall also declined markedly over the course of the first year and the number of people scoring on immediate route and message items fell over the first year. Although we have not carried out comparable analyses of responses to route and message items to those of Huppert and Beardsall (1993), our results suggest that performance on the message items does not deteriorate substantially faster than on the route items in our group. One reason for this difference may be that their results identified people on the borderline of dementia, whereas our participants were already beyond that stage on entry to the study.

The strong correlations between RBMT and MMSE scores both initially and over three years (question 3) indicate that there would be little benefit in routinely administering the longer RBMT for screening purposes but that performance on individual items may provide useful information on preserved abilities as overall MMSE score drops.

Our analyses of the relationship between behavioural changes in AD and memory test performance (question 4) show few significant effects. Whereas memory test performance declines more or less consistently, reports of change in behaviour from premorbid patterns sometimes vary from one visit to another. Although the majority of patients in this study did move from home to institutional care before death, 14 of the 22 whose performance over three years is reported here remained at home throughout that period. Despite high inter-rater and test–retest reliability data for the PBE (Hope & Fairburn, 1992), it is not possible entirely to eliminate the chance element generated by the respondent—a problem common to any questionnaire analysis. As Hope et al. (1999) noted, there is the possibility that some reported behavioural change may be due to differences between carers (e.g., as the patient moves from home to residential care). As noted earlier, interpretations of what constitutes "aggressive" behaviour may differ from one nurse to another. There may also be some effect of within-carer differences. Reports of frequency of checking carer's whereabouts or of verbal aggression, for example, may depend as much on a carer's tolerance levels at the time of being interviewed as on the patient's actual behaviour over the previous four weeks. Nevertheless, results from the present study support the findings of Hope et al. (1999) that, although behaviour changes are a common occurrence, there is neither a consistent link with move from home to institutional care nor a steady pattern of behavioural decline with disease progression. The most straightforward explanation of our results is that the behaviour changes which take place in AD are not primarily the result of specific deficiencies in memory or general cognitive functioning. Instead they may result from an interaction between environment and brain degeneration that affects behaviour directly and is not mediated through cognitive impairment; therefore suggesting separate and distinct channels of cognitive and behavioural decline.

It is also evident from the data in Table 3 that "normal" behaviours (i.e., unchanged from behaviour noted prior to clinical diagnosis of AD) are still quite frequent, thus lessening the likelihood of significant memory test differences being identified in association with differences in reported behaviour. Reported mood changes were few. Incidence of anxiety appeared to change little over the course of these analyses, as did that of apparent sadness, although there is some sign of a decrease in numbers appearing very sad.

Fairly consistent significant relationships were identified between RBMT scores and PBE variables for two behaviours—losing one's way around the home and knowing time of day. We suggest that these behaviours may be the ones most dependent on cognitive status. Nevertheless, because these two behaviours, which appear to be associated with spatial and temporal orientation, are no more closely related to performance on putatively similar RBMT items (route recall and losing one's way; orientation and knowing the time of day) than to performance on other items, we suggest the relationship is with general rather than specific memory attributes.

We did not identify an association between RBMT route recall and getting lost around the house similar to that between route recall and getting lost outside the home reported by McShane et al. (1998). Part of that difference may result from different sample sizes: McShane et al. used data from all 100 participants. However, they only reported results from route recall and one other item, picture recognition, for which no significant effects were found on likelihood of getting lost outside the home. We found significant differences at one or more visits in RBMT scores on picture naming, picture recognition, face gender identification, face recognition, and orientation according to rated change in occurrences of getting lost around the house. Our results suggest that whereas topographical memory may be salient for finding one's way outside the home, getting lost indoors may be more a marker of general cognitive deterioration than of loss of specific topographic or visual perceptual skills.

These analyses are by no means exhaustive, representing as they do only a small subject sample and a subset of information from the PBE. Nevertheless, they confirm our prediction that the augmented version of the RBMT would be a useful tool for measuring memory changes as AD progresses. However, in view of the conclusions of Hope et al. (1999, p.43) that "there was such variation between individuals that no robust timing of onset of a specific type of behaviour and psychiatric change was apparent" and the evidence from analysis presented here of wide variation in RBMT scores within behavioural subcategories, we conclude that there is little evidence for a consistent association between decline in memory test performance and increase in behavioural change from premorbid levels as the disease progresses.

Although we acknowledge that neither objective nor subjective measures of cognition and behaviour can ever be 100% reliable and that our sample is relatively small, our finding of little relationship between specific memory impairments and changes in behaviour is, nevertheless, important. It suggests that, for example, differences between someone who loses their way around the home and someone who does not cannot be explained solely in terms of loss of the specific skill of spatial awareness. We consider, therefore, that cognitive deterioration and behavioural change need to be examined separately when assessing overall status and determining the most appropriate care management for any individual with advanced AD.

REFERENCES

Brandt, J., & Rich, J.B. (1995). Memory disorders in the dementias. In A.D. Baddeley, B.A. Wilson & F.N. Watts (Eds.), *Handbook of memory disorders*. Chichester, UK: Wiley.

Cockburn, J., & Smith, P.T. (1989). *The Rivermead Behavioural Memory Test: Supplement 3: Elderly people*. Bury St. Edmunds, Suffolk: Thames Valley Test Co.

Folstein, M.F., Folstein, S.E., & McHugh, P.R. (1975). Mini-Mental State: A practical method for grading the cognitive state of patients for the clinician. *Journal of Psychiatric Research, 12,* 189–198.

Gilley, D.W., Wilson, R.S., Bennett, D.A., Bernard, B.A., & Fox, J.H. (1991). Predictors of behavioural disturbance in Alzheimer's disease. *Journal of Gerontology; Psychological Sciences, 46,* 362–371.

Hodges, J.R., Salmon, D.P., & Butters, N. (1991). The nature of the naming deficit in Alzheimer's and Huntington's disease. *Brain, 114,* 1547–1558.

Hope, T., & Fairburn, C.G. (1992). The Present Behavioural Examination (PBE): The development of an interview to measure current behavioural abnormalities. *Psychological Medicine, 22,* 223–230.

Hope, T., Keene, J., Gedling, K., Cooper, S., Fairburn, C., & Jacoby, R. (1997a). Behaviour changes in dementia 1: Point of entry data of a prospective study. *International Journal of Geriatric Psychiatry*, *12*, 1062–1073.

Hope, T., Keene, J., Fairburn, C., McShane, R., & Jacoby, R. (1997b). Behaviour changes in dementia 2: Are there behavioural syndromes? *International Journal of Geriatric Psychiatry*, *12*, 1074–1078.

Hope, T., Keene, J., Fairburn, C., Jacoby, R., & McShane, R. (1999). Natural history of behavioural changes and psychiatric symptoms in Alzheimer's disease. *British Journal of Psychiatry*, *174*, 39–44.

Huppert, F.A., & Beardsall, L. (1993). Prospective memory impairment as an early indicator of dementia. *Journal of Clinical and Experimental Neuropsychology*, *15*, 805–821.

Lezak, M.D. (1995) *Neuropsychological assessment*, (3rd Edition). New York: Oxford University Press.

Maylor, E.A. (1995). Prospective memory in normal aging and dementia. *NeuroCase*, *1*, 285–289.

McKhann, G., Drachman, D., Folstein, M., Katzman, R., Price, D., & Stadlan, E.M. (1984). Clinical diagnosis of Alzheimer's disease: Report of the NINCDS-ADRDA Work Group under the auspices of Department of Health and Human Services Task Force on Alzheimer's disease. *Neurology*, *34*, 939–944.

McShane, R., Gedling, K., Keene, J., Fairburn, C., Jacoby, R., & Hope, T. (1998). Getting lost in dementia: A longitudinal study of a behavioural symptom. *International Psychogeriatrics*, *10*, 253–260.

Rabins, P.V., Mace, N.L., & Lucas, M.J. (1982). The impact of dementia on the family. *Journal of the American Medical Association*, *248*, 333–335.

Saxton, J., McGonigle, K.L., Swihart, A.A., & Boller, F. (1993). *The Severe Impairment Battery (SIB)*. Bury St. Edmunds, UK: Thames Valley Test Co.

Steele, C., Rovner, B., Chase, G.A., & Folstein, M. (1990). Psychiatric symptoms and nursing home placements of patients with Alzheimer's disease. *American Journal of Psychiatry*, *147*, 1049–1051.

Welsh, K., Butters, N., Hughes, J., Mohs, R., & Heyman, A. (1991). Detection of abnormal memory decline in mild cases of Alzheimer's disease using CERAD neuropsychological measures. *Archives of Neurology*, *48*, 278–281.

Welsh, K., Butters, N., Hughes, J., Mohs, R., & Heyman, A. (1992). Detection and staging of dementia in Alzheimer's disease. *Archives of Neurology*, *49*, 448–452.

Wilson, B.A., Cockburn, J., & Baddeley, A.D. (1985). *The Rivermead Behavioural Memory Test*. Bury St. Edmunds, UK: Thames Valley Test Co.

Wilson, B.A., Cockburn, J., Baddeley, A.D., & Hiorns, R.W. (1989). The development and validation of a test battery for detecting and monitoring everyday memory problems. *Journal of Clinical and Experimental Neuropsychology*, *11*, 855–870.

Wilson, B.A., & Ivani-Chalian, R. (1995). Performance of adults with Down's syndrome on the children's version of the Rivermead Behavioural Memory Test: A brief report. *British Journal of Clinical Psychology*, *34*, 85–88.

Wilson, B.A., Ivani-Chalian, R., & Aldrich, F. (1991). *The Rivermead Behavioural Memory Test for children aged 5–10 years*. Bury St. Edmunds, UK: Thames Valley Test Co.

Wilson, R.S., Kasniak, A.W., Bacon, L.D., Fox, J.H., & Kelly, M.P. (1982). Facial recognition memory in dementia. *Cortex*, *18*, 329–336.

Manuscript received May 1999
Revised manuscript received February 2000

APPENDIX 1

RBMT items and maximum score for each item

RBMT item	Maximum score
Picture naming	10
Picture recognition	10
Face gender identification	5
Face recognition	5
Immediate route recall	5
Immediate message recall	3
Delayed route recall	5
Delayed message recall	3
Immediate story recall	21
Delayed story recall	21
Name recall	4
Orientation	10
Remembering a hidden belonging	4
Remembering an appointment	2

A set of questions to elicit cued recall of immediate and delayed story was also included in the study and administered after free recall but scores did not significantly improve performance over free recall and have not been reported here.

APPENDIX 2

Percentage frequency of behaviour rating on entry to the study of six PBE variables selected for analysis (*N* = 48)

Behaviour	Description of item	Behaviour absent or no change	Minor change	Marked change
Anxiety	Anxiety or fearfulness (with physical symptoms)	78	16	6
Apparent sadness	Appeared to be particularly sad, miserable or depressed	51	25	25
Checking	Frequently checking carer's whereabouts	69	21	10
Getting lost around the home	Loses way around the home	54	31	13 *
Knowing time of day	Evidence of disruption to diurnal rhythm	63 (knows time of day)	25 (does not know time of day)	12 (diurnal rhythm disrupted)
Verbal aggression	Spoke in an aggressive or angry way	31	29	41

* One person was immobile.

Assessing quality of life in dementia: Preliminary psychometric testing of the Quality of Life Assessment Schedule (QOLAS)

Caroline E. Selai, Michael R. Trimble, Martin N. Rossor, and Richard J. Harvey

National Hospital for Neurology and Neurosurgery, London, UK

We adapted a generic, individualised, patient-centred quality of life (QOL) assessment technique, the Quality of Life Assessment Schedule (QOLAS) for use with patients with dementia. The QOLAS was administered to a group of patients with mild to moderate dementia alongside a number of other measures of well-being to assess its psychometric properties. Each patient's main carer also completed the QOLAS, giving a proxy rating of the QOL of the patient. The patients understood the interview and were able to describe their quality of life both qualitatively and quantitatively. In this preliminary study the QOLAS was demonstrated to have good validity (content, construct, and criterion) and good internal reliability. The carers rated the patients as having a worse QOL than did the patients themselves on all subdomains of the QOLAS. The results suggest that patients with mild to moderate dementia can rate their own QOL and that the QOLAS is a promising method for assessing QOL in this patient group. The discrepancy between the patients' own views and the views of their carers raises important issues about whether the patient or a proxy is the best judge of QOL in patients with dementia.

Correspondence should be sent to Caroline E. Selai, Research Psychologist, Raymond Way Neuropsychiatry Research Group, Institute of Neurology, University College London, National Hospital for Neurology and Neurosurgery, Queen Square, London WC1N 3BG. Telephone: 020 7837 3611, Fax: 020 278 8772; e-mail: c.selai@ion.ucl.ac.uk

The authors thank the Queen Square Dementia Research Group nurses who helped co-ordinate patient recruitment. Caroline Selai acknowledges support from the Raymond Way Neuropsychiatry Research Fund. Richard Harvey acknowledges support from the Alzheimer's Society.

INTRODUCTION

Quality of life (QOL) data are now an established outcome measure in the assessment of therapeutic interventions (Bowling, 1995; Brooks, 1995). Since all pharmacological, and other treatments, have implications for quality of life, the prospect of drug treatment for Alzheimer's disease (AD) raises questions about the most appropriate methods to measure the QOL of this patient group (Burns, 1995; Kelly, Harvey, & Cayton, 1997). By far the most common and best known of the dementias is Alzheimer's disease which is characterised by progressive global deterioration of intellect and personality (Lezak, 1995). Although Alzheimer's is predominantly a disease of old age, some patients have symptoms as early as their fourth decade (Rossor, 1993).

The assessment of QOL in dementia raises a number of complex method-ological issues (Rabins & Kasper, 1997; Whitehouse et al., 1997) and reseach in this patient group is just beginning. Since QOL assessment requires a highly complex procedure of introspection and evaluation, involving several com-ponents of cognition including implicit and explicit memory (Barofsky, 1996), it follows that, at a certain stage of cognitive decline, there will come a point where QOL self-assessment will no longer be possible. It has been suggested, therefore, that both patient self-report and proxy ratings of QOL are important in dementia (Lawton, 1994; Stewart, Sherbourne, & Brod, 1996). A patient's ability to evaluate and communicate aspects of their well-being will be deter-mined by a number of clinical features such as the decline of cognitive skills, insight, denial, anosognosia, and a range of neuropsychiatric symptoms. One question, therefore, is to establish at what stage of the disease self-report is no longer possible (Fletcher, Dickinson, & Philp, 1992).

QOL: Measurement issues

There is a fundamental tension in the measurement of QOL. Since what is deemed important for QOL is acknowledged to be subjective and idiosyncratic, differences being influenced by a variety of personal and cultural factors, an appraisal of QOL should strive to capture the individual's subjectively appraised phenomenological experience. On the other hand, the hallmark of scientific measurement is reliable, "objective", empirical data collection. Researchers have devised QOL measurement techniques at various stages of this "subjective/objective" continuum and there now exist over 1000 instru-ments that have been developed taking a variety of approaches to measurement (Hedrick, Taeuber, & Erickson, 1996). The two poles of the qualitative–quantitative continuum have different strengths. It has been suggested that qualitative methods are more valid whilst quantitative methods are more reliable (Mays & Pope, 1996).

The QOL literature advocates a robust and rigorous programme of instru-ment development and testing, and most QOL measures are developed within the psychometric tradition (Juniper, Guyatt, & Jaeschke, 1996; McDowell & Newell, 1987). Some researchers have argued, however, that since quality of life is a uniquely personal perception, most standardised measurements of QOL in the medical literature seem to aim at the wrong target (Gill, 1995). It is argued that quality of life can be suitably measured only by determining the opinions of patients and by supplementing (or replacing) the instruments developed by "experts" (Gill & Feinstein, 1994). Scales developed within the psychometric tradition often omit items important to the beliefs and values of individual patients (Gill, 1995; Hunt, 1999) and the psychometric aim of internal reli- ability is in conflict with the goals of achieving comprehensiveness and content validity (Brazier & Deverill, 1999). In response to this, a number of "individu- alised", patient-driven techniques have been developed whereby the patient can nominate items of importance to him/herself (Geddes et al., 1990; Guyatt et al., 1987a, b; Fraser et al.,1993; O'Boyle et al., 1993; Ruta et al., 1994; Tugwell et al., 1990). The literature on "individual" QOL assessment techniques has recently been reviewed (Joyce, O'Boyle, & McGee, 1999).

There are strong arguments in favour of a number of approaches to QOL measurement and, since there is no gold standard, this debate is likely to continue. In practice, the choice of QOL assessment technique depends on the goal of the study and the type of data required which, in turn, will depend upon the use to which the data will be put. Uses include the simple description of QOL, screening in the clinical context, population surveys of perceived health problems, medical audit, and cost–utility analyses (Fitzpatrick et al., 1992). Assessment of QOL in dementia is in its infancy and it is likely that, as with other patient groups, a number of approaches will be developed, each appropriate for a different purpose.

QOL in dementia: Recent work

Research in this area has only recently begun and the definition of QOL in dementia and a number of other conceptual, practical, and ethical issues remain the subject of some debate (Rabins & Kasper, 1997; Whitehouse et al., 1997). Several scales, focusing on proxy reports, observational methods, and patient self-reports are in the early stages of development. To date, very little has been published on patient self-reported QOL in dementia although studies are under way (Albert & Logsdon, 1999; Selai & Trimble, 1999; Whitehouse et al., 1998). Patients with dementia were asked to rate their own QOL using the Schedule for the Evaluation of Individual Quality of Life (SEIQoL) a technique based on "judgement analysis". The procedure is complex, however, and in this study only 6 of the 20 patients completed the full assessment (Coen et al., 1993).

A number of scales purporting to measure QOL have been used in clinical trials of anti-dementia drugs but these measures have been criticised for a number of reasons. The QOL scales used in these trials have either not been fully validated for use in dementia (Howard & Rockwood, 1995) and/or have assessed only some aspects of activities of daily living, or affect, rather than comprehensively assessing QOL (Salek, Walker, & Bayer, 1998). To date, no QOL instrument used in clinical trials of anti-dementia drugs appears to be satisfactory (Walker, Salek, & Bayer, 1998).

The development of the Quality of Life Assessment Schedule (QOLAS)

Since so little data have been published on patient self-report, we developed and refined a technique that is subject-driven, i.e., personally tailored to each individual patient, the Quality of Life Assessment Schedule (QOLAS). This approach yields both qualitative and quantitative data. The QOLAS was derived from a technique called Quality of Life Assessment by Construct Analysis (QoLASCA) which in turn was based on Personal Construct Theory (PCT) and the Repertory Grid Technique (RGT) (Kendrick, 1993, 1997; Kendrick & Trimble, 1994; McGuire, 1991).

The Repertory Grid Technique (RGT) is the methodological component of Personal Construct Theory, a theory of personality proposed by George Kelly in the 1950s (Kelly, 1955). The fundamental postulate of this theory is that "a person's processes are psychologically channelized by the ways in which he anticipates events" (Kelly, 1955). According to Kelly, a person can be viewed as a scientist, who formulates theories or hypotheses relating to themselves and the world they inhabit. These theories are based on their personal construction or interpretation of experienced events and thus form a "personal construct system" (Kelly, 1955). The Repertory Grid Technique attempts objectively to explore and measure an individual's construct system.

Four major concepts underpinned the method (QoLASCA) that was developed for the assessment of quality of life. This was designed to be a generic technique but was originally developed to assess QOL in patients with neurological disorders, and the early work was done with patients with epilepsy. First, based on a comprehensive literature review, it was proposed that, in general terms, five areas important to quality of life can be defined. These are physical functioning, psychological/emotional status, social and family life, economic/employment status, and cognitive abilities. Second, it was recognised that within these general areas, specific items of importance will vary from individual to individual. Third, it was hypothesised that QOL is a function of levels of expectation. Thus, it is the discrepancy between current life situation and expectations that is important in determining an individual's QOL, not simply how they are at present. Fourth, it was suggested that QOL is a comparative phenomenon. In judging their QOL, individuals make comparisons concerning their current life situation in relation to other times and people in their lives.

The full QoLASCA interview was lengthy and cumbersome and it was deemed desirable to streamline the method. The brief version has been used in two studies of patients with epilepsy (Selai & Trimble, 1998; Selai, Elstner, & Trimble, 2000) and patients with Gilles de la Tourette syndrome (Elstner, Selai, Trimble, & Robertson, in press). Preliminary results have shown the revised method to be reliable, valid and more sensitive to post-treatment changes than some other QOL measures.

QOLAS interview as used with patients with epilepsy

After initial streamlining, the revised QOLAS interview, as used in the *epilepsy* studies is as follows: (1) introduction and rapport-building; (2) the respondent is invited to recount what is important for his/her QOL and ways in which current health condition is affecting it; (3) in total, 10 "constructs" are elicited, two for each of the following domains of QOL: physical, psychological, social/family, work/economic, and cognitive functioning; (4) the patient is asked to rate how much of a problem each of these is *now* on a 0–5 scale where 0 = no problem; 1 = very slight problem; 2 = mild problem; 3 = moderate problem; 4 = big problem, and 5 = it could not be worse; (5) the patient is asked to rate how much of a problem they would "*like*" each of these to be ideally on a 0–5 scale as above; (6) at follow-up interview, the respondent's individual constructs are read out to them and they are invited to re-rate each on the 0–5 scale for how much of a problem there is with each "now".

Using the QOLAS in dementia: Pilot study

Since it was not clear whether the revised technique would be understood by patients with dementia, a pilot study was carried out.

We recruited 10 patient–carer dyads into a small pilot study to test the feasibility of using the first-stage revised QOLAS used in the epilepsy studies (outlined earlier). The patients all had mild to moderate dementia. The patients and carers were all able to understand the basic interview and to respond. As with the epilepsy patients, the dementia patients sometimes needed prompting. The scoring options for each construct (0–5) needed to be repeated and the patients tended to use the descriptive word answer (e.g., "slight problem" or "big problem") rather than answer with a number from 0–5. Two particular problems emerged from the pilot interviews and these resulted in two further refinements being made.

First, although the element "NOW" was understood by the patients, who could all rate themselves "now", the element "LIKE", i.e., "how you would like to be" raised a number of questions and so this was dropped from the interview.

In the epilepsy interviews, the score for "LIKE" was nearly always "0", i.e., "no problems" and so this resulted in the dementia scoring system being, in fact, virtually the same as that for the epilepsy patients.

Second, although the original five domains from the QoLASCA were kept for the revised QOLAS, as used in patients with epilepsy, it became clear that the question about work/economic functioning was not appropriate for patients with dementia, nor was it relevant to many of the carers . Most of the patients interviewed had been obliged to give up work and take medical retirement some time prior to the interview. Many of the carers had given up work or had never worked. This question was therefore ambiguous and most patients and their carers wanted to answer "not applicable". The interviews yielded much qualitative data and, based on their comments, it became clear that this question would best be substituted by a question concerning whatever the patient or carer did during the day-time, e.g., gardening, going for a walk, or household duties. The domain "work/economic" was therefore substituted by a domain headed "daily activities".

QOLAS interview as used with patients with dementia and their carers

After piloting the QOLAS in dementia, modifications were made and the technique is as follows:

1. Introduction and rapport-building.
2. Respondents are invited to recount what is important for their QOL and ways in which their current health condition is affecting their QOL. Key constructs are extracted from this narrative. Prompting is sometimes required.
3. In total, 10 "constructs" are elicited, two for each of the following domains of QOL: physical, psychological, social/family, daily activities, and cognitive functioning (or well-being).
4. The patient is asked to rate how much of a problem each of these is *now* on a 0–5 scale where 0 = no problem; 1 = very slight problem; 2 = mild problem; 3 = moderate problem; 4 = big problem; and 5 = it could not be worse.
5. At follow-up interview, the respondent's individual constructs are read out to them and they are invited to re-rate each on the 0–5 scale for how much of a problem there is with each "now".

QOLAS as used in dementia: Scoring

The scores for the two constructs per domain are summed to give a domain score out of 10. The total for each of the five domains is summed to give an overall QOLAS score out of 50. An example is shown in Table 1.

TABLE 1
Scoring: An example

Domain	Construct	Construct score	Domain score	Total score
Physical:	Headaches	3		
	Tiredness	2	5	
Psychological:	Anxious	4		
	Feels sad	4	8	
Social/family:	Don't go out any more	4		
	Children no longer visit	5	9	
Work:	Had a lot of time off work	4		
	I am not promoted	3	7	
Cognitive:	Memory	5		
	Finding the right word	3	8	
Total				37

CURRENT STUDY

Aims

The present study had three aims: (1) to develop and test the psychometric properties of the QOLAS for the assessment of QOL of patients with dementia, (2) to compare patients' ratings of their own QOL with the ratings given by the main carers, and (3) to look at which independent variables might predict the total QOLAS score as rated by both the patient and the carer using multivariate regression techniques.

Materials and methods

In consultation with the nursing staff, patient–carer dyads were recruited from the outpatient clinics of the Dementia Research Group, Queen Square. Written informed consent was obtained prior to each interview.

The patient completed: (1) the Quality of Life Assessment Schedule (QOLAS); (2) the Mini-Mental State Examination (MMSE); (3) the EuroQol EQ-5D and a selection of the Dartmouth COOP charts. The carer rated the QOL of the patient using (1) the QOLAS (a semi-structured interview) (2) the Interview to Determine Deterioration in Daily Functioning in Dementia (IDDD); (3) the Neuropsychiatric Inventory (NPI), and (4) the EuroQol EQ-5D. These instruments are briefly described later.

The carers were also asked to rate their *own* QOL on (1) the QOLAS; (2) the Medical Outcomes Study Short-form-36 (MOS SF-36) (Ware & Sherbourne, 1992); (3) the General Health Questionnaire (GHQ-30) (Goldberg & Williams,

1988); and (4) the Profile of Mood States (POMS) Short Form (McNair, Lorr, & Droppleman, 1992). The main focus of this paper is the QOL of the patient.

QOL assessment: Patient on self

Modified QOLAS.   This was described earlier.

Mini-mental state examination (MMSE) (Folstein, Folstein, & McHugh, 1975).   This is probably the most widely used brief screening instrument for dementia (Lezak, 1995). The test consists of two parts: verbal and performance. The scores range from 0–30 with a lower score indicating greater cognitive impairment.

EQ-5D (Brooks, 1996; EuroQol Group, 1990).   This generic instrument, which measures health-related quality of life, has five domains: mobility, self-care, usual activities, pain/discomfort, and anxiety/depression. Respondents also rate their own health today on a visual analogue scale (VAS) from 100 (best imaginable health state) to 0 (worst imaginable health state). The data can be presented descriptively as a health profile and a single index utility score can be calculated. The EQ-5D is designed for self-completion but in the current study it was interviewer-assisted, i.e., a copy was given to patient but it was also read out to the patient.

Dartmouth COOP charts (Nelson et al., 1987).   These generic self-rated health status questions were developed for the assessment of patients' functional health in routine clinical practice. Each chart consists of a question referring to the past month, with five response choices, each illustrated with a drawing. The scoring for each question is from 1 = no difficulty to 5 = cannot do with higher scores representing worse QOL. A sub-set of five questions was chosen which assessed the domains: (1) overall health, (2) daily activities, (3) physical fitness, (4) social activities, and (5) feelings. The questions were presented so that one question filled a page of A4 size paper.

Proxy QOL assessment: Carer describing patient

QOLAS (as earlier).   Carers were asked to nominate the QOL items they perceived to be of most importance for the patient's QOL. The carers were asked to think about how *they* (i.e., the carer) perceived the QOL of the patient. Carers were not asked to think about how they thought *the patient* perceived his/her own QOL. This distinction is of increasing importance in the proxy literature (Jeffrey A. Johnson, personal communication). Carers were reminded that there would be an opportunity later in the interview for them to discuss their *own* QOL.

Interview to Determine Deterioration in Daily Functioning in Dementia (IDDD) (Teunisse, Mayke, & Van Crevel, 1991).   This scale has 33 items concerning changes in patient's daily functioning. The questions refer to self-care and daily activities. A higher score indicates poorer abilities.

The Neuropsychiatric Inventory (NPI) (Cummings et al., 1994).   This scale, which assesses neuropsychiatric problems, has 12 domains. If a positive response is elicited from an initial screening question, further questions about each item are asked and a total score based on frequency and severity can be calculated for each of the 12 items.

EQ-5D (carer on patient).   The EQ-5D was interviewer administered and the question plus response options were read out replacing, for example, "Do you have any problems in walking about?" with "Does you wife/husband (etc.) have any problems in walking about?".

Staging of dementia

The staging of dementia was calculated using cutoffs on the MMSE as follows: scores 0–10 = severe; 11–20 = moderate; 21–30 = mild (Mega, Cummings, Fiorello, & Gornbein, 1996).

DATA ANALYSIS

Psychometric testing of the QOLAS

Any new measure of health status/QOL must undergo full psychometric testing to ascertain its validity, reliability, and responsiveness, or sensitivity to change (Juniper et al., 1996; Streiner & Norman, 1995).

Validity.   There are a number of different types of validity. *Face* or *content* validity simply concerns whether all important aspects of the phenomenon are covered by the scale. Since the QOLAS is tailored to each respondent, it has optimum validity for each individual. *Criterion* validity is the correlation of a scale with some other measure of the trait or disorder under study, ideally a 'gold standard' which has been used and accepted in the field. In this study, we examined the correlations between the QOLAS and other measures assessing similar aspects of well-being.

Construct validation is an ongoing process whereby hypothetical "constructs" or "mini-theories" are tested. One such hypothesis might be that higher disease severity would correlate with lower scores indicating worse QOL. We tested construct validity in two ways. First, we tested the hypothesis that the patients with greater deterioration in skills of daily activities, as measured by the IDDD would have a worse QOL than patients with less deterioration in these skills. We arbitrarily chose a cutoff of 50 on the IDDD and compared the two groups using independent *t*-tests. Second, we tested the hypothesis that the QOLAS total score (patient self-rating) would correlate with the MMSE.

Reliability. The reliability of a measure can be assessed in two ways: (1) internal consistency is assessed by looking at the correlation of each item/domain with the total score and coefficient alpha; (2) test–retest reliability is assessed by a repeat administration of the measure after an interval sufficiently short that genuine changes in QOL/health status would not have occurred and sufficiently long such that similarity in responses is not due to a learning effect.

Most of the interviews were conducted in the patients' homes after considerable negotiation to find a convenient time and there was a high level of emotion expressed by both patients and carers. Although a repeat interview one week later had been planned to assess test–retest reliability, this was felt to have been too intrusive and burdensome. In this study we were able to look at the internal reliability of the QOLAS but not test–retest reliability. We recognise the need to assess the QOLAS for test–retest reliability.

Patient/proxy comparison. We looked at the correlations between the patients' and the carers' scores for each QOLAS domain. Since the QOLAS is in an individual, respondent-tailored technique, one would not expect, *a priori*, as much agreement between any two raters as with a fixed questionnaire with identical wording. We therefore also looked at the head-to-head comparison of the EQ-5D, patient rating self and carer rating patient.

Statistical analysis

In the psychometric testing of a new scale there is debate in the literature as to whether parametric or non-parametric statistics should be used. One criterion is whether the data are normally distributed. Another issue is that whilst the response options give the impression that the Likert is an interval scale, psycho-semantic studies have shown that it is only an ordinal scale of measurement, i.e., the distance between any two adjacent points on the scale cannot be assumed to be the same. Other researchers have argued that this theoretical technicality does not matter in practice (Ware, 1995). We analysed the data using both the Pearson's correlation and the non-parametric Spearman's rank correlation coefficient. The results were almost identical. We report the Spearman's rank correlation coefficient only.

The patients' and carers' scores on the QOLAS were compared using correlations, as were the tests of construct validity. Criterion validity was tested in two ways: The two groups were compared using an independent *t*-test and the hypothesis that decreasing MMSE scores were associated with worse QOL scores was tested by correlation. We assessed internal reliability by looking at correlations between each domain score and the total score and by the coefficient alpha.

In a head-to-head comparison of the responses to the EQ-5D, we compared the level of agreement between the patients and carers using the Cohen's kappa statistic.

Finally, using MINITAB, we investigated the contribution of the various predictor variables assessed (neuropsychiatric symptoms, dementia severity, patient and carer gender, etc.) in determining QOL, i.e., the total QOLAS score as rated by the patient and by the carer. To achieve this, an all-subsets regression technique was used to choose the best subset of predictor variables from all available variables as follows:

All possible (2Pmax-1) regression analyses were performed, with R^2 calculated for each model.

The best models having the largest R^2 with each number of parameters (1, 2, ... , Pmax) were chosen.

Mallows Cp statistic was then used to determine the optimal number of predictor variables to include in the model and hence the optimal model.

Mallows Cp is calculated as follows; for a model with p predictor variables ($1 <= p <=$ Pmax)

$$C_p = \frac{(SS_0)_p}{\hat{\sigma}_2} + 2(p+1) - n$$

Where $(SS_0)p$ = residual sum of squares for the model with p parameters.

We then used Hocking's criteria that the optimal model is the one with the least number of parameters such that $Cp <= 2(p+1) -$ Pmax. The appropriateness of the models chosen were assessed using the overall F-test, normal plots of residuals, and plots of residuals against fitted values.

Since the patient's cognitive ability is likely to affect the results, the results, where appropriate, are shown for the whole group of patients with mild to moderate dementia ($n = 22$) and for the subgroup of patients with mild dementia ($n = 12$).

RESULTS

A total of 37 patient–carer dyads were recruited. The cognitive status of 13 patients precluded interview. These 13 patients, who did not engage in the interview and/or did not give meaningful replies, all had an MMSE score less than 11. A further two patients were subsequently found not to have a regular carer and were excluded from this study. The current paper addresses the QOL of the 22 patients with mild to moderate dementia who could be interviewed and for whom a primary carer was identified and interviewed. The QOL of the 13 patients who could not be interviewed will be reported elsewhere. The interviews took place either at The National Hospital, Queen Square, or at home. Most of the patients had presenile dementia of the Alzheimer's type (DSM-IV criterion of onset before age 65 years) and in this preliminary study the patients were not further subgrouped according to aetiology. Standard sociodemographic data were collected from the carer.

The patients in these 22 patient–carer dyads all had an MMSE score within the range 11–30 and thus were in the mild to moderate stages of dementia (Mega et al., 1996). The mean age of the patients was 65 years, SD = 8, range 48–80. Twelve patients were male and 10 were female. Eighteen of the carers were spouses and all carers were living with the patient at the time of interview. The mean age of the carers was 61 years, SD = 13, range 30–77. Eight of the carers were male and 14 were female. The mean time of onset prior to interview was 5 years, SD = 3 years.

An attempt was made to interview the patients and carers separately so that neither would feel inhibited and discouraged from speaking frankly. All patients and carers were willing and indeed eager to conform to this arrangement. During the patient interviews the carers absented themselves to get a cup of tea or attend to a household chore. When it was the carers' turn to be interviewed they asked the patient to wait in another room or perform an errand such as collecting the newspaper from the local shop.

Qualitative data: QOLAS semi-structured interview

One main advantage of the QOLAS interview is that each respondent can identify the items of importance to their own QOL, thus maximising the validity of the method. The items most frequently mentioned by the patients and by the carers are summarised in Table 2; full details of the constructs elicited can be obtained from the authors. The QOLAS subscale scores for both the patients' and the carers' ratings are shown in Figure 1. For each domain, the carers rated the patients as having a worse QOL than did the patients themselves. We looked at the correlations between the patients' and the carers' scores for each QOLAS domain. There was good agreement in all domains except daily activities and cognitive functioning. As predicted, the correlations were slightly better for the patients with only mild dementia ($n = 12$). These results are summarised in Table 3.

Validity

The results for the assessment of criterion validity are summarised in Table 4. The QOLAS total score as rated by the patient correlated with measures of affect, social life, and activities whereas the carers' rating of the QOL of the

Table 2
QOLAS: Describing the QOL of the patient. The three constructs
most frequently elicited per domain by the patients and by the carers

QOLAS domain	Patients' self-report	Carer on patient
Physical	No problems/healthy	Physical health is good
	Headaches	Tiredness
	Various symptoms, e.g., back/chest pain	Various symptoms, e.g, eczema, deafness
Psychological	No problems/happy	Seems mainly happy
	Depressed/down	Anxious
	Feel vulnerable/unsafe	Up-and-down/agitated
Social/family	Going out	Relationship with family
	Seeing friends/leisure activities	Going out
	Seeing family	Friends backing off
Daily activities	Gardening	Cooking/housework
	Going for walk	D.I.Y
	Doing things round home	Going for walk
Cognitive	Memory/forgetting	Memory
	Concentration, e.g., TV	Concentration
	Thinking and speaking (finding the right words)	Repeatedly asks the same question

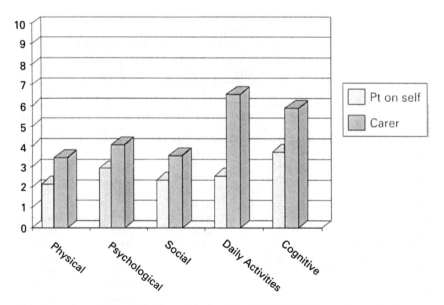

Figure 1.   QOLAS scores for each of the five domains.

TABLE 3

Correlations between patients' self-rating and carers rating
the patient for two groups: mild-to-moderate dementia
(n = 22) and mild dementia (n = 12)

Domain	Mild-to-moderate (MMSE >10)	Mild (MMSE > 20)
Physical	.3787**	.7934**
Psychiatric	.3699**	.6671*
Social	.4252**	.6107*
Daily activities	.4123*	.4045
Cognitive	−.0519	.2906
Total	.4061*	.7349**

Spearman's correlation coefficient. * p = .05; ** p = .01.

patient correlated with more objective measures of mobility, activities of daily living and neuropsychiatric symptoms. As predicted, the correlations were generally slightly better for the subset of patients with only mild dementia (n = 12).

Construct validity was assessed, first, by testing the hypothesis that the patients with greater deterioration in skills of daily activities, as measured by the IDDD, would have a worse QOL than patients with less deterioration in

TABLE 4

Criterion validity: Correlations between the total QOLAS score
and instruments assessing other aspects of well-being.
All (non-parametric) Spearman's correlation coefficients

Scale	Patient rating self		Carer rating patient	
	mild-to-moderate (n = 22)	mild dementia (n = 12)	mild-to-moderate (n = 22)	mild dementia (n = 12)
COOP (overall)	.4060	.4690	–	–
COOP (daily activities)	.3914	.7058**	–	–
COOP (fitness)	.4264*	.8838***	–	–
COOP (social)	.6495***	.8517***	–	–
COOP (feelings)	.6574***	.7900**	–	–
EQ-5D (mobility)	.2253	.2609	.4312*	.5886*
EQ-5D (self-care)	−.0105	.4838	.2551	.3893
EQ-5D (usual activities)	.4076	.5099	.5389	.5731*
EQ-5D (pain/discomfort)	.3862	.5671	−.1530	.2052
EQ-5D (anxiety/depression)	.5170*	.6189*	.3157	.4660
NPI-global	–	–	.6347**	.7005**
IDDD	–	–	.4248*	.5477

*p = .05; **p = .01; ***p = .001.

these skills. We arbitrarily chose a cutoff of 50 on the IDDD and compared the
two groups ($n = 11$ patients per group) using independent t-tests. For the group
where IDDD ≤ 50 the mean total QOLAS score was 18.5 (SD = 7.3) and for the
group with IDDD scores above 50, i.e., with more problems, the mean QOLAS
total score was 28.5 (SD = 9.0), the higher scores indicating a poorer QOL. The
mean scores were significantly different, $t = 2.85$, $p = .01$.

We found that whilst the patient self-rated QOLAS total score for the whole
group ($n = 22$) did not correlate with the MMSE score, when we looked at the
patients with mild dementia only ($n = 12$), the patient self-rated QOLAS total
did correlate with the MMSE score, $r = 0.6$, $p = .05$.

Reliability

Table 5 shows the internal consistency of the QOLAS. Each domain correlated
highly with the total QOLAS score showing good internal consistency. The
coefficient alpha, for patient rating self and carer rating patient was in each case
.78, and this result is well within the acceptable range.

TABLE 5
Internal consistency: Correlation of QOLAS
domain scores with QOLAS total score.
All (non-parametric) Spearman's correlation coefficients.

QOLAS domain	Patient rating self (n = 22)	Carer rating patient (n = 22)
Physical	.5888**	.6657***
Psychological	.8112***	.8065***
Social	.8579***	.6447***
Daily activities	.7941***	.7140***
Cognitive	.8112***	.6996***

** $p = .01$; *** $p = .001$.

Patient self-rating and carer rating patient on the EQ-5D

A head-to-head comparison was made of the results of the patient self-rated
EQ-5D and the EQ-5D rated by the main carer to look at the level of agreement.
The three levels per domain (no problem, some problems, and extreme
problems), yield ordinal scale data and agreement in each domain was assessed
using Cohen's Kappa statistic with the strength of agreement for each value of
K rated using the convention from "poor" to "very good" as per the current literature (Altman, 1991; Landis & Koch, 1977). The results are summarised in
Table 6. The Cohen's weighted kappa, which takes account of the level of

TABLE 6
EQ-5D head-to-head comparison. Cohen's kappa statistic

	Mild to moderate (n = 22)		Mild dementia (n = 12)	
Mobility	.35	Fair	.43	Moderate
Self-care	.67	Good	.63	Good
Usual activities	.09	Poor	.09	Poor
Pain discomfort	.67	Good	.82	Very good
Anxiety depression	.45	Moderate	.47	Moderate

disagreement, was not calculated because it assumes equal intervals between each measurement level, e.g., between "no problems" and "some" and between "some" and "extreme" and a previous study showed this was not the case (Selai, 1998). The results for the "usual activities" domain was poor. Qualitative data revealed that both patient and carer asked what was usual. In cases where the patient had been retired early on medical grounds, sometimes months or years previously, it was not clear whether work was a "usual activity". This finding would suggest that a less ambiguous question would be more appropriate for patients with dementia.

Most patients and carers had problems making a global rating on the EQ-5D visual analogue scale (VAS). The most frequent comment was that the patients' physical health was good but that "mental" or cognitive functioning was poor so the respondents wanted to give a separate score for each of these components of well-being.

TABLE 7
Eleven parameter optimal model for patient self-rated QOL

Predictor	Partial regression coefficient (β)	95% confidence interval	p
Patient Age (years)	0.26	−0.03 to 0.55	.08
Patient Gender (0 = Male, 1 = Female)	−6.38	−10.1 to −2.6	.004
MMSE Score	−1.14	−1.67 to −0.61	.001
IDDD Score	−0.66	−0.91 to −0.42	.001
Co-op Overall	−2.25	−4.95 to 0.44	.09
Co-op Daily Activities	−2.25	−4.84 to 0.33	.08
Co-op Fitness	9.31	5.94 to 12.69	.001
Co-op Social	8.08	5.49 to 10.66	.001
Co-op Feelings	−3.94	−6.58 to −1.29	.009
Profile of mood states	−0.40	−0.70 to −0.1	.01
GHQ Score	0.13	−0.21 to 0.49	.39
Constant (α)	33.6	11.8 to 55.4	.007

$F(11,8) = 18.07, p = .0002, R^2 = .96$, Adjusted $R^2 = .91$

TABLE 8
Six parameter optimal model for carer-rated patient QOL

Predictor	Partial regression coefficient (β)	95% confidence interval	p
Patient gender (0 = Male, 1 = Female)	−7.84	−13.9 to −1.76	.02
Age at onset (years)	0.94	−0.03 to 2.02	.08
IDDD	0.22	−0.03 to 0.48	.08
NPI Global Score	0.26	0.05 to 0.47	.02
Co-op Daily Activities	−2.05	−5.6 to 1.49	.23
Co-op Feelings	3.19	0.79 to 5.61	.01
Constant (α)	3.12	−11.65 to 17.9	.65

$F(6,13) = 7.25, p = .0002, R^2 = .77$, Adjusted $R^2 = .66$

Regression analysis

For *patient self-rated* QOL, the optimal model had 11 parameters: patient age; patient gender; MMSE; IDDD; COOP overall; COOP daily activities; COOP fitness; COOP social; COOP feelings; profile of mood states; and GHQ, and is summarised in Table 7. For *carer-rated* patient QOL a model with six parameters was optimal: patient gender; age at onset; IDDD; NPI; Co-op daily activities; and Co-op feelings (Table 8).

DISCUSSION

We present the results of a study to assess the feasibility of using an individual-ised assessment technique, the QOLAS, to rate the QOL of patients with dementia as rated by both the patients themselves and their main carer. These patients with mild to moderate dementia understood the interview and were able to answer questions about their QOL, providing both qualitative and quan-titative data. It was found during the psychometric testing that the subset of patients with only mild dementia generally did slightly better than the whole group of patients with mild to moderate dementia.

At the time of writing only one previous published study of patient self-reported QOL was found in the literature (Coen et al., 1993) although a number of other studies of patient self-reported QOL are in preparation or in press (Selai & Trimble, 1999; Albert & Logsdon, 1999). In the previous published study of patient self-reported QOL in dementia, the method was complex and only 6 out of 20 patients completed the full interview (Coen et al., 1993).

Although various purported QOL measures have been used in clinical trials of anti-dementia drugs, these instruments have either not been fully validated for dementia or they do not comprehensively assess QOL (Salek et al., 1998; Walker et al., 1998).

Since the QOLAS is a subjective, respondent-driven approach, the method has optimum face (or content) validity. This study demonstrated that the QOLAS had acceptable criterion validity and construct validity. Reliability was good, as assessed by internal consistency and the coefficient alpha. In this study we were not able to address test–retest reliability or sensitivity to change. Test–retest reliability for other individualised approaches has been good. For example, respondents made a mean of 1.7 changes in their choice of constructs on the PGI (Ruta et al., 1994) and changed a mean of 1 construct on the SEIQOL at 2 years follow-up (O'Boyle et al., 1993). We acknowledge the need to assess these measurement properties of the QOLAS in patients with dementia.

There are a number of points for discussion. First, this is a small feasibility study of patients with "dementia", irrespective of aetiology. In future studies, it would be important to look at patients subgrouped according to diagnosis, since factors of importance to both patients and carers might vary considerably according to the type of dementia. For example, patients with frontotemporal dementias have profound alteration in social conduct and personality which might have different implications for the QOL of both patient and carer (Neary & Snowden, 1997).

Some health services researchers are sceptical about the feasibility of asking patients with dementia to rate their own well-being (Bond, 1999). The first question, therefore, concerns the reliability or stability of responses and this raises a number of methodological issues. Since cognitive deterioration will affect the patient's ability to self-report, it is of interest to look at whether the patient's views correspond to those of their main carer. However, there are a number of problems with this approach. First, many studies have documented poor patient-proxy agreement in QOL ratings (Slevin et al., 1988). Poor agreement might be due to a number of factors, such as (1) there might be error inherent in the measuring instrument, e.g., ambiguous wording of an item on a questionnaire, (2) the patient and carer might just have different views on whether something is relevant to QOL, e.g., attending dinner-parties, and (3) an eccentricity identified by the carer might be acknowledged by the patient but not be felt to be a problem by the patient, e.g., choosing to wear orange trousers with a pink shirt. One of the patients in this study felt it was entirely acceptable to wear her nightdress under an anorak to church on Sunday causing her sister much distress. Published studies suggest that there will be less agreement for non-observable things, e.g., pain and psychological problems compared to concrete, observable items such as ability to walk (Magaziner, 1997; Zimmerman & Magaziner, 1994).

Criterion validity can be assessed by comparing answers to items on different questionnaires which are tapping the same QOL domain. However, there are a number of problems with this approach which have been highlighted in the psychometric literature. Research has shown that even an apparently identical question, phrased in a slightly different way, or situated in a different place on the questionnaire page, can lead to quite different responses. Also, the time frames for measures of QOL or health status are often different, with some questions asking how things are today and others asking how things have been in the last week, the last month, or in the last six months.

With no "gold standard", and a paucity of measures of well-being for this patient group, criterion validity was difficult to assess. Our results relied heavily on a comparison with the COOP charts. It could be argued that these are not really appropriate since the precise wording of the questions (and the time frame that the respondent is asked to consider) result in the COOP charts tapping into different aspects of health or well-being when compared to the QOLAS. The pictorial representations (cartoons of "stick-men") will have added to the difference between the questions asked, and thus information being elicited, by the two measures. Bearing in mind these methodological limitations, the QOLAS appeared to have acceptable construct and criterion validity.

The carers rated the patients as having a poorer QOL in all domains of the QOLAS than the patients rated themselves, and this might be due to lack of insight or anosognosia (Whitehouse et al., 1997; Selai & Trimble, 1999). This finding raises a number of technical and ethical issues concerning who is the best "judge" of QOL in cases where patients have poor and diminishing cognitive abilities.

It is interesting to note the similarities in the constructs elicited from the patients and carers (Table 2). The most frequently made comment, by both patients and carers, in the physical domain, was that physical health was good or that the patient was physically fit. Since physical health might not be a problem in the early stages of dementia, especially in younger patients, generic measures of health status might not pick up the subtle early manifestations of the disease and they might be susceptible to ceiling effects.

There is a complex interaction of patient and carer QOL since the two are mutually influential. Carer stress, mood, and psychiatric morbidity, exacerbated by carer burden, will, in turn, affect the patient's QOL (e.g., the carer might be angry, hostile, or emotionally unavailable for the patient). Many carers in this study tearfully recounted how they had, on occasions, shouted, screamed, "bullied", and "punished" the patient whilst feeling under extreme pressure.

This stress will also influence the carer's judgement and perception of the patient's QOL. Since proxy measures yield data that are coloured by the opinion, and biases of another person, it has been suggested that researchers should carefully document their use of proxies and the potential error/bias their use introduces to specific studies (Magaziner, 1997).

The regression analyses provide an intriguing insight into the determinants of QOL from both the patients' and the carers' perspective. The correct interpretation of the regression models are important in understanding these results. The objective of the regression analysis is to select the best combination of predictor variables that together provide a linear prediction of the QOL score. The models presented in Tables 7 and 8 are two of many possible models, but are essentially "optimal" in terms of their ability to predict QOL scores, and the proportion of the variance explained (R^2). The partial regression coefficients represent units on the QOLAS scale, for example in Table 7, for patient gender, a 1 unit increase in gender (i.e., changing from male to female) is associated with a 6.38 unit drop in QOL ($p = .004$) controlling for all other predictors, i.e., female patients report a worse QOL than male patients when controlled for other factors. Similarly, a 1 year increase in patient age is associated with a 0.26 increase in the QOL score, which can be interpreted as older patients experiencing better QOL, when controlled for other factors.

It is however important to realise that these are only two of many possible models, and it is more important to interpret trends in determinants of QOL, than to draw very specific conclusions about particular predictors. Finally, caution in interpreting these findings is particularly important in view of our small sample size.

When multiple statistical comparisons are being made there is the increasing probability that significant results are due to chance and some method of correcting for this, such as Bonferroni corrections is often recommended. Since this study was exploratory we did not apply Bonferroni corrections and our results therefore must be interpreted with caution.

This study has a number of limitations. First, as mentioned previously, we acknowledge the small sample size. A number of patients could not be interviewed themselves and we only had carer proxy QOL data. This small sample precludes definitive psychometric testing in this patient group and our study must be replicated with a larger sample.

A second point for discussion concerns the suitability of the use of a method based on RGT for patients with dementia. We chose an "individualised technique" as the general approach, and the Repertory Grid in particular, because the literature suggests (both theoretically and empirically) that individualised methods are more valid. Instead of a fixed questionnaire, the respondent is invited to think, reflect, judge, and generate items of concern to themselves. As outlined in Kelly's original work, construct theory is based on the idea of the person as a "scientist". By this, he meant that we have our own view of the world (our theories), our expectations of what will happen in given situations (hypotheses), and through our behaviour we continue to experiment with life. Exploring the world like a scientist, however, entails a fairly sophisticated level of cognitive functioning and we might ask whether this theoretical underpinning holds up for the person with increasing cognitive impairment. On the other hand, the vast Personal Construct and Repertory Grid literature has many papers on the use of the Repertory Grid with patients with a range of psychiatric illness including schizophrenia, organic brain injury and suicidal behaviour. The Repertory Grid has also been used with children and adults with low IQ. Most patients with dementia in general, and Alzheimer's disease in particular, have few cognitive problems in the very early stages of their illness and the patients interviewed for this research were fluent and articulate in the mild to moderate stages of the disease. It therefore seems appropriate to continue to tap in to the construct system of the person with dementia until such time as the cognitive complexity of this interview is no longer possible.

There are a number of issues which we would like to address in future research. Although preliminary testing of the psychometric properties of the modified and streamlined QOLAS shows this to be a promising technique, further testing of the method is required in a number of other settings with larger sample sizes. Whilst internal reliability was assessed, and found to be acceptable, test–retest reliability was not assessed and this needs to be addressed in a future study. It was not possible to assess sensitivity to change and this also remains to be tested. A number of new anti-dementia drugs are becoming available and one possibility would be to incorporate the QOLAS alongside other measures into a follow-up study to look at QOL pre- and post-treatment.

The QOLAS is one of a growing number of patient-tailored approaches, which take account of the individual's perspective, in a way that cannot be addressed by the fixed, standardised questionnaire. The need for such an approach has been strongly argued for in the QOL literature (Bowling, 1995; Gill, 1995).

The finding of poor agreement for the EQ-5D domain "usual activities" highlights the problem. The patients and their carers found this question ambiguous and asked what a "usual" activity was. An individualised approach would have allowed the respondent to identify an activity, the performance of which mattered greatly to their QOL.

Attention has only relatively recently turned to the assessment of QOL in dementia. As with the assessment of QOL in other patient groups, the most suitable QOL measure for use in dementia will depend upon the use to which the data will be put and it is likely that a variety of assessment methods will be useful for different purposes. A number of recommendations have been made in the dementia literature, e.g., that QOL measurement should use disease-specific measures which have an individualised outcome. In other words, the baseline and change in each individual patient should be monitored and account taken of the views and values of each patient and his or her family (Rockwood & Wilcock, 1996). The advantage of the QOLAS is its individualised outcome and it is therefore likely to have a role to play in the assessment of QOL in dementia.

CONCLUSION

We tested the feasibility and the psychometric properties of an individualised patient-tailored quality of life assessment technique, the QOLAS, for use as a measure of QOL in patients with dementia. The QOLAS was shown to have good validity and reliability. The results suggest that patients with mild to moderate dementia can rate their own QOL and that the QOLAS is a promising method for assessing QOL in this patient group.

REFERENCES

Albert, S., & Logsdon, R. (1999). Assessing Quality of Life in Alzheimer's disease. *Journal of Mental Health and Aging, 5*(1), 3–6.

Altman, D.G. (1991). *Practical statistics for medical research.* London: Chapman and Hall.

Barofsky, I. (1996). Cognitive aspects of quality of life assessment. In B. Spilker (Ed.), *Quality of life and pharmacoeconomics in clinical trials.* Philadelphia, New York: Lippincott-Raven.

Bond, J. (1999). Assessing quality of life for people with dementia. *Progress in Neurology and Psychiatry, 3,* 29–34.

Bowling, A. (1995). *Measuring disease: A review of disease-specific quality of life measurement scales.* Buckingham, UK: Open University Press.

Brazier, J., & Deverill, M. (1999) A checklist for judging preference-based measures of health related quality of life: Learning from psychometrics. *Health Economics, 8,* 41–51.

Brooks, R.G. (1995). *Health status measurement: A perspective on change.* Basingstoke, UK: Macmillan.

Brooks, R.G. (1996). EuroQol: The current state of play. *Health Policy, 37,* 53–72.

Burns, A. (1995). Alzheimer's disease: Pharmacological developments to the year 2000. *Human Psychopharmacology, 10* (Suppl. 4), S247–S251.

Coen, R., O'Mahoney, D., O'Boyle, C., Joyce, C.R.B., Hiltbrunner, B., Walsh, J.B., & Coakley, D. (1993). Measuring the quality of life of dementia patients using the Schedule for the Evaluation of Individual Quality of Life. *Irish Journal of Psychology, 14,* 154–163.

Cummings, J.L., Mega, M., Gray, K., Rosenberg-Thompson, S., Carusi, D.A., & Gornbein, J. (1994). The Neuropsychiatric Inventory: Comprehensive assessment of psychopathology in dementia. *Neurology, 44,* 2308–2314.

Elstner, K., Selai, C.E., Trimble, M.R., & Robertson, M.M. (in press). Quality of life in Gilles de la Tourette Syndrome. *Acta Psychiatrica Scandinavica.*

EuroQol Group (1990). EuroQol: A new facility for the measurement of health related quality of life. *Health Policy, 16,* 199–208.

Fitzpatrick, R., Fletcher, A., Gore, S., Jones, D., Spiegelhalter, D. & Cox, D. (1992). Quality of life measures in health care, I: Applications and issues in assessment. *British Medical Journal, 305,* 1074–1077.

Fletcher, A.E., Dickinson, E.J., & Philp, I. (1992). Review: Audit measures: Quality of life instruments for everyday use with elderly patients. *Age and Ageing, 21,* 142–150.

Folstein, M.F., Folstein, S.E., & McHugh, P.R. (1975). Mini Mental State: A practical method for grading the cognitive state of patients for the clinician. *Journal of Psychiatric Research, 12,* 189–198.

Fransella, F., & Bannister, D. (1977). *A manual for repertory grid technique.* London: Academic Press. Harcourt Brace Jovanovich.

Fraser, S.C.A., Ramirez, A.J., Ebbs, S.R., Fallowfield, L.J., Dobbs, H.J., Richards, M.A., Bates, T. & Baum, M. (1993). A daily diary card for quality of life measurement in advanced breast cancer trials. *British Journal of Cancer, 67,* 341–346.

Geddes, D.M., Dones, L., Hill, E., Law, K., Harper, P.G., Spiro, S.G., Tobias, J.S., & Souhami, R.L. (1990). Quality of life during chemotherapy for small cell lung cancer: Assessment and use of a daily diary card in a randomised trial. *European Journal of Cancer, 26*, 484–492.

Gill, T.M. (1995). Quality of life assessment: Values and pitfalls. *Journal of the Royal Society of Medicine, 88*, 680–682.

Gill, T.M., & Feinstein, A.R. (1994). A critical appraisal of the quality of quality of life measurements. *Journal of the American Medical Association, 272*, 619–626.

Goldberg, D.P., & Williams, P. (1988). *A user's guide to the General Health Questionnaire.* Windsor, UK: NFER-Nelson.

Guyatt, G.H., Berman, L.B., Townsend, M., Pugsley, S.O. & Chambers, L.W. (1987a). A measure of quality of life for clinical trials in chronic lung disease. *Thorax, 42*, 773–778.

Guyatt, G.H., Townsend, M., Pugsley, S. O., Keller, J.L., Short, H.D., Taylor, W., & Newhouse, M.T. (1987b). Bronchodilators in chronic air-flow limitation. *American Review of Respiratory Disorders, 135*, 1069–1074.

Hedrick, S.C., Taeuber, R.C., & Erickson, P. (1996). On learning and understanding quality of life. In B. Spilker (Ed.), *Quality of life and pharmacoeconomics in clinical trials.* Philadelphia, New York: Lippincott-Raven.

Howard, K., & Rockwood, K. (1995). Quality of life in alzheimer's disease: A review. *Dementia, 6*, 113–116.

Hunt, S.M. (1999). The researcher's tale: A story of virtue lost and regained. In C.R.B. Joyce, C.A. O'Boyle, & H.M. McGee (Eds.), *Individual quality of life: Approaches to conceptualisation and assessment.* Amsterdam: Harwood Academic Publishers.

Joyce, C.R.B., O'Boyle, C.A. & McGee, H.M. (Eds.) (1999). *Individual quality of life: Approaches to conceptualisation and assessment.* Amsterdam: Harwood Academic Publishers.

Juniper, E.F., Guyatt, G.H. & Jaeschke, R. (1996). How to develop and validate a new health-related quality of life instrument. In B. Spilker (Ed.), *Quality of life and pharmacoeconomics in clinical trials* (2nd Edition). Philadelphia, New York: Lippincott-Raven.

Kelly, G.A. (1995). *A theory of personality: The psychology of personal constructs.* New York: W.W. Norton & Co.

Kelly, C.A., Harvey, R.J. & Cayton, H. (1997). Drug treatments for Alzheimer's disease. *British Medical Journal, 314*, 693–694.

Kendrick, A. (1993). *Repertory Grid Technique in the assessment of quality of life in patients with epilepsy.* PhD thesis. University of London.

Kendrick, A. (1997). Quality of life. In C. Cull & L.H. Goldstein (Eds.), *The clinical psychologist's handbook of epilepsy.* London and New York: Routledge.

Kendrick, A.M., & Trimble, M.R. (1994). Repertory Grid in the assessment of quality of life in patients with epilepsy: The Quality of Life Assessment Schedule. In M.R. Trimble & W.E. Dodson (Eds.), *Epilepsy and the quality of life.* New York: Raven Press.

Landis, R.J., & Koch, G.G. (1977). The measurement of observer agreement for categorical data. *Biometrics, 33*, 159–174.

Lawton, M.P (1994). Quality of life in Alzheimer disease. *Alzheimer's Disease and Associated Disorders, 8* (Suppl. 3), 138–150.

Lezak, M.D. (1995). *Neuropsychological assessment* (3rd Edition). Oxford: Oxford University Press.

Magaziner, J. (1997). Use of proxies to measure health and functional outcomes in effectiveness research in persons with Alzheimer's disease and related disorders. *Alzheimer Disease and Associated Disorders, 11* (Suppl. 6), 168–174.

Mays, N., & Pope, C. (1996). Rigour and qualitative research. In N. Mays & C. Pope (Eds.), *Qualitative Research in Health Care.* London: BMJ Publishing Group.

McDowell, I., & Newell, C. (1987). *Measuring health: A guide to rating scales and questionnaires.* Oxford, New York: Oxford University Press.

McGuire, A.M. (1991). Quality of life in women with epilepsy. In M.R. Trimble (Ed.), *Women and Epilepsy*. Chichester, UK: John Wiley.

McNair, D.M., Lorr, M., & Droppleman, L.F. (1992). *EdITS manual for the profile of mood states*. San Diego, CA: EdITS/Educational and Industrial Testing Service.

Mega, M.S., Cummings, J.L., Fiorello, T., & Gornbein, J. (1996). The spectrum of behavioural changes in Alzheimer's disease. *Neurology, 46*, 130–135.

Neary, D. & Snowden, J. (1997). Frontotemporal dementias and unusual dementing syndromes. In M.R. Trimble & J.L. Cummings (Eds.), *Contemporal behavioural neurology*. Oxford, UK: Butterworth-Heinemann.

Nelson E., Wasson, J., Kirk, J., Keller, A., Clark, D., Dietrich, A., Stewart, A., & Zubkoff, M. (1987). Assessment of function in routine clinical practice: Description of the COOP chart method and preliminary findings. *Journal of Chronic Diseases, 40* (Suppl. 1), 55S–63S.

O'Boyle, C.A., McGee, H.M., Hickey, A., Joyce, C.R.B., Browne, J., O'Malley, K., & Hiltbrunner, B. (1993). *The schedule for the evaluation of individual quality of life (SEIQoL). Administration manual*. Department of Psychology, Royal College of Surgeons in Ireland, Dublin.

Rabins, P.V. & Kasper, J.D. (1997). Measuring quality of life in dementia: Conceptual and practical issues. *Alzheimer Disease and Associated Disorders, 11* (Suppl. 6), 100–104.

Rockwood, K., & Wilcock, G.K. (1996). Quality of life. In S. Gauthier (Ed.), *Clinical diagnosis and management of Alzheimer's disease*. Oxford, UK: Butterworth-Heinemann.

Rossor, M. (1993). Alzheimer's disease. *British Medical Journal, 307*, 779–782.

Ruta, D.A., Garratt, A.M., Leng, M., Russell, I.T., & MacDonald, L.M. (1994). A new approach to the measurement of quality of life: The patient-generated index (PGI). *Medical Care, 32*, 1109–1126.

Salek, S.S., Walker, M.D., & Bayer, A.J. (1998). A review of quality of life in Alzheimer's disease. Part 2: issues in assessing drug effects. *Pharmacoeconomics, 14*, 613–627.

Selai, C.E. (1998). Scaling the EQ-5D middle-level quantifiers. In R.E. Rabin, J.J.V. Busschbach, F.Th. de Charro, M.L. Essink-Bot, & G.J. Bonsel (Eds.), Proceedings of the EuroQol Plenary Meeting, 2–3 October 1997, Rotterdam: Erasmus University.

Selai, C.E., Elstner, K. & Trimble, M.R. (2000). Quality of life pre and post epilepsy surgery. *Epilepsy Research, 38*, 67–74.

Selai, C.E., & Trimble, M.R. (1998). Adjunctive therapy in epilepsy with the new antiepileptic drugs: Is it of any value? *Seizure, 7*, 417–418.

Selai, C.E., & Trimble, M.R. (1999). Assessing quality of life in dementia. *Aging and Mental Health, 3*, 101–111.

Slevin, M.L., Plant, H., Lynch, D., Drinkwater, J., & Gregory, W.M. (1988). Who should measure quality of life, the doctor or the patient..? *British Journal of Cancer, 57*, 109–112.

Stewart, A.L., Sherbourne, C.D., & Brod, M. (1996). Measuring health-related quality of life in older and demented populations. In B. Spilker (Ed.), *Quality of life and pharmacoeconomics in clinical trials*. Philadelphia, New York: Lippincott-Raven.

Streiner, D.L., & Norman, G.R. (1995). *Health status measurement* (2nd edition). Oxford: Oxford University Press.

Teunisse, S., Mayke, M.A., & Van Crevel, H. (1991). Interview to Determine Deterioration in Daily Functioning in Dementia (IDDD). *Archives of Neurology, 48*, 274–277.

Tugwell, P., Bombardier, C., Buchanan, W.W., Goldsmith, C., Grace, E., Bennett, K.J., Williams, J., Egger, M., Alarcon, G.S., Guttadauria, M., Yarboro, C., Polisson, R.P., Szydlo, L., Luggen, M.E., Billingsley, L.M., Ward, J.R., & Marks, C. (1990). Methotrexate in rheumatoid arthritis: Impact on quality of life assessed by traditional standard item and individualized patient preference health status questionnaires. *Archive of Internal Medicine, 150*, 59–82.

Walker, M.D., Salek, S.S. & Bayer, A.J. (1998). A review of quality of life in Alzheimer's disease. Part I: issues in assessing disease impact. *Pharmacoeconomics, 14*, 499–530.

Ware, J.E. (1995). *Interpreting SF-36 health status scores.* Workshop held at the second conference of the International Society of Quality of Life (ISOQOL). Montreal, Canada.

Ware, J.E. & Sherbourne, C.D. (1992). The MOS 36-item short form health survey (SF-36): I. Conceptual framework and item selection. *Medical Care, 30,* 473–483.

Whitehouse, P.J., Orgogozo, J-M., Becker, R.E., Gauthier, S., Pontecorvo, M., Erzigkeit, H., Rogers, S., Mohs, R.C., Bodick, N., Bruno, G., & Dal-Bianco, P. (1997). Quality of life assessment in dementia drug development. Position paper from the International Working Group on Harmonization of Dementia Drug Guidelines. *Alzheimer Disease and Associated Disorders, 11,* (Suppl. 3), 56–60.

Whitehouse, P.J., Winblad, B., Shostak, D., Bhattacharjya, A., Brod, M., Brodaty, H., Dor, A., Feldman, H., Forette, F., Gauthier, S. Hay, J.W., Hill, S., Mastey, V. Neumann, P.J., O'Brien, B.J. Pugner, K. Sano, M., Sawada, T., Stone, R., & Wimo, A. (1998). 1st International Pharmacoeconomic Conference on Alzheimer's Disease: Report and Summary. *Alzheimer Disease and Associated Disorders, 12*(4), 266–280.

Zimmerman, S.I. & Magaziner, J. (1994). Methodological issues in measuring the functional status of cognitively impaired nursing home residents: the use of proxies and performance-based measures. *Alzheimer Disease and Associated Disorders,* 8: (Suppl. 1): S281–S290.

Manuscript received May 1999
Revised manuscript received August 2000

Memory training improves cognitive ability in patients with dementia

Stephanie Moore, Curt A. Sandman, Katie McGrady,
and J. Patrick Kesslak

University of California, Irvine, USA

Clinical symptoms of Alzheimer's disease (AD) include a variety of progressive cognitive deficits, particularly memory. Twenty-five patients with mild to moderate AD and their caregivers, who served as controls, participated in a 5 week memory training programme, with a 1 month follow up. Participants were taught strategies that included name–face rehearsal, effortful recall, and a significant event technique. Intervention efficacy was assessed on task specific tests, administered on a weekly basis, and general cognitive measures obtained at the first and last sessions of the intervention. During the memory training programme patients showed improved performance on the recall of names and faces, recognition memory after effortful processing of information, and significant events ($p < .05$). Controls consistently performed better than the AD group, making few errors. Standardised measures for the AD group improved on the Kendrick Digit Copy and had lower scores on the Geriatric Depression Scale ($p < .05$). Caregivers also rated patients higher on the Memory Function Questionnaire (MFQ) ($p < .05$). Thus, a memory training programme can be beneficial for patients with mild to moderate AD to improve some aspects of memory and behaviour. Ultimately, behavioural interventions in conjunction with pharmacological therapies may optimise functional ability and provide a framework to further enhance cognitive function in patients with dementia.

Patients with Alzheimer's disease (AD) can be characterised as having quantitative and qualitative deficits in the acquisition of new information, memory, language, and orientation to time and place, which progressively declines as the

Correspondence should be addressed to Dr Stephanie Moore, 1101 Easy Bryon, Suite A, Tustin, CA 92780-4401, USA, tel: (714) 731-6231, fax: (949) 644-8451.

We would like to thank Malcom Dick, Kristy Nielson, and Carl Cotman for their assistance in patient referrals, evaluations, and helpful discussions. This work has been supported in part by grants NIA 3P50 AG05142 and the state of California Department of Health Services 98-14972.

disease progresses (Cummings & Benson, 1992). As a result of these cognitive deficits patients show deficits in normal activities of daily living skills that can have a detrimental impact on careers, finances, family, and social interactions. Memory deficits are one of the early and prominent symptoms of AD that can result in frustration, depression, and withdrawal. Daily interactions are affected by diminished capacity for name–face recognition, ability to convey information, and recollection of daily events. Behavioural strategies may be helpful in compensating for some of these cognitive deficits.

The development of behavioural and pharmacological interventions for AD can have a significant impact on patient care. Currently in the US cholinesterase inhibitors are the primary pharmacological intervention for the treatment of AD. The benefits of these compounds are modest and may not be effective for all patients. Behavioural strategies, alone or in conjunction with drug interventions, should also be considered for the treatment of dementia. Early attempts to apply behavioural strategies for individuals with AD have had limited success in improving memory. Many procedures for retraining memory and language are designed for healthy volunteers (Cermak, 1975; Lorayne & Lucas, 1974; Minninger, 1984), aged individuals (Poon, 1980; Poon, Fozard, & Treat, 1978; Smith, 1980; Zarit, Cole, & Guider, 1981), and patients with head trauma (Berrol, 1990; Van der Linden & Van der Kaa, 1989; Wilson, 1987). These strategies rely heavily on semantic or phonemic association to facilitate the organisation and manipulation of material. The limited success of these methods in AD may be due to their inability to make associations which is vulnerable in this patient population (Craik & Watkins, 1973; Miller, 1975; Morris & Kopelman, 1986; Rabinowitz, 1984).

Since AD patients are not totally amnesic, particularly in the early to moderate stages of the disorder (Cummings & Benson, 1992), researchers continue to explore compensatory mechanisms that rely on functional neural circuits to sustain cognitive abilities. Unlike healthy elderly patients, Alzheimer's patients do not respond to comprehensive memory enhancement programmes (Mohs et al., 1998). However, by engineering the environment, cognitive support through experimental manipulation can improve memory (Bäckman, 1996). Improvement is particularly powerful if the training focuses on relatively preserved skills that may utilise functional neural circuits.

Hofmann, Hock, and Muller-Spahn (1996) have trained patients to use computers to access personally relevant information at different stages of the disease. This computer-assisted cognitive training requires scanning photographs of each patient's personal surroundings and entering autobiographical data into the computer. With the use of an interactive monitor, performance of patients from mild to advanced stages improved in a variety of behavioural functions. Patients in different stages of AD showed improvement negotiating in a social environment. For example, mildly impaired subjects demonstrated improvement in shopping, moderately impaired subjects improved in orientation, and those severely impaired indicated an enhanced emotional status after treatment (Hofmann, Hock, Kuhler, & Muller-Spahn, 1996). Although patients became faster and made fewer mistakes with practice in using the computer, there was no significant cognitive improvement on standardised measures (Hofmann et al., 1996).

Highly individualised assistance at encoding and at retrieval has been shown to enhance episodic memory (Bäckman, 1996). Organisational strategies that utilise spaced retrieval and/or the use of external memory guides have been especially successful (Bäckman, 1996). For example a calendar that has one page per day is less confusing than multi day calendars for patients with dementia. Other memory aids include post-it pads, beepers, alarm clocks, and tape recorders. These are paired with verbal instructions and physical demonstrations (Bäckman, 1996). Wilson and Moffat (1992) report improved learning when the patient is not allowed to make mistakes ("errorless" learning).

Implicit memory (learning without conscious awareness) and procedural (motor) learning have also been utilised to enhance performance in activities of daily living for AD patients (Zanetti et al., 1997). Mild to moderately impaired AD patients have been trained to perform tasks such as brushing teeth, preparing coffee, and writing a cheque. Each task is paired with verbal support, including prompts and cues and 15 individualised sessions. Improvement was noted in non-trained activities of daily living as well as target areas.

Camp et al. (1997) have developed an intergenerational programme based upon the belief that cognitive abilities deteriorate in reverse order from which they developed in childhood. Developmental sequencing of cognitive events through Montessori techniques is believed to involve implicit memory. As with other programmes, immediate verbal feedback and structured repetition or practice is paired with Montessori-based tasks involving cognitive, sensory, and motor functions. Elderly demented adults are paired with a child to work on skills that are preserved in the adult and new to the child. While serving as mentors to the children, the adult's social skills demonstrated no apathy or agitation. Montessori skills learned by the child were implicitly evident to the adult, who was then able to guide the child through the various tasks.

Initial results from our memory rehabilitation intervention (Kesslak, Nickoul, & Sandman, 1997; Sandman, 1993) suggest that in AD patients, memory can be improved through persistence and specificity of an intervention. The most effective procedures, consistent with enrichment strategies, assumed that performance in AD patients could be enhanced by alteration of the environment (Hirst, 1988; Renner & Rosenzweig, 1987) rather than teaching sophisticated cognitive strategies that required substantial emotional and intellectual resources. The current study was designed to extend the initial study by adding a motor component to the name–face recognition, testing for generalisation of training to external measures of memory, attention and mood, and long-term retention of the information learned in the training sessions.

The memory-training programme was developed with a focus on recall of names, faces, places and events. Procedures designed to "amplify" sensory information were employed with an emphasis on effort, rehearsal and arousal/interest and by engineering the interaction between the patient and the environment. In response to training, patients with dementia showed increased ability to perform situation-specific tasks that addressed the materials covered in the programme and there was general improvement in a set of standard cognitive measures.

METHODS

Subjects

Twenty-five individuals with mild to moderate dementia (mean age 72.5, ±8.04 years SD) and their caregivers (age matched controls with a mean age 70.0, ±10.5 years SD) were recruited from the University of California, Irvine (UCI) Alzheimer's Disease and Aging Clinic and the UCI Health Assessment Program for Seniors. Diagnosis of dementia was determined according to NINCDS-ADRDA guidelines for AD (McKhann et al., 1984). All patients were given a complete diagnostic evaluation by a neurologist or geriatrician and neuropsychologist. Routine laboratory tests were given, such as CBC, chemistry panel, B12, folate, MHA-TP serology, thyroid function, chest X-ray, electrocardiogram, VDRL, urinalysis, and magnetic resonance imaging. Diagnosis was made based on the consensus of the clinical team.

Each patient and his or her caregiver, who acted as an aged-matched control, participated in the memory-training programme. All participants received the same evaluation, instruction and homework. All of the memory training exercises required interaction between the patient, caregiver and instructor and both groups were exposed to approximately the same environmental conditions.

Memory Training Programme

The Memory-Training Programme (MTP) (Kesslak et al., 1997; Sandman, 1993) was devised from common strategies to increase both learning and memory. Our 5-week programme included key concepts in problem solving such as effort, arousal, and interest. The primary training methods such as the Significant Event Technique and other problem solving skills were introduced in the initial sessions and followed up and elaborated on in subsequent sessions. Standardised cognitive tests were administered at week 1 and 5 and included the Kendrick Digit Copy, Geriatric Depression Scale (GDS), Memory

Function Questionnaire (MFQ), Blessed Dementia Scale (BDS), and Relative Stress Scale (RSS). Task specific tests were administered weekly to assess individual performance relative to caregivers. Each member was given immediate feedback. There was enough flexibility in the programme design to aid each participant in his or her specific memory or learning impairment. This application of individualised techniques was considered to enhance the success of the programme. Each strategy was assessed weekly by objective tests administered at the start of each session. The tests covered materials to be learned in each of the following strategies of the training programme.

Lecture.   Each session began with a standardised lecture on memory and an outline of the explicit goals for that week. A review of how memory works was illustrated during the first week. The group was given information on the biological processes of memory as well as the different types of memory problems. Basic information on the brain, aging and behaviour was discussed regularly, explaining biological and psychological aspects of the MTP and its potential benefits. An analogy was made that learning and memory takes effort today just like when first memorising the multiplication tables in primary school. Before introducing and applying each technique the background and implications of the various techniques was discussed.

Name–Face Rehearsal (picture test).   During the first session, a Polaroid picture was taken of each person. Photocopies of individual members were placed on a sheet of paper, four to a page and distributed to every participant. The students were instructed to introduce themselves by name, including a short biography of themselves. To facilitate "deeper processing", relevant details, such as hobbies, interests, accomplishments, children, grandchildren and other pertinent details were told to the group. Each member of the group took notes under the appropriate pictures as the participants spoke. After introductions, the students asked questions of other participants to clarify details. Members also chose a particular motor movement that matched their interest, such as carving a piece of wood, swinging a tennis racket, or flying an airplane.

Pantomiming personal motor movements along with repeating the person's name was practised routinely during each group session and at home with the caregiver. Additional sheets of photos were given to participants if needed to rehearse the names, faces and motor movements during the week. Each couple was given a daily log to keep track of practice time and instructed that there would be a test on names, faces, and motor movements on subsequent weeks. Weekly sessions required all participants to write the first and last names and motor movements of each participant on a sheet of photos similar to the one given in class. After this, a verbal recognition test was administered to group members. Participants were given immediate feedback on their progress during the group sessions. Any failures to name members and/or motor movements were accompanied with encouragement to recall the person's hobbies, interests, and accomplishments. Graphs were presented to participants to determine individual progress immediately after the task. Participants returned a weekly log of how much time each day they practised and rehearsed at home.

Significant Event Technique (SET).   The SET involved planning an event that was novel, unique and unusual. Couples were requested to *plan* this event together. Often older people become isolated and confined by a routine. Creating something unusual to do can thus be fun and fairly easy. Sample activities have included a picnic to an important place with foods never eaten such as exotic fruits and visiting either a new shopping centre or a museum. The next step was to execute or "*do*" the event or activity. Members were asked to *discuss* the activity after participation. To determine how much each participant could recall, a series of objective questions about the SET were asked. In contrast, objective questions were also asked about another day in which there was no planning or novelty (a non-SET or control day). Results of the planned versus non-SET days were graphically displayed for immediate feedback and discussion by the group.

Effortful Recall.   The group was given a video with four television sitcoms of about 20 min each. Instructions were given to watch one sitcom per week and the group was tested weekly on details of the programme. A 10-item-free-recall and 10-item-recognition test was administered on each successive week beginning with the second week of MTP. Additionally, after the recognition test, the group was primed and then took the 10-item-recall test once again. On the third week, participants were asked to develop five questions to ask group members about the video. For the fourth and fifth weeks participants were requested to make up 10 questions about the video, similar to the tests they had taken in the group. Participants then questioned their peers, using the questions that they had developed, during priming. The intention was to activate attention in a high-effort condition. As with other results, test scores were graphically presented to the individual participants immediately after testing.

Support intervention

Support interventions were also included since caregivers have a significant incidence of illness compared to the general population. Caregiver support included education, emotional support and some stress relief. All participants were encouraged to share their experiences and any coping strategies. The influence of the support intervention was not documented in this study, but was examined in an earlier report that treated the support as a separate component (Kesslak et al., 1997).

Long-term follow up

Approximately 1 month after the fifth training session, AD patients and controls returned to the clinic. At this time their ability to recall names and faces was assessed and they were asked for a subjective evaluation of the programme.

Weekly test battery

Brief psychometric tests such as the Geriatric Depression Scale, the Kendrick Digit Copy and the Activities of Daily Living from the Blessed Dementia Rating Scale, and the Memory Functioning Questionnaire (MFQ) were administered at the beginning of sessions one and five. This battery measured attention, cognition and mood (i.e., depression) and was given to both patients and controls. Caregivers were asked to rate the patient's abilities on the Activities of Daily Living (Blessed Dementia Rating Scale). Because patients and caregivers often have different views on the patient's cognitive ability and rate of depression, caregivers were also asked to answer the Geriatric Depression Scale and the Memory Functioning Questionnaire in reference to the patient.

RESULTS

Task specific measures

Ability to recall names on the "picture test" was analysed separately for recall of one name (first or last), both names, and the motor movement associated with a name. Repeated measures analysis of variance (ANOVA) was used to determine if recall of names improved over the weeks of practice after the AD patients and controls were instructed in the name recall strategies. As expected, the control group performed better than did the AD patients in recall of names and motor movement. Performance improved across weeks of training, with the control group reaching asymptotic performance early in the training, while the AD group showed improvement with practice (Figure 1). For the verbal recall of one name there was a significant difference between groups, $F(1, 31)$, $p = .02$; improvement over time, $F(3, 93)$ $p = .0013$; and an interaction, $F(3, 93)$, $p = .04$. Similar results were observed for the ability to recall both the first and last names with a significant difference between groups, $F(1, 31)$, $p = .0002$; improvement over time, $F(3, 93)$, $p = .0003$; but a non-significant interaction, $F(3, 93)$, $p = .08$. Recall of the motor movement associated with the names and faces differed between groups, $F(1, 31)$, $p = .0002$; improved across weeks of training, $F(3, 93)$, $p = .001$; and had a significant interaction, $F(3, 93)$, $p = .007$. When subjects were tested 1 month after the completion of the memory training programme information for name recall and motor

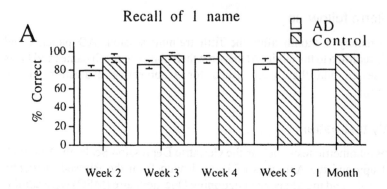

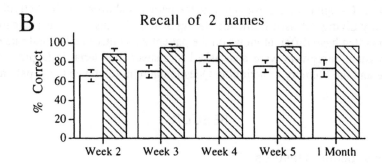

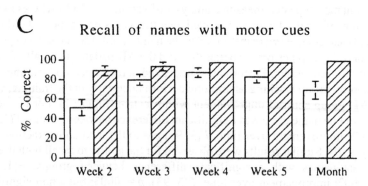

Figure 1. Recall of either one name (A), two names (B), or a motor cue associated with the name (C) all improved across the 5 weeks of memory training for the demented patients. Age-matched controls rapidly learned the names and motor cues during the memory training programme, consistently maintaining a high level of performance for recall. Ability to recall the names and motor cues was retained for at least one month after the completion of the memory training programme.

movements was maintained and did not differ from the level of performance during the last training session ($p < .01$).

The ability to recall information in temporal proximity to a significant event (SET) was assessed relative to a non-SET day. On days when a SET occurred the AD group recalled significantly more information than on a non-SET day, but never attained the same high level of performance as the control group. There was a significant difference between groups on both SET and non-SET days, $F(1, 51)$, $p < .01$; however, the AD group significantly improved on the SET days relative to the non-SET day, $F(2, 92)$, $p = .0017$. Control recall of information on set and non-SET days was typically very good, while the AD group showed marked improvement after planning and executing a significant event (Figure 2).

In the effortful recall tests groups were examined after viewing a video programme during the week and given tests on the programme content that first required free recall, followed by a recognition test and then a second test of free recall. Comparisons were made between weeks when participants were asked to take notes on the programme and to construct their own test questions (high effort) or just view the programme (low effort). On the first free recall tests, the AD group consistently recalled fewer items than the controls, $F(1, 21)$,

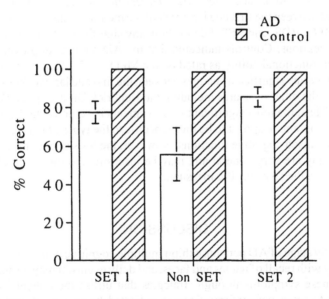

Figure 2. The planning and execution of a significant event (SET) by patients and caregivers improved performance on an objective test pertaining to the SET day. Recall of information on the SET day for patients significantly improved compared to the non-SET day, and approached the performance levels of the control group.

$p = .008$; and both benefited from increased effort to improve performance, $F(3, 63), p < .0001$; with no interaction, $F(3,62), p = .48$. Recognition memory and level of effort showed a similar pattern of differences between groups, $F(1, 21), p = .037$; with both groups benefiting from increased effort $F(3, 63)$, $p = .0007$; and no interaction, $F(3,62)$, $p = .37$. After discussion of the programme a second free recall test was administered. Even after the discussion the AD group had significantly fewer correct answers than the control group, $F(1, 21), p = .005$; but the AD group did improve with increased effort, $F(3, 63), p = .001$; and there was a significant interaction, $F(3, 63), p = .0018$. The significant interaction after the second free recall testing was most likely due to the controls having a ceiling effect in correctly answering the questions after reviewing the programme in both the low and high effort conditions; while the AD group benefited from the review more in the high effort condition compared to the low effort condition (Figure 3).

Standardised measures

The standardised measures of cognitive change showed variable and modest effects for the memory training programme, similar to our previous report (Kesslak et al., 1997). AD patients' scores on the Kendrick Digit Copy, $t = 2.952$, $p = .006$, and Geriatric Depression Scale, $t = 2.071$, $p = .04$, improved between the first and last week of the memory training. Patient scores on the MFQ, BDS, and RSS did not show any significant change between the two test sessions. Controls indicated that the AD patients improved in their perceived functional ability as rated on the MFQ, $t = 2.125, p = .04$. Controls did not have any significant changes between the first and last weeks of training on any of the other measures including the Kendrick Digit Copy, GDS, BDS, or RSS. Thus, the most significant improvements in response to the memory-training programme appear to be more specific to the types of strategies, rather than generalised cognitive functions. However, the tests of cognitive function in this study are very general and may be insensitive to the modest benefits observed on the task specific measures.

DISCUSSION

In the early stage of AD patients exhibit multiple cognitive deficits that include difficulty with recall of names and faces, and daily events. It may be possible to reduce these symptoms through strategies that utilise the patients' retained capacity to learn new information, as indicated by improved performance during participation in a 5-week memory-training programme. Furthermore, the improved capacity to remember information is sustained for at least 1 month after the completion of the memory retraining.

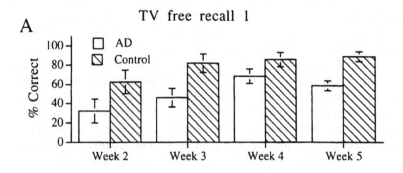

TV free recall 1

A

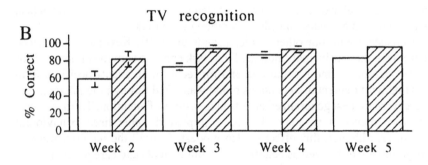

TV recognition

B

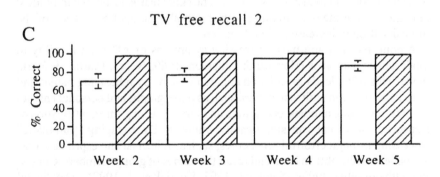

TV free recall 2

C

Figure 3. To increase the amount of effort in processing new information patients and controls were instructed to view a television programme, take notes and construct a test on the programme content. Ability for recall (A) and recognition (B) of information after viewing an assigned television programme improved across the weeks of training. Review of the programme content in class further enhanced the ability to recall information (C). By the end of the training programme performance on the recognition and recall after review tests did not differ for the patient and control groups.

As in our earlier study (Kesslak et al., 1997), enhanced cognitive function showed minimal generalisation to increase performance on standardised tests of general functional ability. No significant changes were seen for caregiver ratings on the Blessed Dementia Scale, Relative Stress Scale, and Geriatric Depression Scale. However, caregivers did rate patients higher on the MFQ, suggesting a slightly higher level of function. On the standardised measures, patients with AD did show improved performance on the Kendrick Digit Copy test, similar to our previous report (Kesslak et al., 1997), which may be due to enhanced attention and/or speed of processing. Patients also rated themselves as less depressed, which may interact with attentional processes to improve performance on the Digit Copy task. There were no changes in the AD patients' ratings on the MFQ, Blessed DRS or RSS. Overall, the results of the standardised tests scores did not show any consistent pattern of improved function; however, the value of these retraining procedures is most likely situation or task dependent and can vary considerably among individuals.

Consistent with our other studies (Sandman, 1993; Kesslak et al., 1997), there were three principal findings. First, task specific activities improved for name–face recall and recognition, and for recall of an event-specific task in patients with dementia. Second, as mood was lifted through the intervention, there were modest generalized effects in measures of attention. Third, our task specific interventions may also have improved generalised behavioural measures, although this effect is also modest. Overall the memory training programme was viewed as beneficial by both patients and caregivers. Examination of retention of material learned during the memory training course one month after completion indicated that information, such as people's names, can be retained for extended periods of time. The skills learned from the individual strategies in the memory training course can also be applied outside of the clinical setting to increase patient function.

Among the first and most distressing symptoms of AD is an inability to recall names and faces (Howard & Patterson, 1989; Nebes, Martin, & Horn, 1984). This often leads to isolation and depression. By rehearsing names and faces in association with visual cues, such as photographs and personal characteristics, including hobbies, occupation and family history, the identification of a specific individual can significantly improve. By engaging "automatic" processing through effortful procedures, such as rehearsal and esprit de corps, AD patients were able to learn and recall the names of group members. Consistent with our other studies (Sandman, 1993; Kesslak et al., 1997) AD patients' recall of one or both names significantly improved during the five-week intervention. In addition, this ability to recall the names and associated motor movements was maintained for over a month after the course was completed. Although there was significant improvement, the dementia patients never reached the same level of performance as the controls, who were able to identify the majority of group members throughout the memory-training programme. The flexibility of recalling a single name, either Mary or Mrs. Jones, allows for versatility of response and places fewer demands on the memory system. Facilitation of memory for names and faces may have been enhanced through semantic elaboration (Scogin & Prohaska, 1993) such as the integrating historical data about group members with their names and faces over time. As the disease progresses compensatory mechanisms become necessary to counteract the now decaying ability for consolidation of new memories. These methods, such as practising the elaboration of details about the group members, may have promoted recall of names and faces. Chaining these cues to new names and faces provides additional information with which to stimulate name recall (Murdock, 1991). Providing immediate feedback or correction during rehearsal and practice strengthened associations, either at home with the caregiver or during group sessions. With the addition of "errorless learning" AD patients will maximise their encoding abilities, without confusing group members' names and faces (Wilson & Moffat, 1992). An increase in ability to identify names and faces may reduce isolation and related stress and facilitate social interactions. It is important to note that these skills can be maintained and the information stored in long-term memory, retained for an extended period of time, as exhibited by the participants' ability to recall names when tested one month after completion of the course.

An inability to recall a movie just seen or information just read is another common complaint of AD patients. From one study to the next (Sandman, 1993; Kesslak et al., 1997), we have had mixed results on the ability to recall information previously presented. Our first study indicated significant improvement in memory when encoding information required effort, such as preparing a 10-item objective test (Sandman, 1993). The results of the second study (Kesslak et al., 1997) were not as promising, patients did not improve in either recall or recognition of facts after the effortful production of a 10-item test. In this study, healthy controls recalled and recognised more information about the video than AD patients. The recognition memory for AD patients did improve with training using effortful recall, although they never reached the level of performance comparable to the healthy controls. The AD patients' memory for facts slightly improved with practice. Compliance appears to be a critical component of these findings. On several occasions throughout the sessions either the AD patients did not create the test questions or did not watch the video, which could significantly impair their test performance. Motivation is a key factor and is often reduced with the progression of dementia. Additionally, interaction between caregiver and patient should be encouraged to facilitate the use of strategies such as effortful recall, with the realisation that additional effort may be required on their part.

Our third strategy utilised a procedure for improving memory through the application of the Significant Event Technique (SET). This has been our most successful method to improve memory. Patients and caregivers are required to discuss, plan and execute an event that is out of their normal routine. By engineering the environment to optimise memories, using activities tinged with emotion, novel events are enhanced, and thus, more easily recalled (Brown & Krulik, 1977; Levin, 1990; Sandman, 1993). In addition, encoding of information may be enhanced by increased information processing during the event due to the planning and discussion of the event. This could also increase antici-pation, orientation or awareness during the time of the event and increase atten-tion to various stimuli. Consistent with our previous research (Sandman, 1993; Kesslak et al., 1997) there was significantly improved recall of information in close temporal proximity to the significant event. The effectiveness of the SET days eliminated differences in recall between healthy controls and AD patients. These "flashbulb" memories, memories that are vivid and coloured by emotion, persist long after the significant event (Brown and Krulik, 1977; Levin, 1990; Sandman, 1993). This strategy was first developed using vivid words in laboratory studies (Brown & Krulik, 1977) where it was discovered that provocative or unusual words elicit "flashbulb" memories. These mem-ories are strengthened by unexpected events, which illuminate the context of the information, such that even minor information surrounding the event can facilitate memory for that event.

In contrast to traditional literature that recommends routine management of patients, our studies confirm that novelty may actually enhance memories. A regimented lifestyle may avoid placing demands on memory. Yet, that same routine may actually dim differences in memory across time, such that days, followed by weeks and months are no longer discrete. This threading of uninterrupted time may ultimately contribute to one's memory impairment. By requiring variety, diverse activities not done before, interest is captivated, greatly improving the recollection of routine facts. The utility of the SET for long-term memory enhancement is unknown with AD patients (Berrol, 1990; Levin, 1990). However, for the short-term, we have found nothing with this patient population that leads to greater improvement. Both patients and care-givers self-efficacy is improved as relationships are enhanced through better recall of events. By stimulating the information, through either positive or negative arousal (LeDoux, 1994; McGaugh et al., 1993) encoding is facilitated. As the pathology progresses, particularly to the amygdala and frontal cortex (Braak & Braak, 1991; Hyman, Van Hoesen, & Damasio, 1990), we anticipate decay in the arousal and memory systems, which will impact the success of the SET. Because of the pathological processes it is also necessary to consider the types of events, a balance must be maintained where the activities involve the individual without overwhelming him or her.

Despite the enhancement of event-specific memory noted from pre and post memory-training tests, it is apparent that the interventions reveal only a modest generalised influence. Intervention response by patients suggests that they perceived themselves as less depressed. As a consequence there was an improved performance on tests of psychomotor speed. There is mild evidence of improved mood; clinically, patients adapted and responded to lectures and assessment more readily as the weeks progressed. It may be that the stimulation through group assignments and social interaction improved higher cognitive or attentional processes.

Consistent with reports in the literature (Sohlberg & Mateer, 1989), primarily tasks that were specific to the memory training were facilitated by the training paradigm. This may be due to insensitivity of the tests used to assess generalisation, or facilitation of function may be restricted to the types of cognitive functions or processes directly manipulated by the memory strategies taught during the course. Regardless, the improved performance on the tasks specifically related to the materials learned during the memory training indicates that new information can be learned and retained for an extended period of time. The challenge will be to adapt and apply these techniques in everyday living to optimise patient function and increase self-esteem. Examples of how the techniques can be incorporated into the daily environment include reducing the daily routine to add stimulating new activities, and review of photo albums of friends, family, and important persons. These seemingly simple processes can serve a two-fold purpose, to improve the memory of the patient and increase the positive interactions between patients and caregivers. It should be noted that these procedures may be time-consuming and require patient–caregiver interaction. The caregiver must be willing and capable of committing to these procedures and share responsibility with the patient. Although not examined in this study, the combination of behavioural and pharmacological interventions in other types of pathology, such as depression, can be more beneficial than either intervention alone. A combination of pharmacological and behavioural interventions, that include a memory training programme, may promote increases in the level of function and provide a framework to develop more effective treatment strategies for dementia.

REFERENCES

Bäckman, L. (1996). Utilizing compensatory task conditions for episodic memory in Alzheimer's disease. *Acta Neurologica Scandinavica*, Suppl, 165, 109–113.

Berrol, S. (1990). Issues in cognitive rehabilitation. *Archives of Neurology*, 47, 219–220.

Black, J.E., Polinsky, M., & Greenough, W.T. (1989). Progressive failure of cerebral angiogenesis supporting neural plasticity in aging rats. *Neurobiology of Aging*, 10, 353–358.

Braak, H., & Braak, E. (1991). Neuropathological staging of Alzheimer-related changes. *Acta Neuropathologica*, 82, 239–259.

Brown, R., & Krulik, J. (1977). Flashbulb memories. *Cognition*, 5, 73–99.

Camp, C., Judge, K.S., Bye, C.A., Fox, K.M., Bowden, J., Bell, M., Valencic, K., & Mattern, J.M. (1997). An intergenerational program for persons with dementia using Montessori methods. *Gerontologist*, 37, 688–692.

Cermak, L.S. (1975). *Improving your memory*. New York: W.W. Norton.

Craik, F.I., & Watkins, M.J. (1973). The role of rehearsal in short-term memory. *Journal of Verbal Learning & Verbal Behavior, 12*, 599–607.

Cummings, J.F., & Benson, D.F. (1992). *Dementia: A clinical approach* (2nd ed.), Stoneham, MA: Butterworth-Heinemann.

Hirst, W. (1988). Improving memory. *Perspectives in memory research* (pp. 219–244). New York: MIT Press.

Hofmann, M., Hock, C., & Muller-Spahn, F. (1996). Computer-based cognitive training in Alzheimer's disease patients. *Annals of the New York Academy of Sciences, 777*, 249–254.

Hofmann, M., Hock, C., Kuhler, A., & Muller-Spahn, F. (1996). Interactive computer-based cognitive training in patients with Alzheimer's disease. *Journal of Psychiatric Research, 30*, 493–501.

Howard, D., & Patterson, K. (1989). Models for therapy. In X. Seron, G. Deloche, (Eds.), *Cognitive approaches in neuropsychological rehabilitation. Neuropsychology and neurolinguistics* (pp. 39–64). Hillsdale, NJ: Lawrence Erlbaum Associates.

Hyman, B.T., Van Hoesen, G.W., & Damasio, A.R. (1990). Memory-related neural systems in Alzheimer's disease: An anatomic study. *Neurology, 40*, 1721–1730.

Kesslak, J.P., Nickoul, K., & Sandman, C. (1997) Memory training for individuals with Alzheimer's disease improves name recall. *Alzheimer's Research, 3*, 151–157.

LeDoux, J. (1994). Emotion, memory and the brain. *Scientific American, June*, 50–57.

Levin, H.S. (1990). Cognitive rehabilitation: Unproved but promising. *Archives of Neurology, 47*, 223–224.

Lorayne, H., & Lucas, J. (1974). *The memory book*, New York: Ballantine.

McGaugh, J.L., Introini-Collison, I.B., Cahill, L.F., Castellano, C., Dalmaz, C., Parent, M.B., & Williams, C.L. (1993). Neuromodulatory systems and memory storage: Role of the amygdala. Special Issue: Emotion and memory. *Behavioral Brain Research, 58*, 81–90.

McKhann, G., Drachman, D., Folstein, M., Katzman, R., Price, D., & Stadlan, E.M. (1984). Clinical diagnosis of Alzheimer's disease: A report of the NINCDS-ADRDA work group under the auspices of Department of Health and Human Services Task Force on Alzheimer's Disease. *Neurology, 34*, 939–944.

Miller, E. (1975). Impaired recall and the memory disturbance in pre-senile dementia. *British Journal of Social and Clinical Psychology, 14*, 73–79.

Minninger, J. (1984). *Total recall—How to boost your memory power*. Easton, PA: Rodale Press.

Morris, R.G., & Kopelman, M.D. (1986). The memory deficits in Alzheimer-type dementia: A review. Special Issue: Human memory. *Quarterly Journal of Experimental Psychology: Human Experimental Psychology, 38*, 575–602.

Mohs, R.C., Ashman, T.A., Jantzen, K., Albert, M., Brandt, J., Gordon, B., Rasmusson, X., Grossman, M., Jacobs, D., & Stern, Y. (1998). A study of the efficacy of a comprehensive memory enhancement program in healthy elderly persons. *Psychiatry Research, 77*, 183–195.

Murdock, B.B. (1991). Serial organization in a distributed memory model. In A.F. Healy, S.M. Kosslyn, & R.M. Shiffrin (Eds.), *Essays in honor of William K. Estes, Vol. 1: From learning theory to connectionist theory; Vol. 2: From learning processes to cognitive processes* (pp. 201–225). Hillsdale, NJ: Lawrence Erlbaum Associates.

Nebes, R.D., Martin, D.C., & Horn, L.C. (1984). Sparing of semantic memory in Alzheimer's disease. *Journal of Abnormal Psychology, 93*, 321–330.

Poon, L.W. (Ed.) (1980). *Aging in the 1980s*. Washington, DC: American Psychological Association.

Poon, L.W., Fozard, J.L., & Treat, N.J. (1978). From clinical and research findings on memory to intervention programs. *Experimental Aging Research, 4*, 235–253.

Rabinowitz, J.C. (1984). Aging and recognition failure. *Journal of Gerontology, 39*, 65–71.

Renner, M.J., & Rosenzweig, M.R. (1987). *Enriched and impoverished environments*. New York: Springer Verlag.

Sandman, C.A. (1993). Memory rehabilitation in Alzheimer's disease: Preliminary findings. *Clinical Gerontologist, 13*, 19–33.

Scogin, F., & Prohaska, M. (1993). *Aiding older adults with memory complaints.* Sarasota, FL: Professional Resource Press.

Smith, A.D. (1980). Age differences in encoding, storage and retrieval. In L.W. Poon, J.L. Fozard, L.S. Cermak, D. Arenberg, & L.W. Thompson (Eds.), *New directions in memory and aging: Proceedings of the George A. Talland Memorial Conference* (pp. 23–46). Hillsdale, NJ: Lawrence Erlbaum Associates.

Sohlberg, M.M., & Mateer, C.A. (1989). Training use of compensatory memory books: A three stage behavioral approach. *Journal of Clinical and Experimental Neuropsychology, 11*, 871–891.

Van der Linden, M., & Van der Kaa, M.-A. (1989). Reorganization therapy for memory impairments. In X. Seron, & G. Deloche (Eds.), *Cognitive approaches in neuropsychological rehabilitation. Neuropsychology and neurolinguistics* (pp. 105–158). Hillsdale, NJ: Lawrence Erlbaum Associates Inc.

Wilson, B.A. (1987). *Rehabilitation of memory.* New York: Guilford Press.

Wilson, B.A., & Moffat, N. (Eds.) (1992). *Clinical management of memory problems* (2nd ed.). San Diego, CA: Singular Publishing Group.

Zanetti, O., Binetti, G., Magni, E., Rozzini, L., Bianchetti, A., & Trabucchi, M. (1997). Procedural memory stimulation in Alzheimer's disease: Impact of a training programme. *Acta Neurologica Scandinavica, 95*(3), 152–157.

Zarit, S.H., Cole, K.D., & Guider, G.L. (1981). Memory training strategies and subjective complaints of memory in the aged. *Gerontologist, 21*, 158–164.

Manuscript received July 1999
Revised manuscript received September 2000

Effectiveness of procedural memory stimulation in mild Alzheimer's disease patients: A controlled study

Orazio Zanetti[1], Gabriele Zanieri[1],
Giuseppina Di Giovanni[1], Luc Pietre De Vreese[1,2],
Alessandra Pezzini[1], Tiziana Metitieri[1],
and Marco Trabucchi[1]

[1]*Alzheimer Unit, IRCCS S. Giovanni di Dio,
S. Cuore-Fatebenefratelli Institute, Brescia, Italy;*
[2]*Department of Geriatrics and Gerontology,
University of Modena, Modena, Italy.*

This study concerns the effectiveness of procedural memory training in mild and mild–moderate probable Alzheimer's disease (AD) patients. Eleven patients with AD (age: 78 ± 8.4 years; MMSE score: 20 ± 3.4; education: 5.7 ± 2.7 years) attending a day hospital, were individually trained, for three consecutive weeks (one hour/day; five days/week), in 13 basic and instrumental activities of daily living such as personal hygiene, using the telephone, dressing, reading, writing, etc. Seven AD patients (age: 74 ± 12 years; MMSE score: 19 ± 4.2; education: 5.3 ± 3.2 years) constituted the control group.

Patients in both groups underwent baseline and follow up assessment (four months later) recording the total mean time employed to perform the 13 activities of daily living. The training group showed a significant reduction ($p < .025$) in the time necessary to perform the activities, while the control group showed a non-significant increase. Our results support the view that procedural memory in mild and mild–moderate AD is relatively well preserved and that training of activities of daily living constitutes a realistic goal for rehabilitation programmes.

Correspondence should be sent to O. Zanetti, Via Pilastroni 4, 25123, Brescia, Italy. Fax: (+39) 30 3501366; e-mail: ozanetti@oh-fbf.it

We wish to thank Silvia Di Cesare, Claudia Ercoli, Filippo Mazzini, Sara Tanelli, Silvia Valent, and Chiara Verzeletti for conducting the memory training.

INTRODUCTION

Notwithstanding the fact that multidisciplinary effort has quickly transformed the area of Alzheimer's Disease (AD) and related disorders, leading to better understanding of clinical manifestation, risk factors, and treatment, definitive knowledge of the pathogenetic mechanisms is still lacking. Recently developed drugs represent significant progress, but mainly in the area of the cholinergic hypothesis, where only partial efficacy can be expected (Zanetti & Trabucchi, 1999). Non-pharmacological interventions can play an important role in addressing the various clinical problems—cognitive, functional, behavioural and affective—of AD (Clark, Lipe, & Bilbrey, 1998; Gwyther, 1990; Koh et al., 1994; Schreiber et al., 1999; Van der Linden & Juillerat, 1998; Zanetti et al., 1995).

Some authors (Bäckman, 1992, 1996) have suggested that, especially during the first stages of the disease, relatively well-preserved skills could be the target of rehabilitative interventions in order to delay the decline of cognitive functions. According to this, in particular, there is evidence that procedural memory, which involves the cognitive use of previous experiences without conscious recognition (Markowitsch, 1998), is relatively well preserved in AD (Perani et al., 1993; Sabe et al., 1995). Patients with AD have been reported to show normal implicit memory abilities in several situations in which no declarative recollection of previous learning is required, such as motor, perceptual, and cognitive skills (Crystal, Grober, & Masur, 1989; Deweer et al., 1994; Poe & Seifert, 1997). Recently, more specific and tailored mental stimulation strategies for patients with dementia have been proposed that rely on the stimulation of procedural learning (Camp & McKitrick, 1992; Ermini-Funfschilling & Meier, 1995; Hirono et al., 1997; Josephsson et al., 1993; Knopman, 1991).

Deweer et al. (1994) demonstrated that AD patients were able to learn and retain motor and perceptual skills normally, even across a long retention interval. Recently, Libon et al. (1998), comparing patients with ischaemic vascular dementia (IVD) with AD patients, found that IVD patients exhibited a higher performance in declarative memory and a lower one in procedural memory, while patients with AD exhibited the opposite profile.

These studies represent important exceptions to a negative pattern which usually indicates how AD patients fail to benefit from a variety of different forms of environmental and cognitive rehabilitative interventions conducted in order to improve cognitive function (Bäckman, 1992, 1996). On the other hand, although these studies clearly show the retention of procedural memory in AD subjects, they have never, or rarely, focused on learning or relearning of activities of daily life, instead emphasising the positive results achieved by participants in accomplishing some activities with little or no ecological validity (e.g., using a pantographic device or a computerised jigsaw puzzle).

The aim of this controlled study is to evaluate the effectiveness of a programme of procedural memory stimulation and its impact on the directly observed performance of everyday activities in two groups of well-selected mild and mild–moderate AD patients (Loewenstein et al., 1989).

METHODS

Subjects

This study was conducted in the Day Hospital of an Alzheimer's Dementia Research and Care Unit, a multidisciplinary care centre providing diagnostic evaluation and treatment of elderly patients with cognitive impairment.

Criteria for eligibility for this study were: (a) diagnosis of probable Alzheimer's disease according to NINCDS-ADRDA criteria (McKhann et al., 1984), (b) mild or mild–moderate cognitive impairments as defined by Mini Mental State Examination (Folstein, Folstein, & McHugh, 1975), and (c) absence of major aphasia, blindness, and relevant behavioural disturbances such as agitation, wandering, or aggressiveness. Eighteen consecutive patients fulfilling the eligibility criteria were enrolled. Of these, 11 subjects (10 females) constituted the training group (TG) while the control group (CG) was formed by seven patients (six females). The main criterion for inclusion in the TG or the CG was the caregivers' availability to take the patient to the day hospital every day for the duration of the programme. Before starting training, all subjects were submitted to a neuropsychological and clinical assessment (Table 1) including: Mini Mental State Examination (MMSE), letter and category fluency tests, ideomotor and oral apraxia tests, visual-spatial span using the Corsi Test, prose recall, forward digit span (Spinnler & Tognoni, 1987), and the Boston Naming Test (Kaplan, Goodglass, & Weintraub, 1978). Functional level was evaluated with the Physical Performance Test (PPT), which assesses multiple domains of physical functioning using observed performance of tasks that simulate activities of daily living of various degrees of difficulty (Reuben & Siu, 1990), and the Direct Assessment of Functional Status (DAFS) (Loewenstein et al., 1989; Zanetti et al., 1998) which is a performance-based measure for evaluating a broad spectrum of behaviours within seven functional domains: orientation, communication abilities, financial skills, shopping skills, transport, dressing, and feeding abilities. At baseline, the only significant difference between the two groups was in forward digit span (Table 1). Medications remained the same for the duration of the study.

TABLE 1
Clinical and neuropsychological characteristics of trained and control patients.
Means (and standard deviations)

	Training Group N = 11	Control Group N = 7	p*
Age	78 (8.4)	74 (12)	.42
Education	5.7 (2.7)	5.3 (3.2)	.78
MMSE	20 (3.4)	19 (4.2)	.58
DAFS	55.5 (8.7)	58.2 (3.8)	.45
PPT	20.9 (3.1)	20 (3.8)	.59
Corsi Test	3.4 (0.8)	3.3 (1)	.81
Boston Naming Test	15.7 (6.7)	14.2 (4.6)	.61
Forward digit span	4.7 (0.8)	4 (0)	.036
Prose recall	5.5 (3.3)	5.4 (4.3)	.95
Verbal fluency for letter	16.3 (4.2)	15.4 (8.8)	.77
Verbal fluency for category	23.7 (8.1)	20.4 (5.5)	.36
Ideomotor apraxia	18.8 (1.7)	18.8 (1.5)	1
Oral apraxia	16.9 (2.3)	17.5 (2.5)	.6

* *T*-test for independent samples

Training

Members of the experimental group were trained in individual sessions, and were exposed to the procedural memory training stimulation for three consecutive weeks (one hour/day; five days/week). Thirteen basic and instrumental activities of daily living (ADLs) were trained: (1) washing face; (2) washing hands; (3) brushing teeth; (4) opening and closing a door; (5) locking a door; (6) putting objects (such as a knife, a fork, or a spoon) in the correct place; (7) preparing a slice of bread with jam; (8) using the telephone; (9) using a calendar; (10) laying the table; (11) reading some brief sentences; (12) using money; and (13) dressing.

An occupational therapist conducted the training sessions, prompting and informing patients about each task to be performed. The activities were trained by inviting the patient to execute a task (e.g., "Please, wash your hands"). Patients were assisted by cues, reinforcement, and verbal (e.g., "Turn on the tap", "Pick up the soap", etc.) and non-verbal prompts, or modelling of the task. The aim of every rehabilitative session was to lead the patient to achieve the tasks in order to allow the learning of specific operational processes.

Training was performed in a setting used for rehabilitative interventions where the rooms resemble a kitchen, a dining room, and a small bathroom and are designed to provide ecological validity.

Training assessment

The effectiveness of the stimulation was assessed by recording the total mean time required to perform all the activities. This was evaluated, for both groups, at baseline and again at follow up four months later (follow up). Two rehabilitation therapists, blind to the stimulation received by the patients, measured the performance time by recording the interval between the verbal command and the completion of the task.

At baseline and at follow up, each task was assessed with a specially designed scorecard which enabled the rater to record the *execution time*, the *number of cues* given to the patient, and a *total score* obtained by adding up subtotal scores ascribed to each intermediate phase (one point for each phase) which served to monitor the execution of the task. Figure 1 shows the scorecard for personal hygiene.

During baseline and follow up the maximum number of cues permitted was two for each task, while during training it was unlimited according to personal needs.

Statistical analysis

Between-group differences in mean performance time necessary to complete all the 13 activities were compared at baseline (two-tailed p) and at follow up (one-tailed p) using the Mann–Whitney U-test. A further analysis compared

---

Personal hygiene

The patient is in the bathroom: There is soap in the washbasin and a bath towel and comb on a sideboard.

Examiner: "Please, wash you hands" (Time 0')

Patient: 1. Turns on the tap
2. Picks up the soap and washes his hands
3. Rinses his hands
4. Turns off the tap
5. Takes the bath towel and dries his hands (Time 1)

Examiner: "And now comb you hair" (Time 0'')
6. The patient combs his hair (Time 2)

(Time 1) _____ (Time 2) _____   Total time _____
Number of cues (max 2) _____   Score (1–6) _____

Figure 1.   Scorecard: Personal hygiene. Time was taken by recording the interval between the verbal command (Time 0'; Time 0'') and completion of the task (Time 1; Time 2).

baseline and follow up scores separately for the training and control groups, using the Wilcoxon Matched-Pairs Signed-Rank Test.

Initial clinical, neuropsychological, and functional characteristics of both groups were compared using an independent samples t-test (Table 1). Statistical significance was defined as a $p \le .05$.

RESULTS

Mean length of time required to perform the 13 ADLs at baseline and follow up are shown in Table 2. Patients in the training group showed an improvement in performance time. The gain of 79 seconds is statistically significant (one-tailed $p < .025$). In contrast, the control group showed a non-significant increase in performance time between baseline and follow up (mean difference: +34 seconds).

The difference between groups at baseline was not statistically significant, whereas at follow up the difference was significant (one-tailed $p < .025$).

DISCUSSION

The results of this study, in accordance with previous research (Zanetti et al. 1997), show that rehabilitation of activities of daily living through developing procedural strategies may be effective in mild and mild–moderate AD patients and that the relative sparing of implicit memory in AD constitutes a good theoretical rationale for the stimulation of procedural skill. Similar results were obtained by Hirono et al. (1997) comparing motor, perceptual, and cognitive skill learning abilities in mild AD. The results showed that in those AD patients who completed the task, skill learning was as good as in normal controls.

TABLE 2
Mean (and standard deviation) time taken to perform all activities
at baseline and follow up (four months post-intervention)

Group	Baseline	Follow up	p^*
Training ($N = 11$)	799 (225)	720 (161)	$< .025^*$
Control ($N = 7$)	898 (100)	932 (281)	n.s.
p^{**}	n.s.	$< .025^{**}$	

Values are expressed in seconds.
   * within-group analysis; by Wilcoxon test (one-tailed); ** baseline and follow up between-group analysis by Mann-Whitney test (one-tailed); n.s. = not significant.

Such data are not surprising since, according to several authors (Deweer et al., 1994), successful performance on implicit tests has a prominent sensorimotor component depending on the integrity of the basal ganglia—particularly the caudate nuclei—and cerebellum (Perani et al., 1993), which are relatively intact in early AD.

The improvement of the trained patients at follow up is probably due to a set of converging variables. It is possible to hypothesise a kind of "circular reaction": (1) effective and evident benefits induced by training on procedural memory which persist over the medium to long term; (2) greater motivation exhibited by the patients, both during training and at home, that could have played an important role in a possible "caregiver effect" due to a growing awareness of the importance of not completely taking over from the patient in the execution of daily activities. This last aspect is important considering that caregivers have been indirectly involved through daily contacts in gathering information about patients, in explaining the stimulation, and in informing them about results. If so, one important consideration for future research may be to involve families in rehabilitative programmes. Quayhagen and Quayhagen (1989) assessed the efficacy of a home-based programme of cognitive stimulation for the functional status of patients with Alzheimer's disease. Ten family dyads (caregiver and patient) participated in the intervention and six family dyads formed the comparison group. They found that patients in the programme maintained their level of cognitive and behavioural functioning, whereas the comparison group patients deteriorated.

Some limitations of the present study need to be considered:

1. At baseline there was a statistically significant difference between the groups on forward digit span.

   According to the model proposed by Baddeley (Baddeley & Hitch, 1974), working memory is conceptualised as an active system for temporarily storing and manipulating information needed in the execution of complex cognitive tasks (e.g., learning). The model has a subcomponent, the phonological loop, that is assumed to be responsible for the temporary maintenance of acoustic or speech-based information, and which is most characteristically measured by the digit span test, involving the immediate serial recall of strings of numbers. Consequently, a statistical difference in digit span between groups may assume importance in a learning task, in particular, it is possible to suppose, when giving instructions. Notwithstanding this consideration, forward digit span scores were not impaired in either group and the performance time was measured by recording the interval *between the end* of the verbal command *and the completion of the task*.

2. From a neuropsychological point of view, the results of this study can be considered as an indication that procedural memory is preserved, or

relatively well preserved, in mild and mild–moderate AD patients and its stimulation could represent an effective rehabilitation approach. In fact, the training described here improved performance time and not the ability to execute an action which was given as a prerequisite. Future studies will need to focus mainly on clinical relevance, considering personal needs and stimulating in particular those activities of daily living whose maintenance will extend the autonomy of AD patients in their home environment.

The rehabilitative interventions proposed for AD are usually lacking in a specific approach aimed at improving functions that are preserved. Some authors (Ory & Cox, 1994) suggest that health professionals have been reluctant to target older adults in preventive programmes, assuming that this population would fail to benefit significantly from such efforts. However, the results of this study demonstrated that rehabilitative programmes designed for older adults with dementia can be effective.

In conclusion, the present study indicates the efficacy of a programme of procedural memory stimulation in a group of mild–moderate AD patients.

REFERENCES

Bäckman, L. (1992). Memory training and memory improvement in Alzheimer's disease: rules and exceptions. *Acta Neurologica Scandinavica, 139* (suppl.), 84–89.

Bäckman, L. (1996). Utilizing compensatory task conditions for episodic memory in Alzheimer's disease. *Acta Neurologica Scandinavica, 165* (suppl.), 109–113.

Baddeley, A.D., & Hitch, G.J. (1974). Working memory. In G. Bower (Ed.), *The psychology of learning and motivation*. San Diego, CA: Academic Press.

Camp, C.J., & McKitrick, L.A. (1992). Memory interventions in Alzheimer's-type dementia populations: Methodological and theoretical issues. In R.L. West & J.D. Sinnot (Eds.), *Everyday memory and aging: Current research and methodology*. New York: Springer.

Clark, M.E., Lipe, A.W., & Bilbrey, M. (1998). Use of music to decrease aggressive behaviors in people with dementia. *Journal of Gerontological Nursing, 24*, 10–17.

Crystal, H., Grober, E., & Masur, D. (1989). Preservation of musical memory in Alzheimer's disease. *Journal of Neurology, Neurosurgery, and Psychiatry, 52*, 1415–1416.

Deweer, B., Ergis, A., Fossati, P., Pillon, B., Boller, F., Agid, Y., & Dubois B. (1994). Explicit memory, procedural learning and lexical priming in Alzheimer's disease. *Cortex, 30*, 113–126.

Ermini-Funfschilling, D., & Meier, D. (1995). Memory training: An important constituent of milieu therapy in senile dementia. *Zeitschrift fur Gerontologie und Geriatrie, 28*, 190–194.

Folstein, M.F., Folstein, S., & McHugh, P.R. (1975). Mini Mental State: A practical method for grading the cognitive state of patients for the clinician. *Journal of Psychiatric Research, 121*, 189–198.

Gwyther, L.P. (1990). Milestoning: Evoking memories for resocialization through group reminiscence. *Gerontologist, 30*, 269–272.

Hirono, N., Mori, E., Ikejiri, Y., Imamura, T., Shimomura, T., Ikeda, M., Yamashita, H., Takatsuki, Y., Tokimasa, A., & Yamadory, A. (1997). Procedural memory in patients with mild Alzheimer's disease. *Dementia and Geriatric Cognitive Disorders, 8*, 210–216.

Josephsson, S., Bäckman, L., Borrell, L., Bernspang, B., Nygard, L., & Ronnberg L. (1993). Supporting everyday activities in dementia: An intervention study. *International Journal of Geriatric Psychiatry, 8*, 395–400.

Kaplan, E., Goodglass, H., & Weintraub, S. (1978). *The Boston Naming Test.* Boston: Veterans Administration Medical Center.

Knopman, D. (1991). Long-term retention of implicitly acquired learning in patients with Alzheimer's disease. *Journal of Clinical and Experimental Neuropsychology, 13*, 880–894.

Koh, K., Ray, R., Lee, J., Nair, A., Ho, T., & Ang, P. (1994). Dementia in elderly patients: Can the 3R mental stimulation programme improve mental status? *Age and Ageing, 23*, 195–199.

Libon, D.J., Bogdanoff, B., Cloud, B.S., Skalina, S., Giovannetti, T., Gitlin, H.L., & Bonavita, J. (1998). Declarative and procedural learning, quantitative measures of the hippocampus, and subcortical white alterations in Alzheimer's disease and ischaemic vascular dementia. *Journal of Clinical and Experimental Neuropsychology, 20*, 30–41.

Loewenstein, D.A., Amigo, E., Duara, R., Guterman, A., Hurwitz, D., Berkowitz, N., Wilkie, F., Weinberg, G., Black, B., Gittelman, B., & Eisdorfer, C. (1989). A new scale for the assessment of functional status in Alzheimer's disease and related disorders. *Journal of Gerontology, 44*, P114–121.

Markowitsch, H.J. (1998). Cognitive neuroscience of memory. *Neurocase, 4*, 429–435.

McKhann, G., Drachman, D., Folstein, M., Katzman, R., Price, D., & Stadlan, E.M. (1984). Clinical diagnosis of Alzheimer's disease: Report of the NINCDS-ADRDA work group under the auspices of Department of Health and Human Services Task Force on Alzheimer's disease. *Neurology, 34*, 939–944.

Ory, M.G., & Cox, D.M. (1994). Forging ahead: Linking health and behavior to improve quality of life in older people. *Social Indicators Research, 33*, 89–120.

Perani, D., Bressi, S., Cappa, S.F., Vallar, G., Alberini, M., Grassi, F., Caltagirone, C., Cipollotti, L., Franceschi, M., Lenzi, G.L., & Fazio, F. (1993). Evidence of multiple memory systems in the human brain: A [18F] FDG PET metabolic study. *Brain, 116*, 903–919.

Poe, M., & Seifert, L. (1997). Implicit and explicit tests: Evidence for dissociable motor skills in probable Alzheimer's dementia. *Perceptual and Motor Skills, 85*, 631–634.

Quayhagen, M.P., & Quayhagen, M. (1989). Differential effects of family-based strategies on Alzheimer's disease. *Gerontologist*, 29, 150–155.

Reuben, D.B., & Siu, A.L. (1990). An objective measure of physical function of elderly out-patients. *Journal of American Geriatrics Society, 38*, 1105–1112.

Sabe, L., Jason, L., Juejati, M., Leiguarda, R., & Starkstein, S.E. (1995). Dissociation between declarative and procedural learning in dementia and depression. *Journal of Clinical and Experimental Neuropsychology, 17*, 841–848.

Schreiber, M., Schweizer, A., Lutz, K., Kalveram, K.T., & Jäncke, L. (1999). Potential of an interactive computer-based training in the rehabilitation of dementia: An initial study. *Neuropsychological Rehabilitation, 9*, 155–167.

Spinnler, H., & Tognoni, G. (1987). Standardizzazione e taratura Italiana di test neuropsicologici. *Italian Journal of Neurological Sciences,* Suppl. 8/to n. 6.

Van der Linden, M., & Juillerat, A.C. (1998). Prise en charge des déficits cognitifs chez les patients atteints de maladie d'Alzheimer. *Revue Neurologique, 154*, 2S, 137–143.

Zanetti, O., Binetti, G., Magni, E., Rozzini, L., Bianchetti, A., & Trabucchi, M. (1997). Procedural memory stimulation in Alzheimer's disease: Impact of a training programme. *Acta Neurologica Scandinavica, 95*, 152–157.

Zanetti, O., Frisoni, G.B., De Leo, D., Dello Buono, M., Bianchetti, A., & Trabucchi, M. (1995). Reality orientation therapy in Alzheimer's disease: Useful or not? A controlled study. *Alzheimer Disease and Associated Disorders, 9*, 132–138.

Zanetti, O., Frisoni, G.B., Rozzini, L., Bianchetti, A., & Trabucchi, M. (1998). Validity of direct assessment of functional status as a tool for measuring Alzheimer's disease severity. *Age and Ageing, 27*, 615–622.

Zanetti, O., & Trabucchi, M. (1999). Non-pharmacological treatment of Alzheimer's disease and related disorders. In S. Govoni, C.L. Bolis, & M. Trabucchi (Eds.), *Dementias: Biological bases and clinical approach to treatment*. New York: Springer.

Manuscript received August 1999
Revised manuscript received January 2000

Alzheimer rehabilitation by students:
Interventions and outcomes

Sharon M. Arkin

University of Arizona, USA

This article advocates proactive Alzheimer treatment, describes rehab interventions implemented by students, and reports positive first year outcomes for 11 mild to moderate Alzheimer's disease (AD) patients who experienced these interventions in a longitudinal Alzheimer rehabilitation research programme. Students supervised physical fitness training and volunteer work sessions for all participants and administered specific memory and language stimulation exercises to 7 of them (experimental group). Outcomes were measured by standardised and project-related tests before and after two semesters (about 28 weeks) of participation. It was hypothesised that (1) the experimental group would outperform the control group at post-testing on standardised and project-specific cognitive and language measures; that both the experimental and control group would (2) maintain or improve the quality of their spontaneous discourse, (3) improve on measures of mood, and (4) improve on measures of physical fitness. Hypothesis 1 was only partially supported. The experimental group improved significantly from pre- to post-test on two measures, substantially on one measure, and showed no change on eleven measures. The control group declined significantly on three measures and showed no change on eleven measures. However, between group differences were only significant on one measure. Hypotheses 2, 3, and 4 were supported. The major conclusion was that: multi-modal interventions by students can temporarily maintain or improve cognitive, language, social, and physical functioning of Alzheimer's patients.

Correspondence should be sent to Sharon Arkin, University of Arizona, Department of Speech and Hearing Sciences, PO Box 210071, Tucson, Arizona 85721, USA. Fax (520) 760 5596. Email: arkinaz@earthlink.net

The programme is known in the community as Elder Rehab because some participants and/or their families do not acknowledge an Alzheimer's disease (AD) diagnosis or prefer not to be publicly identified with AD.

This research was made possible by a Mentored Research Scientist Development (K01) Award from the US National Institute on Aging. Name of project: AD rehab by students: Effects on functioning and decline.

PROLOGUE

In 1988, when I was in the first year of my doctoral studies in psychology, my mother, Bee Schultz, was diagnosed with probable Alzheimer's disease. Bee had always helped me with my homework when I was a child and teenager. At age 79, she rose to the occasion once again. Bee became my "guinea-pig" in countless experiments, practice testing sessions, and activities I dreamed up in attempts to buttress her failing memory and maintain her highly developed and nearly intact language skills. With unfailing good humour, she co-operated, travelling with me to Boston and California to meet with Alzheimer's experts, demonstrating her accomplishments in live presentations before groups, and always hamming it up for the ever-present video camera I used to record our odyssey.

Bee remained at the mild level of dementia for about 4 years. During the latter two of those years, I stage-managed her activities from afar, a local college student serving "in loco daughteris" to carry them out. I like to think my ministrations had something to do with the longevity of her "plateau". However, I am scientist enough to know that an "n" of 1 proves nothing. Nevertheless, my experiences with her were sufficiently encouraging to motivate me to try them with others in similar circumstances. The rehabilitation programme described here owes three of its four elements to work begun with or inspired by Bee—memory training, language stimulation activities, and "partnered volunteering". The capable and enthusiastic "therapy" provided by her student companion was the inspiration for the programme model I developed at the University of Arizona and which is the subject of this article.

BACKGROUND

The study described here is an outgrowth of two one-semester pilot studies conducted by the author as a post-doctoral project at the Department of Speech and Hearing Sciences and National Center for Neurogenic Communication Disorders at the University of Arizona (Arkin, 1996) and of a series of successful memory training experiments (Arkin, 1992, 1997, 1998).

It is significant for three important reasons: (1) It is the first study to monitor the effects of long-term non-pharmacological rehabilitation intervention on Alzheimer's patients;[1] (2) it trains and uses students as primary interveners, establishing a model that has worldwide replicability; and (3) it gives service in exchange for data.

---

[1] One study (Quayhagen & Quayhagen, 1989) provided eight months of daily caregiver-administered cognitive stimulation to 10 AD patients, with encouraging results.

In the pilot studies, undergraduate students were assigned to administer a variety of memory and language stimulation activities to early stage Alzheimer's disease (AD) patients, and to supervise them in a weekly volunteer service task. A discourse battery, a picture description task, and a proverb interpretation task were administered pre- and post-participation. Outcomes were positive enough to warrant attempts to replicate and expand the programme: Seven out of twelve participants improved in the number of relevant statements (topic comments) produced on the discourse battery; seven improved and four maintained performance on proverb interpretation; eight improved on a picture description task.

The present programme was made possible by a 5-year grant from the US National Institute on Aging. An exercise component, which is the most visible activity and the one most valued by caregivers, was added after the grant was awarded to take advantage of a new state-of-the-art cardiopulmonary rehab and employee wellness facility that opened at the University Medical Center (Wellness Center). The rationale was that participants would most certainly experience physical fitness and mood benefits from regular exercise, and that exercise might have a booster effect on the cognitive and social interventions being implemented.

RATIONALE AND LITERATURE REVIEW

This section reviews the literature on and presents the rationale for the four interventions used in this study: exercise, memory training, language therapy, and supervised volunteer work.

Exercise

The positive role of exercise on health, mood, maintenance of function, and disease prevention in elderly persons has been widely reported (Arkin, 1999; Bonder & Wagner, 1994; Evans & Rosenberg, 1991; Lamb, Gisolfi, & Nadel, 1995; Spirduso, 1995), yet fewer than 20% of Americans over age 65 are as physically active as they should be for optimal health (Vertinsky, 1991). No longer an activity just for the young and fit, exercise is demonstrating especially dramatic improvements among the very old, the very frail, and the cognitively impaired subgroups of seniors (Buchner & de Lateur, 1992; Fiatarone, 1996; Lindenmuth & Lindenmuth, 1994; Pitetti, 1993).

At the time the present study began, only one published study was found that documented benefits of exercise specifically for non-institutionalised dementia patients. Researchers at La Sapienza University Institute of Medicine in Rome (Palleschi et al., 1996), reported a significant improvement on four cognitive measures, including the Folstein, Folstein, and McHugh (1975) Mini-Mental State Exam (MMSE), in 15 male mild to moderate AD patients

(MMSE: 18–21) after 3 months of thrice-weekly 20 min workouts on a cyclo-ergometer (arms-only stationary bicycle).

The obstacles to exercise participation commonly cited by the elderly—inconvenience, lack of time, orthopaedic or other health problems, and beliefs that they get enough exercise elsewhere (Whaley & Ebbeck, 1997)—are multiplied for persons with dementia. Unable to travel, initiate and sustain an organised exercise programme on their own, they typically have caregivers that are too overburdened to organise and supervise such a programme for them (Bonner & Cousins, 1996). Elderly caregivers, like elderly people in general, are not likely to be familiar with the "high tech" atmosphere and equipment of contemporary fitness facilities. Student partners can provide people with dementia access to all the benefits of exercise that were previously unavailable to them.

Memory training

The memory training approach used is unique in that it focuses on biographical information pertaining to each individual participant, rather than on word lists, standardised stories, or other impersonal material. The rationale for this was that, because new learning (or relearning forgotten material) is difficult for Alzheimer's patients, motivation would be increased if the to-be-learned information were personally significant to the participant and his or her family. In fact, both participant and caregiver input were solicited as the content of each individual memory training protocol was being developed.

The technique stems from a discovery that repeated presentation of a video-tape in which an AD patient observed himself taking a quiz about a recent event—with the correct answer supplied for each missed question—led to eventual recall of most of the facts about the event (Arkin, 1991). The method was adapted to audiotape and modified to include brief factual paragraphs, with a question following each statement of fact, a pause for the patient to answer, if able, and the correct answer. The questions were repeated at the end of the paragraph (Arkin, 1992).

Later, it was found that the audiotaped training method was utilising a form of learning described in the literature as spaced retrieval, and which had been found by other researchers (e.g., Camp, Foss, O'Hanlon, & Stevens, 1995) to help AD patients learn via their relatively spared implicit memory system (Bäckman, 1992). The present method uses a "fixed interval" type of spaced retrieval (Foss & Camp, 1994) rather than the "expanding interval" type which has been more widely used. (For information on the use of expanding interval spaced retrieval to teach a variety of activities of daily living (ADLs), and compensatory rehabilitation strategies, see Brush & Camp, 1998.)

Between 1989 and 1994, the author used the audiotaped training method with 14 AD patients and one undiagnosed amnestic in a total of 18 single subject studies. Three of the subjects were trained with several sets of material. Substantial learning occurred in 13 of the 15 patients. MMSE scores of the successful learners ranged from 10 to 27 at treatment onset. One or two week follow-up was done in 12 studies. In 11 of those 12 studies, 78–100% of questions answered correctly at one-hour delayed post-test were answered correctly on the long delay follow-up test (Arkin, 1992, 1998). For a detailed description of the intervention as used in the present programme, see Arkin, 2000a. An excerpt from a sample memory tape script is presented in Appendix B.

Language therapy

Decline in language function is widely recognised as an early and prevalent symptom of AD (Bayles & Kaszniak, 1987, Kempler, 1995; Molloy & Lubinski, 1995; Salmon, Heindel, & Butters, 1995). Yet, a recent national conference devoted to defining and measuring outcomes in AD research (Maslow & Whitehouse, 1997), failed to include language function among the seven outcome domains considered.

Holland et al. (1985) commented on the lack of longitudinal studies that document the progressive language loss associated with degenerative conditions. Bourgeois (1991) reviewed the literature on communication treatment for adults with dementia and found that, in the prior 20 years, not a single treatment study had been published in the journals of the American Speech–Language–Hearing Association.

The present study is the first to do a comprehensive longitudinal assessment of linguistic competence of AD patients and to provide language and other interventions between assessments.

People with dementia have difficulty producing linguistic information because they have trouble thinking, generating, and ordering ideas. They have trouble comprehending linguistic information because of deteriorated inferential capabilities and difficulty accessing semantic memory (Bayles & Kaszniak, 1987). Schacter (1996, p. 135) defined semantic memory as "the vast network of associations and concepts that underlies our general knowledge of the world". Semantic memory deficits develop gradually in AD patients and impair their ability to stay on topic and make coherent conversation. Conversational ability is further hampered by diminished ability to maintain thematic structure (Ripich & Terrell, 1988).

The language interventions administered to the experimental group were selected to address deficits common to AD patients, by activating semantic memory and providing thematic structure. The building blocks of ideas that constitute semantic memory are related to each other and may be accessed via various routes. Activation of one may trigger a chain reaction (Bayles &

Kaszniak, 1987; Collins & Loftus, 1975). The student is the orchestrator and facilitator in this process, providing his or her partner with emotionally charged, sensorily rich experiences, and using a variety of tasks, games, props, and exercises, all aimed at stimulating or reviving connections between the various building blocks of semantic memory. Several of the interventions are adaptations of activities used for language assessment; one is an adaptation of a children's game.

Kagan and Gailey's (1993) observation that people with aphasia often find their conversational opportunities limited to discussions of food preferences and ADLs is true of dementia patients, as well. For this reason, participants were asked for their opinions or advice on controversial situations, in which a moral issue was involved. It is validating for people with dementia to have their opinion or advice sought on adult issues, particularly by a young student. This activity was successfully used in a geropsychiatric hospital in Germany to counteract the loss of social roles and functions that accompanies institutionalisation (Muller, 1993). Muller reported that patients with various degrees of dementia were able to understand hypothetical conflict situations and take a position on complex issues, and that the exercise "activated participants' stores of experience and knowledge and appears to have increased their self-esteem". (Quote from English language abstract in Psycinfo.)

Partnered volunteering

The volunteer service idea derived from my clinical observations that people with dementia seemed to remember a responsibility they had for someone else better than they did their own schedule and experiences. They also felt good about themselves when they were able to be of service to others.

Life satisfaction among the elderly has been linked to level of activity (Havighurst, 1961) and there is evidence that the elderly reap mental and physical health benefits from paid or volunteer work (Abramson, Ritter, Gofin, & Kark, 1992: Soumeri & Avorn, 1983). Successful work therapy programmes have been reported for discharged psychiatric patients (Keys, 1982) and institutionalised dementia patients (Griffin & Mouheb, 1987) and as core elements of nursing home and residential treatment centre programmes (Butin & Heaney, 1991; Voeks & Drinka, 1990). No articles were found in professional journals about volunteer or work programmes for community dwelling people with dementia. However a recent article in Chicago's Rush Alzheimer's Disease Center newsletter (Swanson, Levi, & Matano, 1999) reported that, since 1996, the Center has been involving a small group of early stage patients in monthly volunteer activities, the most notable being tutoring first graders in reading. According to the authors: "people with early stage dementia take pride in accomplishing tasks and providing comfort to others in need. These successful volunteer experiences affect the way professionals and others view the capabilities of people with early stage dementia" (p. 8).

The Elder Rehab programme's "partnered volunteering" activity meets two of the criteria outlined by occupational therapist Jitka Zgola (1990) for therapeutic activity for dementia sufferers: It contributes to maintenance of function, and enhances quality of life—for both the providers and the recipients of the volunteer services.

METHOD

Research participants

Research participants in the present study were 11 very mild to moderate stage AD patients. Some were referred by an adult day-care centre, the Alzheimer's Association, the University Medical Center's memory disorders clinic, and several group homes and assisted living facilities, in response to recruiting visits by the author. Others were referred by family members and physicians who had seen newspaper articles about the programme. All enrolled participants received the benefits of transportation and supervised therapeutic activities from students, membership for themselves and their caregivers in the University Medical Center's Health and Wellness Center, expert neurological and neuropsychological testing, bone density and laboratory testing, attendance at two awards banquets per year, Elder Rehab t-shirts and, during the summer, participation in 10 weekly sessions at an adult day-care centre, with special group cognitive stimulation programmes led by former student rehabilitation partners. No monetary remuneration was provided.

Baseline MMSE scores ranged from 15–29, with a mean of 23 (SD = 4.75). The participant with a score of 29 scored in the demented range on the Mattis Dementia Rating Scale (1988), was rated as a mild stage patient (Clinical Dementia Rating 1) by a Consortium to Establish a Registry for AD (CERAD)-certified clinician, and had an APOE[2] genetic test profile of 4/4, the highest probability score for an AD diagnosis. (Although there was no change in her cognitive performance in her first year of participation, her second year pattern was consistent with an AD progression.)

The age of participants at treatment onset ranged from 59–86 years, with a mean of 79 (SD = 7.33). (See Table 1 for other demographic data.)

These 11 individuals were the first cohort to complete two semesters of participation in the ongoing rehabilitation research programme. As of May, 1999, there were 14 participants in the programme. Ten of the original eleven had completed four semesters of participation and were about to begin

---

[2] APOE = Apolipoprotein, a susceptibility gene for AD.

TABLE 1
Participant demographic characteristics

Subject	Sex	Age[1]	MMSE[1]	Education (in years)	Residence	Primary occupation
Experimental group						
AB	M	78	23	15	Group home	Musician/drummer
DC	F	79	26	12	Home alone	Sales person
HC	F	82	15	18	Assisted living	Nurse
DK	F	84	26	12	Group home	School bus driver for handicapped
IJ	F	83	17	14	Assisted living	Homemaker
WM	F	79	22	12	Home with relatives	Cook's helper
BM	F	86	29	12	Home alone	Mobile home park operator
Control group						
LA	F	78	18	10	Assisted living	Factory worker
MD	M	85	29	12	With spouse	Farmer, maintenance
EMc	F	78	26	12	With relatives	Clerical, sales, waitress
NM	M	59	23	12	With spouse	Electrician

[1] Age and MMSE score at baseline CERAD testing

end-of-second-year testing; two later entrants had completed three semesters; two had completed two and were scheduled for end-of-first-year testing. Unless otherwise specified, persons referred to as participants in this article are the original cohort of 11.

Participants were selected according to criteria used by the CERAD, which did annual assessments of AD patients at 21 co-operating US Alzheimer's research centres (Morris et al., 1989). CERAD criteria correspond to the NINCDS-ADRDA (National Institute of Neurological and Communicative Disorders and Stroke-Alzheimer's Disease and Related Disorders Association) criteria, (McKhann et al., 1984). CERAD criteria also require subjects to be at least 50 years old, community dwelling (not in a nursing home), English speaking, and not on an Alzheimer drug at intake. Three of the 11 participants had a current or recent history of depression when they entered the present study. This was the only deviation from the CERAD criteria, which excluded subjects with depression. This exception was made because of the hypothesis that participation in the programme would improve mood.

Reported MMSE scores were obtained as part of baseline testing with the neuropsychological test battery used by the CERAD (Morris et al., 1989). Subjects were independently diagnosed and staged (10 with probable, one with possible AD) by a CERAD-certified neuropsychologist, using the Clinical Dementia Rating interview (CDR; Berg, 1988), and by the head of the University Medical Center's Department of Neurology, using CERAD's neurological exam protocol (Morris et al., 1989). CERAD tests were administered by psychology doctoral students who were trained and certified by CERAD staff and supervised by the CERAD-certified neuropsychologist who did the CDR interview.

Attempted random assignment to the experimental and control groups resulted in one group having all higher mental status subjects and the other all lower mental status subjects. Non-random switching of subjects based on their mental status and on logistical factors resulted in groups that were statistically equivalent in terms of age and MMSE scores.

Student rehab partners

Student rehab partners were 22 undergraduate students—11 each semester—who were recruited via video-illustrated presentations in speech and hearing and psychology classes. The video shown was a 6-min feature by a local news magazine show which demonstrated the pilot programme in action. An illustrated feature story in the university's student newspaper also attracted several applicants. In subsequent semesters, students were drawn from chemistry and exercise physiology classes and in response to an email message that was sent to honours students. During the first year of the programme, all of the student participants were female. In subsequent semesters, there were typically one to three male participants.

Student partners were selected on a "first come first served" basis, the only requirements being access to a car, a valid driver's licence, and proof of insurance. Students used their own cars to transport their partners to and from activities and were covered under the University's liability insurance plan.

Students earned three undergraduate credits for their participation and were required to attend an exercise training session and six seminars on topics such as the physiology of AD, Alzheimer's assessment, language and memory interventions, community resources, caregiver issues, and exercise and the elderly. They also viewed the prize-winning films *Do You Remember Love?* with Joanne Woodward (Dave Bell Productions, 1987)—about a college professor who gets early onset AD—and the prize-winning *Complaints of a Dutiful Daughter* by caregiver and film-maker Debbie Hoffman (1994). Students working with the experimental participants prepared weekly reports about their partner's performance on the various memory and language exercises, which were used in preparation of a final report which was passed on to their participant's subsequent semester's student partner. Students working with the control participants prepared memory books for their partners. These contained photos of important persons and events of their life, captioned with text written in the first person, so that the subject could read from it in conversational style to a listener. For information on the rationale, use, and benefits of memory books, see Bourgeois, 1990. All students read and summarised five assigned journal articles and transcribed a lengthy discourse sample at the end of the semester. They also took the standardised AD Knowledge Test (Zarit et al., 1988) at the beginning and at the end of the semester.

Pre- and post-participation assessment

In addition to the CERAD neuropsychological battery, cognitive, language, physical fitness, and mood tests were administered—prior to treatment onset and at the end of the second semester of participation. (The same tests were administered at the end of the second and third years, as well.)

Cognitive tests

Standardised cognitive tests used were the Comprehension, Picture Completion, and Similarities subtests of the Wechsler Adult Intelligence Scale—Revised (WAIS-R; Wechsler, 1981) and the Logical Memory subtest of the Wechsler Memory Scale—Revised (Wechsler, 1987). A 30-item biographical knowledge test was also administered, the correct answers having been supplied by caregivers. The test covered basic facts about home town, schools attended, parents and grandparents, siblings, places lived, occupations of self and/or spouse, etc. Substitute questions were created for never-married people and people without siblings.

Functional status assessment

Functional status was assessed by an experienced CERAD-certified neuropsychologist, using CERAD's Clinical Dementia Rating (CDR), a scale which rates four stages of dementia: questionable, mild, moderate, and severe. The scale assesses six domains via interview with both the subject and the primary caregiver: (1) Memory; (2) Orientation; (3) Judgement and Problem Solving; (4) Community Affairs; (5) Home and Hobbies; and (6) Personal Care.

Language tests

Participants were administered a standardised language battery, two language tests on the CERAD battery, and a comprehensive discourse battery. The Arizona Battery for Communication Disorders of Dementia (ABCD; Bayles & Tomoeda, 1991) is a standardised battery of tests which assesses the functional linguistic communication abilities of mild to moderate AD patients. The ABCD was standardized on 86 individuals with AD and is reported to have high internal consistency, test–retest reliability, criterion validity and construct validity (Bayles & Tomoeda, 1991). The test comprises 14 subtests which provide information about five constructs: Mental Status, Episodic Memory,

Linguistic Expression, Linguistic Comprehension, and Visuospatial Construction. The five construct scores are summed to arrive at a total score.

The two CERAD language tests used were an abbreviated (15-item) form of the Boston Naming Test (Kaplan, Goodglass, & Weintraub, 1983) and a 60-s verbal fluency test for the category "animals".

Quantity and quality of discourse were measured by (1) eliciting, tape recording, transcribing, coding, and analysing verbal responses to eight stimulus prompts or questions; (2) counting the number of information units produced on description of the grocery store picture from the Aphasia Diagnostic Battery (Helm-Estabrooks, 1992), and evaluating interpretations of five familiar proverbs from Delis, Kramer, and Kaplan's unpublished California Proverbs Test (1984). Stimulus prompts and questions used to assess spontaneous discourse were: (1) Tell me what you know about John F. Kennedy and his family. (2) Tell me what you know about Alzheimer's disease—this item was also used as one of three indicators of insight (Arkin, 2000c). (3) Tell me about your daily activities, the things you do nearly every day. (4) What are some things you do once in a while? (5) What childhood thoughts and memories does the word "play" remind you of? (6) What adult thoughts and memories does the word "play" remind you of? (7) How would you go about planning a picnic for your family or some friends? (8) Supposing the 13-year-old daughter of your neighbour told you she was pregnant, but was afraid to tell her mother. What would you do? What are some ways a family could handle a situation like that? Stimulus items used represent each discourse type described by Shadden (1995).

Proverb interpretation is frequently used as a test of abstract reasoning ability and as an aid in the diagnosis of dementia (Chapman et al., 1997; Strub & Black, 1985; Van Lancker, 1990).

Proverbs used were:

1. They see eye to eye.
2. Too many cooks spoil the broth.
3. Rome wasn't built in a day.
4. Don't count your chickens before they're hatched.
5. You can't tell a book by its cover.

Fitness measures

Aerobic fitness was assessed by measuring the distance covered during a 6-min walk, a commonly used and reliable measure of fitness in the elderly and disabled (Tappen et al., 1997), and by comparing the duration of aerobic exercise at the first exercise session with that of the last session of the second semester. The 6-min walk test was done in the aerobics room of the Wellness Center where all of the exercise interventions took place. Upper and lower body strength was assessed by comparing the amount of weight lifted on the chest press and leg press machines, respectively, during the first and last sessions of participation each semester.

Mood assessment

Mood was objectively assessed using the 30-item Geriatric Depression Scale (Yesavage et al., 1983) and by obtaining caregiver responses to a project-specific questionnaire. Subjectively, it can be assessed by watching hours of videotaped images of participants happily exercising, conversing, and engaging in volunteer work!

INTERVENTIONS

Four types of interventions were used during the two semesters of the study described here: physical exercise, memory training, language stimulation activities, and supervised volunteer work. Each of these is described below.

Exercise

All 11 participants experienced two physical fitness training sessions per week for 10 weeks during both semesters. One weekly session was supervised by a student partner, the other by a family member or friend. The fitness session consisted of a warm-up walk from the car park, a series of stretches, an aerobic workout on the treadmill followed by one on a stationary bicycle, and two sets of 10–12 repetitions on five different weight training machines. Participants were started at five minutes on each of the aerobic machines, with a goal of 10 min on each machine by the end of the semester. In addition, a brisk 20-min walk was built into the weekly volunteer work session. A detailed description of the exercise programme may be found in the Practice Concepts section of Arkin (1999).

Biographical memory training

The biographical memory training exercise was administered via a tape-recorder to the seven experimental subjects at their home by their respective student partners, before leaving for their weekly exercise session together. Thus, each participant was exposed to the interactive tape-recorded exercise 10 times per semester. Each subject's customised tape-recorded exercise consisted of a series of paragraphs containing factual statements about his or her life history, followed by strategically placed quiz questions about the statements, a pause for his or her response, and the correct answer (Arkin, 2000a). A sample portion of a memory tape script is presented in Appendix B.

Language stimulation activities

Seven participants (experimental group) were administered a series of language stimulation activities during their student-supervised exercise sessions; the four control participants experienced unstructured conversation with their student partners during those sessions.

Students who were partners with an experimental subject were given a resource packet containing stimulus items for each activity category, as well as forms for the recording of participants' free and prompted responses. All participants were given pre- and post-tests on language activities to which only the experimental group was exposed during sessions. Specific language activities that were used are described below. An example of each is provided in Appendix A.

Picture description

Selected pictures from Norman Rockwell[3] calendars were used for this activity. Norman Rockwell pictures have been used as stimulus items by previous researchers for eliciting descriptive discourse (Tomoeda & Bayles, 1993). Examinees are asked to describe what they see in the picture. In testing situations, free responses are sought, with only neutral prompts provided. In the present programme, the pictures were used first to elicit spontaneous responses, but then as a reference point for a series of elaborative prompt questions. This "script" strategy (Clark & Witte, 1991; Penn, Jones, & Joffe, 1997) was designed to elicit inferences—about events, setting, season, relationships, emotions—discernible from details in the pictures, as well as personal experiences suggested by the picture. This task was done at the start of the exercise session, after a resting pulse measure was taken. Example: "The homecoming" picture shows a soldier in uniform carrying a small bag approaching a tenement backyard filled with red-haired people of all ages, obviously his family and neighbours, and a shy teenaged girl hiding along the side of the building, apparently his girlfriend. (See Appendix A for related prompt questions.)

Word association

In this activity (typically conducted while the participant was walking on a treadmill) the student selected an evocative word from a prepared list and asked the participant to tell about some memories from childhood, then later, from adulthood, that the word brought to mind. The student was instructed to

---

[3] Norman Rockwell is a beloved American artist and illustrator who portrayed typical American life in magazine covers and calendars from the 1930s through the mid-1960s.

contribute associated memories and experiences to keep the conversation going. This activity was suggested by the work of Crovitz (1986), who used a random set of words "not for any theoretical reason, but because they were easily accessible in my files" (p. 274) to elicit a specific elusive memory in a head-injured patient. Repeated use of a word that is particularly meaningful to an individual patient, such as "school" for a former teacher, or "war" for a Jewish holocaust survivor tends to produce a relatively rich outpouring of memories. However, repeated use of the word elicits the same stories over and over again. Introducing a variety of cue words has proven to be a good way to elicit novel utterances on topics not in the usual repertoire of Alzheimer's patients left to their own devices.

Advice and opinion questions

In this activity, participants were presented each week with a different "what if" question about a controversial or value-laden problem or situation and were asked to offer an opinion or solution. Following opportunity for free response, a series of prompt questions was presented. Example 1: What if you found out that your best friend's husband were having an affair. What would you do? Example 2: What if your brother were sick with cancer and needed some illegal marijuana to help fight nausea. What would you do? (See Appendix A for follow-up prompt questions.)

The rationale for this activity is that the personalities and values of Alzheimer's patients remain relatively intact well into the disease, and permit them to express opinions and give advice even if they are compromised in their ability to discuss issues or events that depend on episodic or autobiographical memory. One patient from the pilot project, an 88-year-old retired social worker, became so concerned over the plight of her student's (hypothetical) pregnant teenage friend that she cornered the director of the day care centre where she and her student partner did volunteer work to ask her assistance in finding help for the girl. The next week, when the student asked her what she should do after learning her friend's husband was having an affair, the patient commented: "You sure have a lot of problem friends!"

Category fluency

Timed category fluency tests are a standard component of test batteries that assess cognitive and language abilities (Lezak, 1995; Morris et al., 1989); scores on this task are a highly sensitive measure of the deficiencies in semantic memory associated with AD (Butters et al., 1987). As a retrieval activity, category fluency tests are considered more effortful than object or picture naming because they lack visual stimuli (Huff, Corkin, & Growdon, 1986).

When using category fluency tests as a programme activity, the student named various superordinate categories and asked participants to name items that belong to the category. Some patients did well on the task itself. Several sometimes digressed to discuss topics suggested by words that they named. In the first semester, different categories were used each session. In the second semester, one new category and one constant category, "things people wear, such as clothing and jewellery" were presented at each session. The repeated presentation was to elicit multiple lists in order to approximate each participant's repertoire for that category. These repertoire lists were later used in an experiment to determine whether exposure to repeated sessions of a study task involving words from the constant category resulted in post-exposure production of words from the study task (exposure words) that had never been named during the pre-exposure tests—evidence of implicit learning (Camp et al., 1995; Schacter, 1987, 1992). Six of seven participants in the experiment did produce "exposure" words that had never been produced on the pre-exposure tests. Unexpectedly, all of them produced novel words (words never named in their pre-exposure fluency tests and that were not encountered on the study task)—evidence of semantic activation (Arkin, Rose, & Hopper, 2000; Collins & Loftus, 1975).

A related activity, administered during a rest period at some sessions, was the presentation of pairs of related exemplars, such as "Coke and Pepsi" or "bridge and poker" and asking subjects to name the category to which they belong. This task corresponds to the WAIS-R Similarities subtest (Wechsler, 1981); categories from that test were avoided in the practice sessions.

Proverb interpretation

Students were provided with lists and abstract interpretations of selected proverbs from the Dictionary of Cultural Literacy (Hirsch, Kett, & Trefil, 1988). Six proverbs were presented at each session. The student read the beginning of each one and the participant was asked to complete it, if able. Then the student asked the participant what the proverb meant. If the participant did not know, reiterated the proverb, or gave a concrete response, the student read the correct abstract interpretation and asked the participant to repeat it. Several students have reported learning from their elderly partners during this activity!

"A, my name is . . ." game

This activity is derived from a children's ball bouncing game. It provides excellent practice in naming on demand and switching set, two abilities that are compromised in AD patients (Bayles & Kaszniak, 1987; Kempler, 1991). It was administered during a rest period at some sessions. The framework for responding is as follows: A, my name is (name beginning with A) _____, and my husband's/wife's name is (name beginning with A) _____, and we come from (place beginning with A) _____, and we're going down town to buy (object beginning with A) _____. B, my name is _____, etc. The game was modified for one participant, who found it too easy, by having her change letters sequentially for each word produced, i.e., A, my name is Alice and my husband's name is Bob and we come from Chicago, etc.

Famous names

In this activity, done at some sessions during a rest period, students read first names from a prepared list and asked participants to think of a famous person's last name that went with each first name. Several examples were provided for each first name. Sometimes, the participant just named the name. Other times, they were asked to tell something about the person named. Students reported that their elderly partners were often pleased to be able to name and explain about people who were unfamiliar to the students.

Car bingo

This activity was conducted in the student's car on the way between the participant's home and the fitness centre. A large cardboard square with boxes made from five horizontal and five vertical rows was filled in—one per square—with names of objects one might see while riding in the car, such as school bus, dead animal, driver wearing hat, etc. Most participants could not focus on the whole card at once, so the student would suggest one or two objects at a time to be looked for on a given trip and the participant would put a mark in the square when the object was spotted. Many students reported that the drive time was particularly productive for spontaneous conversation initiated by participants. Such conversations were always given priority over the game.

Partnered volunteering

Beginning with semester 2, all participants experienced a session of weekly volunteer service or other personally meaningful community activity plus a brisk walk with their student partner. Most popular activities were reading to preschool age children at a local day-care centre and packaging bulk rice or beans at a community food bank. One participant who had been reluctant to leave her dog at home to go places with a student became an enthusiastic and welcome visitor to a nursing home where she and her partner brought her dog each week. Several participants groomed or walked dogs or socialised with cats at an animal shelter. On nice days, some volunteer pairs went walking in local parks or the university campus and picked up litter. Two participants did not "click" with volunteer activities that were tried with them. One of them played miniature golf, another went bowling with their respective student partner. Students were encouraged to vary the activities and sometimes took their partner to a musical performance, art exhibit, or museum. One student took her partner along on a date to the zoo; another to a women's basketball game on campus.

DATA ANALYSIS AND RESULTS

Hypothesis 1: That the experimental group would outperform the control group at post-testing on standardised and project-specific cognitive and language measures.   This is defined as either a significant or substantial non-significant difference in performance in the positive direction by the experimental group as compared to the control group. This could be either a score indicative of an improvement in performance or one indicative of a lesser decline. Non-significant mean change score differences of less than one point are not reported as differences.

This hypothesis was only partially supported. The experimental group outperformed the control group on the MMSE, on a project-specific biographical memory test, on the ratio of topic comments to total utterances, and on the ratio of different nouns to total nouns. The two groups performed equivalently, showing no change from pre- to post-test, on short story immediate recall (WMS-R, Logical Memory I), WAIS-R Comprehension, WAIS-R Similarities, WAIS-R Picture Completion, the CERAD Boston Naming and Verbal Fluency tests, the ABCD language battery, the ratio of vague nouns to total nouns, and on proverb interpretation. (Difference scores on the ADP picture description were the same for both groups, but showed up as a significant decline only for the control group.) (See Tables 2 and 3 for all individual and group change scores.)

Mental status

Two out of seven experimental participants increased their score and two had the same MMSE score at the end of one year as they did at baseline; three had scores that declined: by 2, 6, and 6 points, respectively. All four control participants' scores declined: by 3, 4, 4, and 6 points, respectively. (Reported annual rate of change on the MMSE cited by the CERAD team, Morris et al., 1989, was 3.9 + 0.7. Range of annual rates of decline on the MMSE reported in nine studies reviewed by Aguero-Torres, Fratiglioni, & Winblad, 1998, was 2.7 + 2.4 to 4.0 + 2.4.)

Decline in scores of the group as a whole and of the control group, as measured by a paired *t*-test was significant: $t(10) = -2.9$, *p < .01 and $t(3) = -6.8$, *p < .01, respectively. Decline in scores of the experimental group was not significant: $t(6) = -1.3$, $p = .12$. A comparison of the mean difference scores of the experimental and control groups, using a two-sample *t*-test

TABLE 2

Individual and group cognitive test scores before and after one year of treatment

Test	Results							Group mean		Mean difference score (SE)
								Pre (SE)	Post (SE)	
Experimental group										
Participant/age at baseline	AB/78	DC/79	HC/82	DK/84	IJ/83	WM/79	BM/86			
MMSE Pre/Post	23/25	26/24	15/9	26/26	17/18	22/16	29/29	22.7 (1.9)	21.0 (2.6)	−1.7 (1.2)
CDR Pre/Post	1/2	1/0.5	2/3	0.5/1	2/2	1/2	1/1			
WMS Logical Memory 1 Pre/Post	4/12	10/8	0/0	5/10	2/5	6/0	16/20	6.1 (2.0)	7.9 (2.7)	1.8 (1.8)
WAIS-R Comp.[2] Pre/Post	12/14	14/13	5/5	12/11	9/12	9/5	11/14	10.3 (1.0)	10.6 (1.5)	0.3 (1.0)
Percentile Rank Pre/Post	75/91	91/84	5/5	75/63	37/75	37/5	63/91			
WAIS-R Similar[2] Pre/Post	14/14	16/14	6/10	8/11	5/8	10/7	15/16	10.6 (1.7)	11.4 (1.3)	0.86 (1.0)
Percentile Rank Pre/Post	91/91	98/91	9/50	75/63	5/25	50/16	95/98			
WAIS-R Pict. Comp.[2] Pre/Post	9/12	12/15	5/7	14/7	9/10	8/5	12/12	9.9 (1.1)	9.7 (1.3)	−0.14 (1.4)
Percentile Rank Pre/Post	37/75	75/95	5/16	91/16	37/50	25/5	75/75			

Test	Results				Group mean		Mean difference score (SE)
					Pre (SE)	Post (SE)	
Control group							
Participant/age at baseline	LA/78	MD/85	EMc/78	NM/59			
MMSE Pre/Post	18/14	29/25	26/20	23/20	24.0 (2.3)	19.8 (2.35)	-4.2* (0.6)
CDR Pre/Post	1/2	1/0.5	1/1	1/1			
WMS Logical Memory I Pre/Post	5/5	18/18	2/4	11/16	9 (3.5)	10.8 (3.6)	1.8 (1.2)
WAIS-R Comp.[2] Pre/Post	9/9	18/14	11/10	16/15	13.5 (2.1)	12 (1.5)	-1.5 (0.9)
Percentile Rank Pre/Post	37/37	99/91	63/50	98/95			
WAIS-R Similar[2] Pre/Post	8/11	11/11	9/7	16/16	11 (1.8)	11.25 (1.8)	0.25 (1.0)
Percentile Rank Pre/Post	25/63	63/63	37/16	98/98			
WAIS-R Pict. Com.p[2] Pre/Post	5/5	11/11	9/9	12/11	9.25 (1.5)	9.0 (1.4)	-0.25 (0.25)
Percentile Rank Pre/Post	5/5	63/63	37/37	75/63			

[1] Stage 0.5 = questionable dementia, Stage 1 mild dementia, Stage 2 = moderate dementia, Stage 3 = severe dementia, [2] Age adjusted scaled scores, SE = standard error.

TABLE 3
Individual and group language test scores before and after one year of treatment

Test	Results							Group mean		Mean difference score (SE)
								Pre (SE)[1]	Post (SE)	
Experimental group										
Participants/MMSE at baseline	AB/23	DC/26	HC/15	DK/26	IJ/17	WM/22	BM/29			
ABCD Total Score Pre/Post	18/17	19/19	12/11	19/19	17/17	18/15	21/22	17.7 (1.1)	17.1 (1.3)	0.6 (0.5)
Boston Naming[2] Pre/Post	15/15	15/15	11/9	12/14	14/11	11/12	15/14	13.3 (0.7)	12.9 (0.9)	0.4 (0.6)
Verbal Fluency (Animals) Pre/Post	12/14	12/11	5/4	13/9	2/7	5/3	14/15	9 (1.8)	9 (1.8)	0 (1.1)
Ratio (%) of Topic Comments/ Utterances Pre/Post	60/57	43/59	48/63	92/86	77/78	63/47	65/73	64 (6.3)	66.1 (5.2)	–2.1 (4.4)
Ratio (%) of Different Nouns/ Total Nouns Pre/Post	69/60	57/55	54/78	46/59	53/48	61/64	56/54	56.6 (2.7)	59.7 (3.6)	–3.1* (4.4)
Ratio (%) of Vague[3] Nouns/ Total Nouns Pre/Post	6/3	7/5	13/20	1/0.9	5/5	5/0	1/2	5.3 (1.6)	5.1 (2.6)	0.23 (1.4)
Proverb Interpretation Pre/Post	25/28	30/29	18/8	25/27	17/19	16/11	19/21	21 (1.8)	20 (2.8)	1 (1.6)
Picture Description[4] No. of Information Units Pre/Post	20/23	48/48	24/19	58/33	31/33	17/23	52/48	35.7 (6.3)	32.4 (4.5)	–3.29 (3.9)

| Test | Results | | | | Group mean | | Mean difference score (SE) |
	LA/18	MD/29	EMc/26	NM/23	Pre (SE)[1]	Post (SE)	
Control group							
Participants/MMSE at baseline							
ABCD Total Score Pre/Post	13/14	18/16	17/17	21/20	17.25 (1.7)	16.75 (1.3)	0.5 (0.65)
Boston Naming[2] Pre/Post	13/8	14/14	13/14	15/15	13.75 (0.5)	12.75 (1.6)	1 (1.4)
Verbal Fluency (Animals) Pre/Post	12/7	5/7	7/9	17/21	10.25 (2.7)	11 (3.4)	-0.75 (2.0)
Ratio (%) of Topic Comments/ Utterances Pre/Post	80/58	48/79	77/76	77/79	70.5 (7.5)	7.3 (5.0)	-2.5 (10.9)
Ratio (%) of Different Nouns/ Total Nouns Pre/Post	52/49	77/70	64/56	79/74	68 (6.3)	62.5 (5.9)	5.75* (1.1)
Ratio (%) of Vague[3] Nouns/ Total Nouns Pre/Post	5/6	2/1	9/7	2/1	4.35 (1.7)	3.6 (1.6)	0.7 (0.8)
Proverb Interpretation Pre/Post	19/21	16/19	25/25	27/25	23.4 (2.6)	24 (1.9)	-0.6 (0.9)
Picture Description[4] No. of Information Units Pre/Post	18/17	16/14	22/18	29/23	21.25 (1.87)	18 (1.87)	-3.5* (1.1)

* Mean group difference score is significant. [1] Scores rounded to the nearest tenth. [2] 15-item CERAD version. [3] Decline in ratio means improvement. [4] Grocery store picture from the Aphasia Diagnostic Battery (Helm-Estabrooks, 1992), Note: Group mean scores and group difference scores include scores of one experimental and one control subject whose individual scores are not on this table. SE = standard error.

with equal variances, showed the difference between the scores to be non-significant, $t(9) = 1.5, p = .07$.

Other cognitive outcomes

Logical Memory I

On the Logical Memory I (immediate story recall) subtest of the WMS-R, there was no significant change in whole group performance from baseline to end of one year: $t(6) = 1.5, p = .085$. There was no upward or downward trend for either group, as measured by mean change scores (see Table 2). A comparison of the mean difference scores of the two groups, using a t-test with equal variances found no difference between the groups: $t(9) = -0.01, p = .50$.

WAIS-R subtests

Seven of the 11 participants—five experimentals and two controls—demonstrated post-test intellectual functioning on two or three of the WAIS-R subtests that was above the 50th percentile for normal people aged 74 or below in the WAIS-R standardisation sample (Wechsler, 1981). Five scored above the 90th percentile on one or two of the tests. This is even more remarkable considering that six of these seven high achievers were 4–12 years older than the oldest age group in the WAIS-R standardisation sample. Individual subtest outcomes are discussed below (see Table 2).

WAIS-R comprehension

On the WAIS-R Comprehension subtest, which measures problem-solving ability, common sense, and abstract reasoning, there was no significant decline in whole group performance: $t(10) = -.5, p = .31$. The experimental group's pre to post mean difference score was a non-significant 1.8 points higher than the control group's score, with the experimental group showing a slight upward trend and the control group a slight downward trend: $t(6) = .2, p = .40$ vs. $t(3) = -1.7, p = .09$. A between group comparison of the mean difference scores showed the difference to be non-significant: $t(9) = 1.2, p = .125$.

WAIS-R similarities

On the WAIS-R Similarities subtest, which is a test of verbal concept formation—explaining what pairs of words have in common—there was no significant decline in whole group performance: $t(10) = 0.89, p = .80$. There was also no difference in performance between the two groups: $t(9) = 0.39, p = .35$.

WAIS-R picture completion

On the WAIS-R Picture Completion subtest—which measures visual reasoning by having examinees note important missing parts in pictures of people or familiar objects—there was no significant decline in whole group performance: $t(10) = -0.02$, $p = .42$. There was also no difference in performance between the two groups: $t(9) = 0.05$, $p = .48$.

Biographical memory outcomes

These results have been previously reported in the *American Journal of Alzheimer's Disease* (Arkin, 2000a, b).

Highly significant learning was achieved during the first 10 sessions of biographical memory training experienced by the experimental group, as measured by the difference between the group's mean score on the (32-item) pre-test and on the one hour delayed post-test following the final training session: $t(6) = 11.268$, $*p < .001$. Five of the seven experimental participants learned or relearned between 10 and 13 personal facts; two learned or relearned seven facts (see Figure 1). The memory training exercise included items still remembered by participants, so that the task would not be too discouraging; this accounts for the high pre-test scores.

Five of the seven participants, who took another post-test two months later, correctly answered between 65 and 93% of the questions which had been answered correctly at the 1-hour delayed post-test (Arkin, 2000b) (see Figure 1). Group mean post-test score was 27.

The same mean post-test score was achieved by the seven experimental participants after another 10 training sessions (see Figure 2). A delayed post-test administered to all seven experimental participants one month after the end

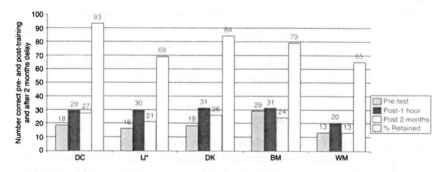

Figure 1. Student-administered Alzheimer memory training: Learning after 10 sessions and retention two months after training. (Values rounded to the nearest whole number.) * IJ's training tape inadvertently contained only 31 items.

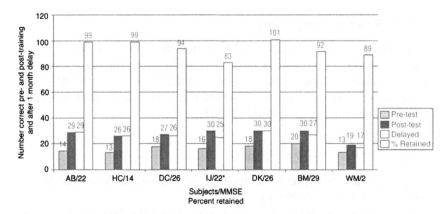

Figure 2. Student-administered Alzheimer memory training: Recall 1 month after 20 sessions. (Values rounded to the nearest whole number.) Training consisted of 20 weekly training sessions, 10 during the fall, 1997 academic semester and 10 during the spring, 1998 semester. Post-test was administered one distraction-filled hour after the 20th training session. * IJ's training tape inadvertently contained only 31 items.

of 20 weeks of training resulted in correct recall of between 89 and 100% of items answered correctly one hour after the end of training (Arkin, 2000b) (see Figure 2).

The amount retained by the five for whom both delayed post-test scores are available was significantly greater after the 10 extra sessions, $t = 2.6044$, *$p < .03$. It is not clear whether the gain was because of the additional sessions or the shorter time period between training and long-delay post-testing.

It is noteworthy that the number of participant AB's correct answers on the first training exercise of the new semester was 27 out of 32, whereas at his first training session of the prior semester, his score was 20. Thus, there was a substantial "savings" effect from the prior semester's training.

The experimental group's mean score on the generic biographical knowledge test significantly increased from baseline to one-year post-test, $t(6) = 2.913$, *$p < .02$. The control group's mean score remained the same. However, according to a t-test comparing the two groups, the difference between them was not significant: $t(9) = 1.4588, p = .91$.

Functional status outcomes

Six of the eleven 1-year completers—three experimental and three control participants—maintained or improved functional status, as measured by the CDR. Two of the six, one experimental and one control, improved from mild to questionable. Five declined: one from questionable to mild, three from mild to moderate, and one from moderate to severe (see Table 2).

Hypothesis 2: That both the experimental and control group would maintain or improve the quality of their spontaneous discourse, as assessed by three different measures. This hypothesis was largely supported. The total group showed no significant decline from pre-test to post-test on any of the three discourse measures. The experimental group significantly outperformed the control group on one measure. The groups performed equally on two measures.

Discourse battery

Responses to the prompt questions were coded and analysed for percentage of content-filled utterances (topic comments) to total utterances, for percentage of different nouns to total nouns, and for percentage of vague nouns to total nouns. An utterance was defined as a clause, a prepositional or infinitive phrase that provided specific information, and each of multiple verbs associated with a single subject. A vague noun was defined as a non-specific noun such as "stuff" or "thing." A paper describing the discourse analysis method has been accepted by *Aphasiology* (Arkin & Mahendra, in press) and may be requested from Arkin. The scores achieved on the three measures are presented in Table 3.

The total group showed no significant change in performance from pre- to post-test on the ratio of topic comments to total utterances: $t(10) = 0.84, p = .21$. The trend was in the improved direction. There was no difference in performance between the experimental and control groups, as measured by a t-test with equal variances: $t(9) = 0.37, p = .36$.

On the ratio of different nouns to total nouns, the group as a whole showed no significant change: $t(10) = -0.03, p = .49$. However, the control group declined significantly: $t(3) = -5.2, *p < .01$, while the experimental group showed a substantial, but non-significant improvement: $t(6) = 0.72, p = .25$ (see Table 3). A comparison of the two groups via a t-test with unequal variances showed the difference between the two groups to be significant: $t(6.7) = 2.0, p < .05$.

The total group showed no change in the percentage of vague nouns to total nouns $t(10) = -0.4375, p = .34$. There was no difference in performance between the two groups: $t(9) = 0.2431, p = .59$.

Other language outcomes

All of the language test scores discussed below are presented in Table 3.

Standardised battery—ABCD

The participants' performance on the ABCD at baseline and after 1 year of participation was compared. A t-test for paired samples was used to determine if total scores on the ABCD were significantly different from time 1 to time 2.

Results showed that the 11 participants demonstrated no significant difference in total test scores from baseline to one year later: $t(10) = -1.5, p = .08$.

A t-test for independent samples was conducted to answer the question of a difference in performance between the group of seven experimental participants—those who received specific language interventions, and the group of four control participants—those who experienced normal conversation with their student partners. The results showed no significant difference between the two groups: $t(9) = -0.1, p = .47$ (see Table 3).

CERAD Boston Naming Test

There was no significant difference in performance for the total group from pre- to post-test on the CERAD's 15-item Boston Naming Test: $t(10) = -1.0$, $p = .16$. There was also no difference in performance between the experimental and the control group, as measured by a t-test with unequal variances: $t(4.4) = 0.38, p = .36$.

CERAD's Verbal Fluency Test

There was no significant difference in performance for the total group from pre- to post-test on the CERAD's 60-s verbal fluency test (for the category "animals"): $t(10) = 0.29, p = .39$. There was also no difference in performance between the experimental and control groups: $t(9) = -0.36, p = .36$.

Picture description

The total group, including one experimental and one control subject who entered the programme during the second semester, produced 3.7 fewer information units at post-test than at pre-test; the decrease just missed significance ($p = .0517$). The control group's decrease was significant: $t(4) = 3.72$, $*p < .05$. The experimental group's was not. However, a between-groups comparison, using a two-sample t-test for unequal variances, showed the difference in performance between the two groups to be non-significant.

Scoring of the picture description task was done according to guidelines and the list of sample acceptable information units in the manual of the ADP (Helm-Estabrooks, 1992). Several transcripts were scored by Helm-Estabrooks and a former graduate student who had worked with her. Information units are typically smaller than topic comments, mostly single nouns, verbs, and adjectives. Exceptions are prepositional phrases (e.g., behind the; next to) and multiple word verb forms (e.g., going to fall over; about to make; shouldn't have done that).

All of the post-test scores were within the normal range for non-demented persons in the standardisation sample of the Aphasia Diagnostic Profile (ADP), the test battery of which the grocery store picture description subtest is a part (mean = 21.6, SD = 8.8) (Helm-Estabrooks, 1992). Four participants' scores were one standard deviation above the mean for non-demented people (see Table 3).

Four participants increased and three maintained the number of main ideas produced in their responses from pre- to post-test. Six produced five of six possible main ideas. Of five normal people (aged 36–74) to whom the author administered this task, only two produced five main ideas.

Proverb interpretation

Expert assistance was obtained for the scoring of proverbs. Sandra Chapman, who has had years of research experience with this task (e.g., Chapman et al., 1997; Ulatowska, Chapman, & Johnson, 1993), and several of her graduate students scored our subjects' interpretations according to a six-point scale (three levels of abstractness and three levels of concreteness), adapted from that of Delis et al. (1984) and described by Chapman and colleagues (1997). The maximum score for five proverbs was 30.

Pre- and end-of-semester 2 post-test scores were available for the original 11 participants, plus two later entrants to the programme. The group as a whole showed no significant change from pre- to post-test: $t(12) = -0.38$, $p = .36$. The control group slightly outperformed the experimental group. However, the difference between the two groups was non-significant: $t(11) = -0.75, p = .24$.

Hypothesis 3. That both the experimental and the control group would improve in mood.   This was assessed using the Geriatric Depression Scale (Yesavage et al., 1983). Additional information on participant gains in well-being was supplied by caregiver responses to an evaluation questionnaire (available from the author).

Mood outcomes

Three subjects who had scored in the depressed range (12 or more out of 30) on the Geriatric Depression Scale at pre-test improved after two or three semesters of participation, two of them substantially (from 19 to 11 and from 11 to 6 responses, respectively, in the non-depressed direction). The improvement in mood for the whole group was significant: $t(10) = -3.271, *p < .01$ (see Figure 3).

Ten of 16 caregivers who responded to an evaluation questionnaire endorsed improvement in mood/morale as a specific benefit of the programme to their care recipient. Other specific benefits endorsed were: opportunities to socialise (14 respondents); feelings of usefulness, energy level, general quality of life (10 respondents each); connectedness to others (9 respondents); and conversation quality (8 respondents). Of the four programme components,

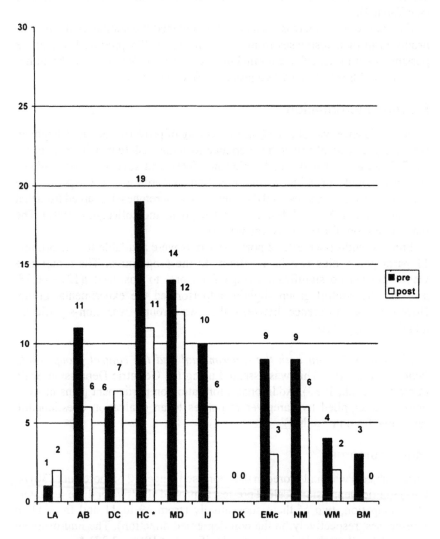

Figure 3. Geriatric Depression Scale scores before and after two semesters in AD Rehab programme. Eleven and below signifies non-depressed, reduction in score means improvement in mood. * Score after 3rd semester of participation.

exercise was ranked the highest, in terms of perceived benefit to participants, followed by volunteer work, conversation stimulation, and memory training.

Hypothesis 4. That both the experimental and control groups would improve on measures of physical fitness. This hypothesis was overwhelmingly supported, with highly significant results in the positive direction on all measures.

Fitness outcomes

These outcomes (minus the figures) have been reported previously (Arkin, 1999).

Aerobics

At the end of their second semester of participation, 10 of the 11 original participants had met or exceeded the programme's goal of doing 20 min of aerobic exercise (treadmill and bicycle combined) per session. Four were doing 30 min or more; one woman, age 85, was doing 44 min. Pre- to post-participation duration gain for the complete group plus three one-semester completers, as measured by a paired t-test, was significant: $t(13) = 6.516$, *$p < .001$ (see Figure 4).

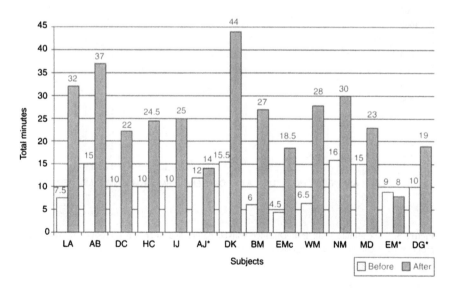

Figure 4.   Minutes of aerobic exercise per session: Beginning and end of first two semesters in AD Rehab programme. Minutes on the bike and treadmill combined. * Only 1 semester of training.

Thirteen out of 14 participants increased the distance walked in the "6-minute walk test" from before treatment to post-test, including three one-semester completers. Pre- to post-participation distance gain for the total group, as measured by a paired *t*-test, was significant: $t(13) = 2.790$, $*p < .01$ (see Figure 5).

Weight training[4]

All participants who completed two semesters, except one with severe arthritis, increased the amount of weight pressed on the MedX leg press machine (see Figure 6). Three doubled or tripled the amount of weight pressed (167%, 150%, 138% increases, respectively). Five increased the amount pressed by between 47% and 84%. Two participants were routinely pressing 400 pounds or more—one a 79-year-old woman. One 84-year-old woman pressed 448 pounds 13 times on a one-time test; her 21-year-old student partner could only do it twice! The feat was videotaped and witnessed by the author and a staff member. Pre- to post-participation increase for the group, except for the

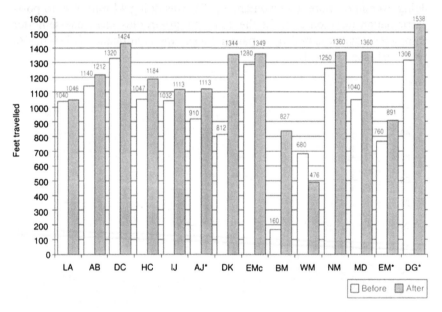

Figure 5. Six minute walk test: Distance walked before and after two semesters of AD Rehab programme. * One semester completers.

---

[4] Because of the way MedX equipment is constructed, a given weight is equivalent to about half that amount if lifted on the more familiar, but less suitable for frail elderly, Nautilus machine.

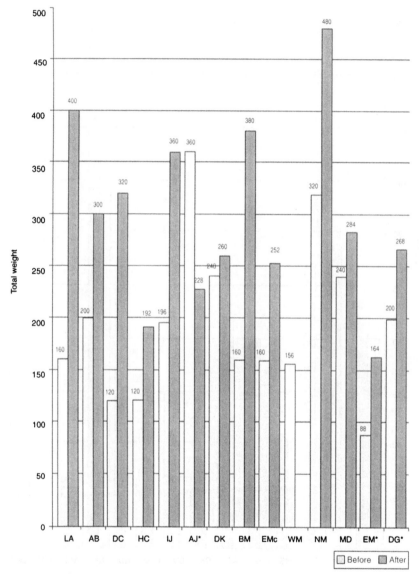

Figure 6. Lower body strength: Weight pressed on the leg press machine per session at the beginning and end of first two semesters in AD Rehab programme. * One semester completers.

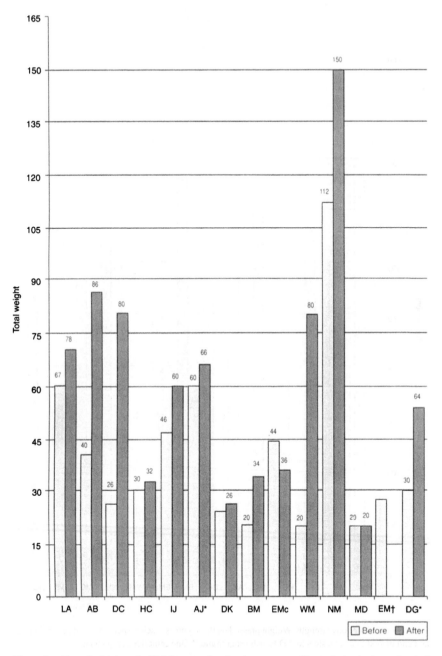

Figure 7. Upper body strength: Weight pressed on the chest press machine at the beginning and end of one year of treatment. * One semester completers. † Did not participate due to shoulder pain.

participant with the arthritic knees who did not participate, as measured by a paired t-test, was significant: $t(12) = 3.712$, *$p < .01$.

On the Chest Press machine, nine of the 11 increased the amount of weight pressed. One, the arthritic woman who could not do the leg press, had a 300% increase. Two 80-year-old women and a 79-year-old man were pressing more than 80 pounds. Four were pressing between 50 and 70 pounds. The pre- to post-participation increase for the group of 13 one and two semester completers, minus a woman with a shoulder injury who did not participate, was significant, as measured by a paired t-test: $t(12) = 3.26$, *$p < .01$ (see Figure 7).

DISCUSSION

Two semesters of intensive physical exercise, and cognitive, language and social interventions administered by students and supplemented by caregivers resulted in maintenance of function (no significant decline) on 13 out of 14 cognitive and language measures for a group of 11 mild to moderate Alzheimer's patients. These same study participants also made significant physical fitness and mood gains.

These positive results are largely consistent with the hypotheses put forth and have explanations that are supported by the literature. What is counter-intuitive is the fact that participants who experienced regular and intensive language activities which had them practice skills most compromised in Alzheimer's disease did not do significantly better on post-intervention language testing than control participants who engaged in normal unstructured conversation with their student rehab partners. The time spent with a student was the same for both groups.

Exercise and language

The fact that subjects who had no specific language interventions did as well at post-test as experimental subjects who did have them was puzzling. However, there is some evidence that the act of engaging in exercise during conversation has a booster effect on language performance. Such an effect was found by Friedman and Tappen (1991) who compared conversational output of nursing home residents while walking with a conversation partner with that of residents who conversed while seated. Thus, the unstructured conversation engaged in with a student during and between exercise seems to have been just as benefi-cial as the specific language exercises the experimental group experienced during and between their exercise activities. Although the sample is too small to allow conclusions to be drawn—the results may have been because of chance factors—the outcomes suggest that it was the exercise that was the salient factor in maintaining language performance. Because the language exercises were stimulating for the participants and had didactic value for the students, they were administered to all participants from the third semester onwards.

The largely positive cognitive and language outcomes in the present study are consistent with the research literature on exercise and cognition. A meta-analysis of 200 studies found that exercise has a small positive influence on cognition (Etnier et al., 1997). Another study found that elderly persons who exercise do better on measures of reasoning, working memory, and reaction time than sedentary older adults (Clarkson-Smith & Hartley, 1989). Exercise has also been found to correlate with better performance on timed tasks in older subjects (Christensen & MacKinnon, 1993), and to maintain cerebral perfusion and cognition in retirees (Rogers, Meyer, & Mortel, 1990).

Memory training results

The following discussion of possible reasons for the success of the memory training aspect of the programme is taken from a previous article in the *American Journal of Alzheimer's Disease* (Arkin, 2000a).

The memory training technique described has three features that may account for its success: (1) It facilitates memory formation and consolidation through structured, automatic rehearsal processes; (2) it provides practice in retrieving information; and (3) it minimises the making of mistakes.

Memory formation and consolidation

The predictable and repetitive pattern of the tape-recorded biographical information that is presented soon becomes familiar. Subjects soon anticipate and begin to talk back to the tape recorder and subvocally rehearse information they hear. Apparently, the material enters the better-preserved long-term memory system without conscious effort on the part of the learner. For more information on unconscious or implicit learning, see Bäckmann (1992), Camp et al. (1996); Schacter (1992), and Schacter, Rich, and Stampp (1985).

Retrieval practice facilitates learning

Prior research with amnesic patients (Glisky and Schacter, 1986; Schacter et al., 1985) and college students (Bjork, 1988) demonstrated that successful retrieval of information upon being questioned increases the likelihood that the success will be repeated upon subsequent presentation of the same question. A prior study by Arkin (1997) found quizzing more effective than repeating to-be-learned information in bringing about new learning in Alzheimer's patients. The memory training tapes in the present study used a fixed interval form of spaced retrieval, which was successfully used by Foss and Camp (1994) in bringing about new learning in Alzheimer's patients. Spaced retrieval is an example of priming, which has been defined as the improved facility for detecting or processing stimuli on the basis of recent experience (Squire, 1994). The narrative, with its embedded questions on the memory tapes, serves as priming for the questions that re-occur after a delay.

Errorless learning produces experiences of success

The memory tapes are structured to maximise success in answering the quiz questions. In the body of the narrative, the question is posed immediately after the related fact is stated, so that a correct response is virtually assured. The question is then given again after a delay during which other information is introduced. The tape always provides the correct answer, after a pause, which reduces anxiety and models the appropriate response for the patient. Wilson, Baddeley, Evans, and Shiel (1994) point out that once errors are produced or elicited, memory-impaired people have great difficulty eliminating them. Clare and colleagues successfully applied this technique specifically to Alzheimer's patients (Clare, Wilson, Breen, & Hodges, 1999; Clare et al., 2000).

Neurobiological hypotheses

Several possible neurobiological explanations for success with this memory training technique are suggested by the research literature. Animal research linking enhanced memory with emotional arousal has been replicated with human subjects and was found to result from an activation of beta-adrenergic hormone systems (Cahill, Prins, Weber, & McGaugh, 1994). The emotional arousal provided by out-of-the-ordinary experiences such as children's embraces at a daycare centre, may be stimulating this or other, as yet unexplored, hormone systems. Sandman (1993) found enhanced memory for days on which out-of-the-ordinary events occurred among Alzheimer patients.

Environmental stimulation in animal research has been linked to increases in dendritic growth and branching (Diamond, 1988; Wallace, Kilman, Withers, & Greenough, 1992) and in synapse formation (Weiler, Hawrylak, & Greenough, 1995). Related research with humans found that "exposure to complex experi-ence can generate new synapses in the cerebral cortex and cerebellum" (Black, Isaacs, & Greenough, 1991). In a review of the arguments for the "wear and tear" vs. "use it or lose it" theories of brain ageing and Alzheimer's disease, Swaab (1991) cites 10 examples to illustrate that activation of neurones may have a beneficial effect on neuronal function and survival during ageing and Alzhei-mer's disease. He concludes that for brain areas that show degenerative alter-ations, one should search for sensory, neurotransmitter, and other stimuli that have disappeared, and attempt to effect recovery via "restoration of the missing stimuli," (pp. 321–322). He quotes Millard (1984), "until better evidence is available, I think I shall tell my mother to go on doing the crossword".

Individual differences in response to programme

Not all AD programme participants benefited equally. Seven of the eight participants who were classified as early stage at programme entry (MMSE of 22–29) improved or maintained function on 9 or 10 of the 14 measures presented in Tables 2 and 3.[5] Two early stage participants improved on eight of the measures. Only one early stage participant declined markedly—on 11 out of 14 measures. This participant, WM, suffered from hearing loss and painful arthritis that worsened since she entered the programme and it is difficult to evaluate how much these two factors contributed to her poor test performance. For two subsequent semesters, she continued to read to and sing with children at the day-care centre where she volunteered, and did a twice weekly regimen of regular and some adapted exercises at the Wellness Center, despite severe pain in her right knee. Her daughter has stated that, without the rehabilitation programme, she would probably have been bedridden and in a nursing home.

One of the three moderate stage participants did better than all of the early stage participants. IJ, with a baseline MMSE score of 17, maintained or improved her scores on 11 of the 14 measures. This participant suffered severe injuries from a fall that occurred after her first year of participation. After a semester of weekly walks and the cognitive/language interventions by a student, this resilient woman's MMSE score, which had dropped following hospitalisation and subsequent stay at a rehabilitation facility, was back to baseline.

One moderate stage patient, LA, who went from 18 to 14 points on her MMSE score, nevertheless maintained or improved on seven other measures, and declined on six.

HC, who entered the programme with an MMSE score of 15 which had declined to 9 by the end of the first year, nevertheless improved or maintained performance on 6 of the 14 measures (on one test, she scored 0 on both testing occasions), plus showed a dramatic improvement in mood (from 19 to 11 on the GDS). A retired Air Force lieutenant colonel and nurse with no family, HC talked herself into the programme after having been screened and rejected for scoring below the desired MMSE cutoff of 18. She found a flyer in her drawer several weeks after her interview, called me and said, "They tell me I have Alzheimer's. I think I should be in your programme!" She was one of six of the

---

[5] Score differences of one point on proverb interpretation and up to five points on picture description are not regarded as changes by individuals. Score differences of 5% or less on ratios of topic comments to utterances and on ratios of different nouns to total nouns are also not regarded as changes. As these scores depend on scorers' subjective judgements, small differences may be the result of scorer inconsistency. (For reliability information on the discourse analysis data, see Arkin & Mahendra, in press.)

original cohort to complete three full years of participation, despite severe language impairment.

Benefits to students

Students benefited academically through increased knowledge about Alzheimer's disease, as measured by improvement on the Alzheimer's Disease Knowledge Test (Dieckmann et al., 1988) from pre- to post-participation. Mean score on the 20-item pre-test was 11 (range 6–19) and on the post-test was 17 (range 12–20). They also benefited from the acquisition of hands-on clinical experience, which is rarely available to undergraduates. Students were given a standardised course evaluation form to complete at the end of the semester. The form had a 5-point scale for the various elements. Twelve of 23 respondents gave the course the highest rating ("one of the best") and 8 rated it "better than average", the second highest rating. As to amount learned, 11 reported "exceptional amount", the highest ranking, and 8 "more than usual", the second highest ranking. A card from a student stated: "I wanted to tell you how much I have enjoyed working for your programme. N has touched my life and I hope that I impacted his as well. The work you are doing is incredible and worth while. Thank you for allowing me to be a part of it."

EPILOGUE

Because of the lack of comparable intervention studies of accurately diagnosed and staged Alzheimer's patients and the small sample sizes of the studies that do exist, it is not possible to draw clear conclusions from the outcomes of this study. Future research with much larger samples is planned to compare the effects on cognition and language of (1) exercise at a fitness facility plus structured memory and language stimulation activities, versus (2) exercise at a fitness facility and just unstructured conversation with a student. These would be compared to control groups that would experience outings—attendance at community cultural and recreational events and volunteer work sessions—plus unstructured conversation with a student. This would dissociate various components of the present programme, with the amount of time spent with a student held constant. University researchers interested in testing these interventions are invited to contact the author, who plans to seek funding for a multiple-site longitudinal study.

The primary value of this study is that it may serve as a tentative benchmark against which the cognitive, language, and functional performance, over time, of other groups of treated and untreated AD patients can be compared. It is the author's hope that it will also stimulate other researchers, clinicians, and caregivers to tap the vast resources of our communities and the reservoirs of good will of our high school and college students to improve the "here and now" for people with Alzheimer's disease and other conditions that prevent them from active involvement in their communities.

REFERENCES

Abramson, J.H., Ritter, M., Gofin, J., & Kark, J.D. (1992). Work-health relationships in middle-aged and elderly residents of Jerusalem. *Social Science and Medicine, 34,* 747–755.

Aguero-Torres, H., Fratiglioni, L., & Winblad, B. (1998). Natural history of Alzheimer's disease and other dementias: Review of the literature in the light of the findings from the Kungsholmen Project. *International Journal of Geriatric Psychiatry, 13,* 755–766.

Arkin, S. (1991) Memory training in early Alzheimer's disease: An optimistic look at the field. *American Journal of Alzheimer's & Related Disorders Care & Research, 6,* 17–25.

Arkin, S. (1992). Audio-assisted memory training with early Alzheimer's patients: Two single subject experiments. *Clinical Gerontologist, 12,* 77–95.

Arkin, S. (1996) Volunteers in partnership: An Alzheimer's rehabilitation program delivered by students. *American Journal of Alzheimer's Disease, 11,* 12–22.

Arkin, S. (1997). Alzheimer memory training: Quiz beats repetition, especially for more impaired. *American Journal of Alzheimer's Disease, 12,* 147–158.

Arkin, S. (1998). Alzheimer memory training: Positive results replicated. *American Journal of Alzheimer's Disease, 13,* 102–104.

Arkin, S. (1998a) Alzheimer memory training: Longterm retention achieved. Paper presented at the 51st Annual Scientific Meeting of the Gerontological Society of America., October, 1998. Accepted for publication by *American Journal of Alzheimer's Disease.*

Arkin, S. (1999). Elder rehab: A student-supervised exercise program for Alzheimer's patients. *The Gerontologist, 39,* 729–735.

Arkin, S. (2000a). Alzheimer memory training: Students replicate learning successes. *American Journal of Alzheimer's Disease, 15,* 152–162.

Arkin, S. (2000b). Alzheimer memory training: Addendum on longterm retention. *American Journal of Alzheimer's Disease, 15,* 314–315.

Arkin, S. (2000c). Insight in Alzheimer's patients: Them that has keeps! Presentation at Symposium on Insight and Dementia at the PSIGE (Psychologists' Special Interest Group in the Elderly of the British Psychological Association) 2000 Conference, Birmingham, UK (Linda Clare, moderator). Synopsis available from author.

Arkin, S., & Mahendra, N. (in press). Discourse analysis of Alzheimer's patients before and after intervention: Methodology and outcomes. *Aphasiology.*

Arkin, S., Rose, C., & Hopper, T. (2000). Implicit and explicit learning gains in Alzheimer's patients: Effects of naming and information retrieval training. *Aphasiology, 14,* 723–742.

Bäckman, L. (1992). Memory training and memory improvement in Alzheimer's disease: Rules and exceptions. *Acta Neurologica Scandinavica, 84,* 84–89.

Bayles, K.A., & Kaszniak, A.W. (1987). *Communication and cognition in normal aging and dementia.* Boston: College-Hill.

Bayles, K.A., & Tomoeda, C.K. (1991). *Arizona Battery for Comunication Disorders of Dementia (ABCD). Research Edition Manual.* Tucson, AZ: Canyonlands Publishing.

Berg, L. (1988). Clinical Dementia Rating (CDR). *Psychopharmacology Bulletin, 24,* 637–639.

Bjork, R.A. (1988). Retrieval practice and the maintenance of knowledge. In M. Gruneberg, P. Morris, & R. Sykes (Eds.), *Practical aspects of memory* (Vol. 2, pp. 396–401). London: Academic Press.

Black, J.E., Isaacs, K.R., & Greenough, W.T. (1991). Usual vs. successful aging: Some notes on experiential factors. Comment. *Neurobiology of Aging, 12,* 325–328; Discussion 352–355.

Bonder, B.R., & Wagner, M.B. (Eds.) (1994). *Functional performance in older adults.* Philadelphia: P.A. Davis.

Bonner, A.P., & Cousins, S.O. (1996). Exercise and Alzheimer's disease: Benefits and barriers. *Activities, Adaptation, & Aging, 20,* 21–32.

Bourgeois, M.S. (1990). Enhancing conversation skills in patients with Alzheimer's disease using a prosthetic memory aid. *Journal of Applied Behavior Analysis, 23,* 31–64.

Bourgeois, M.S. (1991). Communication treatment for adults with dementia. *Journal of Speech and Hearing Research, 34,* 831–844.

Brush, J.A., & Camp, C.J. (1998). *A therapy technique for improving memory: Spaced retrieval.* Beachwood, Ohio: Menorah Park Center for the Aging.

Buchner, D.M., & deLateur, B.J. (1992). The importance of skeletal muscle strength to physical function in older adults. *Annals of Behavioral Medicine, 13,* 91–98.

Butin, D.N., & Heaney, C. (1991). Program planning in geriatric psychiatry: A model for psychosocial rehabilitation. In E.D. Taira (Ed.), *The mentally impaired elderly: Strategies and interventions to maintain function.* New York: Haworth Press.

Butters, N., Granholm, E., Salmon, D. P., Grant, I., & Wolfe, J. (1987). Episodic and semantic memory: A comparison of amnesic and demented patients. *Journal of Clinical and Experimental Neuropsychology, 9,* 479–497

Cahill, L., Prins, B., Weber, M., & McGaugh, J. (1994). Beta-adrenergic activation and memory for emotional events. *Nature, 371,* 702–704.

Camp, C.J., Foss, J.W., O'Hanlon, A.M., & Stevens, A.B. (1995). Memory interventions for persons with dementia. *Applied Cognitive Psychology, 9,* 1–18.

Chapman, S., & Ulatowska, H.K. (1989). Discourse in aphasia: Integration deficits in processing reference. *Brain and Language, 36,* 651–668.

Chapman, S., Ulatowska, H.K., Franklin, L.R., Shobe, A.E., Thompson, J.L., & McIntire, D.D. (1997). Proverb interpretation in fluent aphasia and Alzheimer's disease: Implications beyond abstract thinking. *Aphasiology, 11,* 337–350.

Christensen, H., & MacKinnon, A. (1993). The association between mental, social, and physical activity in young and old subjects. *Age and Aging, 22,* 175–182.

Clare, L., Wilson, B.A., Breen, K., & Hodges, J.R. (1999). Errorless learning of face–name associations in early Alzheimer's disease. *Neurocase, 5,* 37–46

Clare, L., Wilson, B.A., Carter, G., Breen, K., Gosses, A., & Hodges, J.R. (2000). Intervening with everyday memory problems in dementia of the Alzheimer type: An errorless learning approach. *Journal of Clinical and Experimental Neuropsychology, 22,* 132–146.

Clark, C.M., Sheppard, L., Fillenbaum, G., Galasko, D., Morris, J.C., Koss, E., Mohs, R., & Heyman, A. (1999). Variability in annual Mini-Mental State Examination score in patients with probable Alzheimer disease: A clinical perspective of data from the Consortium to Establish a Registry for Alzheimer Disease. *Archives of Neurology, 56,* 857–862.

Clark, L.W., & Witte, K. (1991). Nature and efficacy of communication mangagement in Alzheimer's disease. In R. Lubinski (Ed.), *Dementia and communication* (pp. 238–256). Philadelphia: B.C. Decker.

Clarkson-Smith, L., & Hartley, A.A. (1989). Relationships between physical and cognitive abilities in older adults. *Psychology and Aging, 4,* 183–189.

Collins, A.M., & Loftus, E.F. (1975). A spreading-activation theory of semantic processing. *Psychological Review, 82,* 407–428.

Crovitz, H.F. (1986). Loss and recovery of autobiographical memory after head injury. In D.C. Rubin (Ed.), *Autobiographical memory.* Cambridge, UK: Cambridge University Press.

Dave Bell Productions (1987). *Do You Remember Love?* Available from the Alzheimer Association library in Chicago: greenfield@alz.org

Delis, D.C., Kramer, J., & Kaplan, E. (1984). *The California Proverb Test.* Unpublished protocol.

Diamond, M. (1988) *Enriching heredity: The impact of the environment on the anatomy of the brain.* New York: Free Press.

Dieckmann, L., Zarit, S., Zarit, J., & Gatz, M. (1988). Alzheimer's Disease Knowledge Test. *Gerontologist, 28*, 402–406.

Etnier, J.L., Salazar, W., Landers, D.M., Petruzzello, S.J., Han, M., & Nowell, P. (1997). The influence of physical fitness and exercise upon cognitive functioning: A meta-analysis. *Journal of Sport & Exercise Psychology, 19*, 249–277.

Evans, W., & Rosenberg, I.H. (1991). *Biomarkers: The 10 determinants of aging you can control.* New York: Simon & Schuster.

Fiatarone, M.A. (1996). Physical activity and functional independence in aging. *Research Quarterly for Exercise and Sport, 67* (3 Suppl.), S70.

Folstein, M.F., Folstein, S.E., & McHugh, P.R. (1975). "Mini-Mental State," a practical method for grading the cognitive state of patients for the clinician. *Journal of Psychiatric Research, 12*, 189–198.

Foss, J.W., & Camp, C.J. (1994). *"Effortless" learning in Alzheimer's disease: Evidence that spaced-retrieval training engages implicit memory.* Poster presented at the Fifth Biennial Cognitive Aging Conference, Atlanta, Georgia.

Friedman, R., & Tappen, R.M. (1991). The effect of planned walking on communication in Alzheimer's disease. *Journal of the American Geriatrics Society, 39*, 670–654.

Glisky, E.L., & Schacter, D.L. (1986). Remediation of organic memory disorder: Current status and future prospects. *Journal of Head Trauma Rehabilitation, 1*, 54–63.

Griffin, R.M., & Mouheb, F. (1987). Work therapy as a treatment modality for the elderly patient with dementia. *Physical & Occupational Therapy in Geriatrics, 5*, 67–72.

Havighurst, R.J. (1961). Successful aging. *Gerontologist, 1*, 8–13.

Helm-Estabrooks, N. (1992). *Aphasia Diagnostic Profiles.* New York: Riverside Publishing.

Hirsch, E.D., Kett, J.F., & Trefil, J. (1988). *Dictionary of cultural literacy: What every American needs to know.* Boston: Houghton Mifflin.

Hoffman, D. (1994). *Complaints of a dutiful daughter.* New York, NY: Women Make Movies. Available from the Alzheimer Association library in Chicago: greenfield@alz.org

Holland, A., Miller, J., Reinmuth, O.M., Bartlett, C., Fromm, D., Pashek, G., Stein, D., & Swindell, C. (1985). Rapid recovery from aphasia: A detailed language analysis. *Brain and Language, 24*, 156–173.

Huff, F.J., Corkin, S., & Growdon, J.H. (1986). Semantic impairment and anomia in Alzheimer's disease. *Brain and Language, 28*, 235–249.

Kagan, A., & Gailey, G.F. (1993). Functional is not enough: Training conversation partners for aphasic adults. In A.L. Holland & M.M. Forbes (Eds.), *Aphasia treatment: World perspectives.* San Diego, CA: Singular Publishing Group, Inc.

Kaplan, E., Goodglass, H., & Weintraub, S. (1983). *The Boston Naming Test* (2nd ed.). Philadelphia: Lea & Febiger.

Kempler, D. (1995). Language changes in dementia of the Alzheimer type. In R. Lubinski (Ed.), *Dementia and communication* (pp. 98–114). Philadelphia: B.C. Decker, Inc.

Keys, L.M. (1982). Former patients as volunteers in community agencies: A model work program. *Hospital & Community Psychiatry, 33*, 1017–1018.

Lamb, D.R., Gisolfi, C.V., & Nadel, E. (Eds.) (1995). *Exercise in older adults.* Carmel, IN: Cooper Publishing.

Lezak, M.D. (1995). *Neuropsychological assessment* (3rd ed). New York: Oxford University Press.

Lindenmuth, G.F., & Lindenmuth, E.B. (1994). Effects of a three-year exercise therapy program on cognitive functioning of elderly personal care home residents. *American Journal of Alzheimer's Care and Related Disorders & Research, Jan./Feb.*, 20–24.

Maslow, K. & Whitehouse, P. (1997). Defining and measuring outcomes in Alzheimer disease research: Conference findings. *Alzheimer's Disease and Associated Disorders, 11*, Suppl. 6, 186–195.

Mattis, S. (1988). *Dementia Rating Scale.* Odessa, FL: Psychological Assessment Resources.

McKhann, G., Drachman, D., Folstein, M., Katzman, R., Price, D., & Stadlan, E.M. (1984). Clinical diagnosis of Alzheimer's disease: Report of the NINCDS-ADRDA Work Group under the auspices of Department of Health and Human Services Task Force on Alzheimer's Disease. *Neurology, 34*, 939–944.

Millard, P.H. (1984). Cited in Swaab, D.F. (1991). Brain aging and Alzheimer's disease: "Wear and tear" versus "use it or lose it." *Neurobiology of Aging, 12*, 317–324.

Molloy, D.W., & Lubinski, R. (1995). Dementia: Impact and clinical perspectives. In R. Lubinski (Ed.), *Dementia and Communication*. San Diego: Singular Publishing Group.

Morris, J.C., Heyman, A., Mohs, R.C., Hughes, M.S., van Belle, G., Fillenbaum, G., Mellits, E.D., Clark, C., & the CERAD investigators. (1989). The Consortium to Establish a Registry for Alzheimer's Disease (CERAD). Part I. Clinical and neuropsychological assessment of Alzheimer's disease. *Neurology, 39*, 1159–1165.

Muller, A-A. (1993). Ressourcensicherung durch Aktivierung der Ratgeberfunktion des älteren Menschen—Ein neues Konzept in der Gerontopsychiatrie (Maintaining resources by activating the advisory function of the elderly: A new concept in gerontopsychiatry). *Zeitschrift fur Gerontopsychologie & Psychiatrie, 6*, 119–125.

Netz, Y., & Argov, E. (1997). Assessment of functional fitness among independent older adults: A preliminary report. *Perceptual and Motor Skills, 84*, 1059–1074.

Palleschi, L., Vetta, F., deGennaro, E., Idone, G., Sottosanti, G., Gianni, W., & Marigliano, V. (1996). Effects of aerobic training on the cognitive performance of elderly patients with senile dementia of Alzheimer type. *Archives of Gerontology and Geriatrics, Supplement 5*, 47–50.

Penn, C., Jones, D., & Joffe, V. (1997). Hierarchical discourse therapy: A method for the mild patient. *Aphasiology, 11*, 601–618.

Pitetti, K.H. (1993). Introduction: exercise capacities and adaptation of people with chronic disabilities: Current research, future direction, and widespread applicability. *Medical Science Sports Exercise, 25*, 421–422.

Quayhagen, M., & Quayhagen, M.P. (1989). Differential effects of family-based strategies in Alzheimer's disease. *Gerontologist, 29*, 1150–1155.

Ripich, D.N., & Terrell, B.Y. (1988). Patterns of discourse cohesion and coherence in Alzheimer's disease. *Journal of Speech and Hearing Disorders, 53*, 8–15.

Rogers, R. L., Meyer, J. S., & Mortel, K. F. (1990). After reaching retirement age physical activity (sic!) sustains cerebral perfusion and cognition. *Journal of the American Geriatrics Society, 38*, 123–128.

Salmon, D.P., Heindel, W.C., & Butters, N. (1995). Patterns of cognitive impairment in Alzheimer's disease. In R. Lubinski (Ed.), *Dementia and Communication*. San Diego: Singular Publishing.

Sandman, C.A. (1993). Memory rehabilitation in Alzheimer's disease: Preliminary findings. *Clinical Gerontologist, 13*, 19–33.

Schacter, D.L. (1987). Implicit memory: History and current status. *Journal of Experimental Psychology: Learning, Memory, and Cognition, 13*, 501–517.

Schacter, D.L. (1992). Understanding implicit memory. *American Psychologist, 47*, 559–569.

Schacter, D.L. (1996). *Searching for memory*. New York: Basic Books.

Schacter, D.L., Rich, S.A., & Stampp, M.S. (1985). Remediation of memory disorders: Experimental evaluation of the spaced-retrieval technique. *Journal of Clinical and Experimental Neuropsychology, 7*, 79–96.

Schmand, B., Linderboom, J., Launer, L., & Dinkgreve, M., et al. (1995). *International Journal of Geriatric Psychiatry, 10*, 411–414.

Shadden, B.B. (1995). The use of discourse analyses and procedures for communication programming in long-term care facilities. *Topics in Language Disorders, 15*, 75–86.

Soumeri, S.B., & Avorn, J. (1983). Perceived health, life satisfaction, and activity in urban elderly: A controlled study of the impact of part-time work. *Journal of Gerontology, 38*, 356–362.

Spirduso, W.W. (1995). *Physical dimensions of aging*. Champaign, IL: Human Kinetics.

Strub, R.L., & Black, F.W. (1985). *Mental status examination in neurology* (2nd ed.). Philadelphia: F. A. Davis.

Swaab, D.F. (1991). Brain aging and Alzheimer's disease: "Wear and tear" versus "use it or lose it." *Neurobiology of Aging, 12*, 317–324.

Swanson, N., Levi, G., & Matano, T. (1999) *Rush Alzheimer's Disease Center News* (Spring issue). Chicago: Rush Alzheimer's Disease Center.

Tappen, R.M., Roach, K.E., Buchner, D., Barry, C., & Edelstein, J. (1997). Reliability of physical performance measures in nursing home residents with Alzheimer's disease. *Journals of Gerontology*, Medical Sciences, Series A. Biological Sciences & Medical Sciences, *52A*, M52–M55.

Tomoeda, C.K., & Bayles, K.A. (1993). Longitudinal effects of Alzheimer disease on discourse production. *Alzheimer Disease and Associated Disorders, 7*: 223–236.

Ulatowska, H., Chapman, S., & Johnson, J. (1993) Processing of proverbs in aphasia and old elderly. *Clinical Aphasiology, 23*, 179–193.

Van Lancker, D. (1990). The neurology of proverbs. *Behavioral Neurology, 3*, 169–187.

Vertinsky, P. (1991). Old age, gender, and physical activity: The biomedicalization of aging. *Journal of Sport History, 18*, 64–80.

Voeks, S.K., & Drinka, P.J. (1990). Participants' perception of a work therapy program in a nursing home. *Activities, Adaptation & Aging, 14*, 27–34.

Wallace, C.S., Kilman, V.L., Withers, G.S., & Greenough, W.T. (1992). Increases in dendritic length in occipital cortex after 4 days of differential housing in weanling rats. *Behavioral Neural Biology, 58*, 64–68. .

Wechsler, D. (1981). *Manual for the WAIS-R*. San Antonio, TX: Psychological Corporation.

Wechsler, D. (1987). *Wechsler Memory Scale—Revised*. New York: Psychological Corporation.

Weiler, I.J., Hawrylak, N., & Greenough, W.T. (1995). Morphogenesis in memory formation: Synaptic and cellular mechanisms. *Behavioral Brain Research, 66*, 1–6.

Whaley, D.E., & Ebbeck, V. (1997). Older adults' constraints to participation in structured exercise classes. *Journal of Aging and Physical Activity, 5*, 190–213.

Wilson, B.A., & Baddeley, A. (1994) When implicit learning fails: Amnesia and the problem of error elimination. *Neuropsychologia*, in press.

Yesavage, J., Brink, T., Rose, T., Lum, O., Huang, V., Adey, M., & Leirer, V. (1983). Development and validation of a geriatric depression screening scale: A preliminary report. *Journal of Psychiatric Research, 17*, 37–49.

Zgola, J. (1990). Therapeutic activity. In N. Mace (Ed.), *Dementia care: Patient, family, and community*. Baltimore, MD: Johns Hopkins University Press.

APPENDIX A

AD Rehab activities summary: Examples of each

1. *Biographical Memory Tape*—Excerpt of script attached. At subject's home, before fitness workout.

2. *Category Fluency exercise*. Name as many _____ (fruits, modes of transportation, types of clothing, etc.) in 60 s. Alternative: Tell subject you will name a category and count to 10, during which he or she is to name something from that category. Use a series of categories. Have subject give categories for you to name from.

3. *Picture description*. Present Norman Rockwell or other evocative picture. Say: "Tell me what you see in that picture—what's going on?" Record free response. Then ask prompt questions. Example:

Homecoming (prompt questions after free response is recorded)
What is the occupation of the young man in the picture with his back to us? How can you tell?

(uniform). Who are the people on the back porch? What kind of emotion are the people in the picture feeling? How can you tell? Do you think he's home for a short visit or for good? (small bag— probably short visit). What kind of neighbourhood does this soldier live in? How can you tell? Who do you suppose the young woman is who is leaning against the side of the house? How do you think she is feeling? What do the mother and all of her children in the picture have in common? (red hair). About how old would you guess that mother is? What could be causing her legs to be so fat? (fluid retention from heart problems). Do women of that age look like that nowadays? How does being well-to-do financially help a woman look younger than poor women of the same age? Did you ever have a loved one in the service? Who? What was that like? If you were in the service, what were short visits home like? How did you and your family keep in touch? Have you saved any letters from those years? What famous entertainer used to give shows at overseas military bases at Christmas time?

4. *Word Associations* (While on treadmill). Tell me all the (childhood) (adult) thoughts and memories the word reminds you of . . . (e.g., birthday, garden, graduation, funeral, thunderstorm). Student shares stories from his/her life on same topic).

5. *Opinion and Advice Questions* (While on exercise bike) A situation involving a moral issue or personal values is presented to subject and his/her opinion is solicited. A series of probing questions is asked after free response is recorded. Example:

Affair: Suppose you found out that your best friend's husband was having an affair and spending a lot of money on an attractive widow living in your community. Your friend and her husband are living on a limited retirement income, half of it from the wife's pension. You're afraid for her financial well-being, but don't want to hurt her. What would you do?
Would you say anything to the cheating husband? What? Would you say anything to your friend? What? What would you advise her to do? Do you think trust can be rebuilt in a marriage after one partner has been unfaithful? How? If it were your husband (or wife) having an affair, would you want to be told about it? Would you feel appreciative or resentful towards the friend who told you about the affair?

6. *Story Recall Exercise* (During rest after bike) Student reads brief story containing six to seven facts and asks subject to repeat story. Student then rereads story, posing a question about each fact after it is stated, pausing for the subject to answer, if able, then gives the correct answer. Student then repeats the six questions that were embedded in the story. Subject is then asked to re-tell the story again. When all six questions are answered correctly and subject recalls four major facts about the story, a new story is introduced for the following session. Example:

Poor puppy: A cocker spaniel puppy that is usually kept in the basement got into the living room when the owner was at work. When the puppy's owner got home, she found a wet spot on the carpet. She spanked the puppy with a newspaper. Then she noticed water dripping from the ceiling right over the wet spot on the carpet. She apologised to the puppy and gave him a biscuit.

This story is about a cocker spaniel puppy. What kind of puppy is the story about? _____ (cocker spaniel). The cocker spaniel puppy is usually kept in the basement. Where is the puppy usually kept? _____ (in the basement). One day, the puppy got into the living room when the owner was at work. Where did the puppy go while the owner was at work? _____ (into the living room). When the puppy's owner got home, she found a wet spot on the carpet. What did the puppy's owner find on the carpet when she got home? _____ (a wet spot). She spanked the puppy with a newspaper. What did the owner do to the puppy? _____ (spanked him with a newspaper.) Then she noticed water dripping from the ceiling right over the wet spot on the carpet. What really caused the wet spot on the carpet that the puppy was blamed for? _____ (water dripping from the ceiling).

7. *Proverb Interpretation* (During rest after bike). First five sessions, work with first five proverbs; sessions 6–10, work with remaining five: Read proverb beginning to see if the know the ending. Write down what they say. Ask them the meaning of it and write down what they say. If subject gives a

concrete or incorrect response, then read the abstract interpretation. Then read proverb *again* and ask subject to interpret it. Write it on record sheet. Example:

A bird in the hand _____ (is worth two in the bush).
(The things we already have are more valuable than the things we only hope to get. Better to hang on to what you have than take a chance on something you might not be able to get.)

Final Rest Period Activities

8. *A, My Name is game.* Subject is told that this exercise is to practise producing words quickly. Have subject read or say the framework phrase with the student and produce a word beginning with the target letter for each blank

A, My Name is . . . _____ and my (husband's/wife's) name is _____ and we come from _____ and we're going downtown to buy some _____, B my name is _____, etc.

9. *Similarities.* Subjects are asked what the two words in each pair of items have in common—how they are alike.

Cup and plate _____
Shark and tuna _____
Vodka and gin _____

10. *Famous Names.* Subjects are read a series of first names and are asked to name a famous person with that first name. Student then asks if the subject can tell something about that person.

George _____ (Washington/Jessel/Burns)
Jimmy _____ (Carter/Stewart/Hoffa/Durante)

11. *Travelling Bingo.* A card is created that contains 12 or 16 squares, each containing the name of something one might see from a car window, e.g., red pick-up truck, school bus, police car, driver with a beard, passenger with a pony tail, pizza delivery truck. Depending on capability of subject, whole card is played or one or more objects are targeted for a particular trip. Involve subjects in the creation of items to put in the squares.

APPENDIX B

Sample of a memory tape script

Hello Irene. This is Debbie Bernstein speaking to you by tape recorder. Can you repeat my name? (5 s pause) _____ Again, my name is *Debbie Bernstein*.

The purpose of this tape is help you relearn some things you may have forgotten about your life and to help you keep remembering the things you do remember. First I will give you some information. Then I will ask you questions about it. If you don't know the answer, don't worry, I'll give you the correct answer right away. Eventually, you should learn most of the information. Before we begin, let me repeat my name. My name is *Debbie Bernstein*. Say my name if you can (5 s pause) _____ *Debbie Bernstein*. (2 s pause) Ready? Let's begin.

I spoke with your daughter, Sarah, and she told me a little bit about you and your family. Let's see if I have it right. You were born in Santiago, Chile on *September 10, 1913*. What was the date and year of your birth? (5 s pause) _____ September 10, 1913. (2 s pause) Your father's name was Edward Steele

---

* Questions preceded by an asterisk were not known by the subject at baseline; the script should contain 12–15 known and 12–15 not known facts.

and he was born in Liverpool, England. Where was your father born? (5 s pause) _____ *Liverpool, England.* (2 s pause) Your father worked as a writer for Kennecott Copper company *What company did your father work for? (5 s pause) _____ *Kennecott Copper company.* (2 s pause) Your mother was a homemaker. Her maiden name was Mary Edwards. *What was your mother's maiden name? (5 s pause) _____ *Mary Edwards.* (2 s pause) Your mother had eight children, four boys and four girls. You were child number five. What was your birth position in your family? _____ (5 s pause) *Number five.* (2 s pause)

Now for some review questions. First question:

1. On what date and year were you born? (5 s pause) _____
   The correct answer is *September 10, 1913.* (2 s pause) Next question
2. Where was your father born? (5 s pause) _____
   The correct answer is *Liverpool, England.* (2 s pause) Next question
3.* What company did your father work for? (5 s pause) _____
   The correct answer is Kennecott Copper Company. (2 s pause) Next question
4.* What was your mother's maiden name? (5 s pause) _____
   The correct answer is *Mary Edwards.* (2 s pause) Next question
5. What was your birth position in your family? (5 s pause) _____
   The correct answer is *Number 5.* (2 s pause)

You attended Santiago College in Santiago Chile. What was the name of the college you attended? _____ (5 s pause) *Santiago College.* (2 s pause) You met your husband at a dance at the El Teniente Country Club. *What was the name of the Country Club where you met your husband? _____ (5 s pause) *El Teniente Country Club.* (2 s pause) Your husband was a metallurgical engineer. What was your husband's occupation? _____ (5 s pause) Metallurgical engineer. (2 s pause). When he retired, he was working for the US Steel Corporation. *What company was your husband working for when he retired? _____ (5 s pause) *US Steel.* (2 s pause). Your daughter Sarah lives near you in Tucson. She works as a school psychologist. What is your daughter's occupation? _____ (5 s pause). *School psychologist.* (2 s pause). Sarah works with 3 and 4-year-old children. *What ages are the children that Sarah works with? _____ (5 s pause) *3 and 4 years old.* (2 s pause)

Now for some review questions. First question

6. What was the name of the college you attended? (5 s pause) _____
   The correct answer is Santiago College (2 s pause) Next question
7.* What was the name of the country club where you met your husband? (5 s pause) _____
   The correct answer is El Teniente. (2 s pause) Next question et cetera.

Manuscript received July 1999
Revised manuscript received June 2000

Testing of a cognitive stimulation intervention for dementia caregiving dyads

Mary P. Quayhagen and Margaret Quayhagen

University of San Diego, USA

Two experimental studies are presented which compare the effect of one home-based cognitive stimulation intervention for the caregiving dyad with a subsequent modification of that intervention on outcomes for spouses coping with dementia of the Alzheimer's type. In each experiment, samples were drawn from a larger study and were selected on common criteria relative to initial level of cognitive functioning and if they were spousal units. The 56 couples in the first study and the 30 couples in the subsequent study had all been randomised to either experimental, control, or placebo groups. Data had been collected initially and post-intervention (3 months) on measures of immediate and delayed memory, verbal fluency, and problem solving, along with marital interaction. The interventions varied in length of time (12 vs. 8 weeks) and direction of weekly focus (single vs. integrated). Results showed improvement in immediate memory for patients in the first study, in problem solving in the second study, and in verbal fluency for patients in both studies, with decline in the respective control groups. These findings support the inclusion of spousal caregivers as active participants in cognitive remediation for dementia.

During the past decade, there has been a movement towards the use of more environmentally relevant tasks and stimuli for remediating and/or enhancing cognitive function in persons with early to middle stage dementia. Lawton

Requests for reprints should be sent to Mary P. Quayhagen, Professor and Director of Research, School of Nursing, University of San Diego, 5998 Alcala Park, San Diego, CA 92110, (619) 260-4562, Fax (858) 458-0863, e-mail: mquay@acusd.edu.

The research studies were supported by grants awarded to Mary P. Quayhagen from the National Institute of Nursing Research, National Institutes of Health, Grant No. RO1-NR01931 and Grant No. R01-NR03239, with supplemental funding from Shelia Davis Lawrence and M. Larry Lawrence of the Lawrence Family Foundation.

Gratitude is expressed to Robert R. Corbeil, for statistical consultation, to Robert Katzman, for neurological interpretation, to Marcia Borgie, Jo Ann Butler, and Margaret DeBon, for their assistance with data collection, and to Janet A. Rodgers, Patricia A. Roth, Carol Hamilton, and Colleen Smith, for their assistance in implementation of the interventions.

(1996) documented the importance of continuing research to improve cognitive functioning since even modest improvement may enhance the feelings of competence in the person with dementia (patient). Further, Bäckman (1992) noted that intelligently designed cognitive stimulation studies have the ability to slow manifestations of the disease, while Woods (1996) concluded the need for attention to the type of memory used, the cognitive load, and the retrieval/cueing support addressed in cognitive rehabilitation studies.

Although the memory stimulation intervention studies have differed in length and specific training techniques and foci, they have all documented some degree of improvement in selected memory components. Sandman (1993) tested a memory rehabilitation programme for patients with mild to moderate Alzheimer's disease. Using two specific techniques, rehearsal and elaboration to stimulate deep processing, and emotional and flashbulb memories, he noted improvement in face–name associations and recall of significant events. Abrahams and Camp (1993) and Camp, Foss, O'Hanlon, and Stevens (1996) have successfully trained family caregivers to use the cognitive stimulation techniques (object naming training through spaced retrieval) to enhance memory and recall in their family members with dementia thereby reducing repetitive verbalisations and behaviours. These techniques were time-limited and task-specific. Quayhagen et al. (1995) used various memory techniques as part of a multi-strategy approach to improve memory. In contrast to the task-specific findings of Camp and associates, they noted modest post-test improvement on a greater range of cognitive abilities indicating a potential transfer of training effect. Also, in the Quayhagen study, patients had maintained baseline cognitive levels at nine months as compared to a decline in controls. The transfer of training effect was a finding similar to that of Butti, Buzzelli, Fiori, and Giaquinto (1998) who found their computerised cognitive rehabilitation programme generalised to life situations for patients with vascular dementia. Using a procedural memory stimulation programme with senile dementia of Alzheimer's type patients, Zanetti et al. (1997) noted that patients in the earlier stages of dementia improved for daily living activities on which they were not trained as well as those targeted for training.

Researchers have also documented the importance of meaning and motivation for intervention research. Camp and associates (1997) provided meaningful tasks in a pilot study of the effect of Montessori-based activities for persons with dementia. The authors had the participants serve in a mentoring role for the children. This approach compensated for memory and executive function deficits and succeeded in increasing environmental involvement and competence through use of social skills and longer-term memory. By using a hierarchy of activities, Quayhagen and associates (1995) found meaning and motivation were enhanced through self-selection of the specific activity or task to use for meeting the focus within the intervention guidelines. Similarly, with an interactive computer-based training programme, Hofmann, Hock, Kuhler, and Muller-Spahn (1996) noted that the familiar environmental stimuli were motivating and emotionally rewarding for the patient with dementia even though, contrary to the Quayhagen study, general cognitive improvement did not occur.

Cognitive stimulation has also been achieved through problem solving and communication techniques. Cavanaugh et al. (1989) found that when caregiver/patient dyads completed a cognitive problem solving task together, the caregivers gave motivating and positive feedback to the patients which increased the competence of the patients. The positive effect of the joint problem solving task on the patient/caregiver relationship was similar to that documented by Quayhagen and Quayhagen (1996), where working together through obstacles enhanced life quality for the dyad. Some cognitively challenging activities (Bourgeois, 1992; Friedman & Tappen, 1991), along with behaviour management techniques for verbalisation (Bourgeois et al. 1997) have been used to improve communication deficits. The persons with dementia were generally more cognitively debilitated than those in the Quayhagen et al. (1995) study where improvement was also noted in verbal fluency.

Cohn, Smyer, and Horgas (1995) emphasised the importance of assisting family caregivers living with dementia patients to examine life long communication patterns, so that the tone of voice does not become a trigger which fosters behaviour problems. Similarly, Montgomery (1996) supported measuring the quality of the caregiver/patient interaction since change in the patient impacts their relationship. Dal Canto, Darnley, Jacob, and Gallagher-Thompson (1997) explored the spousal interaction in the home and found the conflicted caregivers were less validating and less supportive of their dementia-diagnosed spouse, and reported a greater degree of patient behavioural impairment. In addition, Phillips et al. (1995) found that interactional process variables were strong predictors of the quality of care in the caregiving situation, while Woods (1999) noted the implicit assumption that increased interaction would be associated with increased quality of life for the patient.

The purpose of this report is to compare the effect of the cognitive stimulation intervention programme developed and used in an initial experimental research project (Quayhagen et al., 1995) with the effect of a modified version of the intervention designed for use in a subsequent experimental research project (Quayhagen et al., in press). In both of these original studies, all participants were randomised to their respective conditions using a stratified condition by level of impairment format so as to reduce pre-test differences in cognitive functioning between groups. In the first study there was a 9 month follow-up in addition to the pre- and immediate post-treatment assessments, and the Alzheimer-diagnosed participants had a score of 85 or above on the Dementia Rating Scale (DRS; Mattis, 1988) in initial testing. On the other hand, in the second original study, only pre- and immediate post-treatment assessments were done, dementia diagnosis was not limited to possible or probable Alzheimer's disease, criterion for the DRS score was 100 or greater, and caregivers could be either a spouse or an adult child caring for a demented parent. Although this second project included a comparison of multiple treatments (Quayhagen et al., in press), only the active cognitive stimulation group data and the control group data were deemed appropriate to answer the research question of relevance here, since no placebo group had been used in this project.

The research question of interest for this paper was whether the shorter version of the active cognitive stimulation programme was as effective as the initial version. Although the larger research studies differed in scope, level of cognitive impairment of the patient, and length of follow-up, only comparable samples and common procedures were used for the analyses in each of the two studies reported in this paper. Specifically, the participant samples (derived from their respective larger data sets) were limited to caregivers who were caring for spouses diagnosed with possible or probable Alzheimer's disease in accord with the clinical criteria of Reisberg, Ferris, De Leon, and Crook (1988), and who scored at or above 100 on the DRS at the first time of testing. Likewise, only the initial pre-test and immediate post-treatment assessments (baseline and at 12 weeks) using measures common to both studies were included in the analyses reported in this paper.

In each study, once the Institutional Review Board (IRB) approved consents had been signed, the patients were assessed in the home on the neuropsychological measures while the caregivers completed their evaluation packets in a different room. All measures were administered in the same order in both studies. Also, for both studies, all the research assistants were college educated in the health sciences and trained for their respective tasks by the licensed investigative team. In each study, the assessment team was blind to the condition to which the unit was randomised. In addition, different teams of the research assistants conducted either the intervention or the placebo programmes so as to reduce cross-treatment as well as testing/treatment confounds.

EXPERIMENTAL STUDY 1

Method

Design and procedure

In order to make comparisons across the studies, the analysis presented here was limited to data for participants from the Quayhagen et al. (1995) study who met the inclusion criteria noted above. Also, the repeated measures design was limited to two occasions of testing, namely, pre- and post-intervention (at 3 months). Participant units (patient and caregiver) had been randomly assigned to one of three conditions in this study (i.e., cognitive stimulation, placebo, control) following the initial assessment.

Participants

For this analysis, 56 caregiving units (patients, spousal caregivers) met the criteria for comparison of the initial intervention with the modified version used in the subsequent project. The patients (44 men; 12 women) had an average age of 73.18 (SEM = 1.05) years, and education of 15.93 (SEM = 2.23) years, while their spouses who were caregivers (12 men; 44 women) had an average age of 67.75 (SEM = 1.41) years and education of 13.82 (SEM = 0.38) years. Ninety-one percent were Caucasian, with the remaining 9% primarily of Hispanic or African–American ethnic origin. None of the groups differed on age or education, and ethnic participants were randomly distributed across groups.

Intervention

Experimental treatment. The active cognitive stimulation intervention of Quayhagen et al. (1995) was constructed for use in the home with the family caregiver as the intervening agent who helped to cognitively stimulate the patient through memory provoking, conversational fluency, and problem solving activities, with the actual intervention being one hour daily for five days each week of active cognitive stimulation. Each week had a specific cognitive focus, with seven weeks targeted to memory components, three weeks to problem solving skills, and two weeks to fluency and communication skills. Stimuli in all three cognitive components were selected from a taxonomy of tasks and activities which ranged from simple to complex in order to accommodate a range of ability in the patients. This allowed for adjustment of sensory stimuli to the patient as advocated by Gerdner, Hall, and Buckwalter (1996). Also, all stimuli had been previously found by Quayhagen and Quayhagen (1989) to be meaningful to the patients and caregivers, and all were financially feasible for continued use by caregiving units after the study was completed. The caregiver was assisted to interact more effectively with the patient through observation and modelling of the interaction of the research team with the patient during the one hour per week in which the weekly instruction was given in the home. In this way success could be achieved and frustration avoided for both the caregiver and the patient. This cognitive stimulation programme was adapted from the original intervention conceptualised and developed by Quayhagen and Quayhagen (1989).

The memory component was based on the model of Craik (1977). Using this model the attention to stimuli was sustained through active participation in the cognitively stimulating activities which were selected for their interest, thereby maintaining motivation. Since implicit memory or priming tasks show less decline, the tasks during the early weeks of intervention addressed long-term and recognition memory or more permanently stored knowledge and its retrieval. Rehearsal, association, and elaboration of detail were used with such activities as reminiscing. Recognition memory tasks included such activities as search-a-word puzzles and picture recognition. The work of Wilson (1987) also influenced the selection of memory remediation activities. Tasks later in the programme addressed the consolidation and retrieval of short-term information through association and free recall of information such as television news and book passages, and cueing techniques for remembering dates and time. An important ingredient in all components of the cognitive stimulation programme was emphasis on positive feedback and encouragement.

The conversation fluency component of the intervention was directed toward remediation of language deficits in word finding and topic mainte-nance, and based on the work of Feier and Leight (1981). The focus was on word fluency and communication skills required for eliciting facts, opinions and rationale or justification for opinions, with attention to the conversational discourse patterns noted by Ripich et al. (1991). The more complex activities for this component were frequently integrated with short-term memory recall tasks of the memory component (e.g., recall of newspaper and TV news items).

The problem solving component was theoretically rooted in the problem solving approach of D'Zurilla (1986), with techniques also influenced by the work of Spivack, Platt, and Shure (1976). This approach included problem orientation (perception, appraisal, and causal attribution), problem identifica-tion and goal setting, generation of alternative solutions, decision making with evaluation of outcomes and consequences for the selected alternative solutions, and implementation and verification of the solution through feedback. The cognitive stimulation activities for this component included practical problems (e.g., a fire in the home) with practice in generating alternative solutions, and identifying possible causes of the problem and consequences of different solutions. Initially, non-threatening neutral situations were used but as the intervention progressed the tasks increased in complexity to include real-life problems which affected spousal interaction.

Placebo treatment.   The placebo treatment consisted of passive activities for the caregiving unit such as watching television games and other shows of interest, as well as having the caregiver read news items to the patient but not encouraging discussion of the items. The participation of the research team and of the spousal units randomly assigned to the placebo condition was equal to the time frame for the experimental group.

Controls.   All caregiving units randomly assigned to the control group were put on a waiting list to receive instruction in the experimental intervention if they wished, after the completion of the time frame for formal participation in their condition. During the waiting list period, there was no initiated contact between the control group and the researchers.

Measures

Composite scores were used for analysis of patient outcomes of immediate and delayed memory, verbal fluency, and problem solving, with all composites having interscale correlations ranging from .52 to .67. The *immediate memory* score was derived from a composite of three tests: the 25-point Logical Memory I and Visual Reproduction I subscales of the Wechsler Memory Scale—Revised (WMS-R; Wechsler, 1987), and the 25-point memory factor from the Dementia Rating Scale (DRS; Mattis, 1988). The *delayed memory* score (30-minute delayed recall) was a combination of the WMS-R subscales of Logical Memory II and Visual Reproduction II (0–25 points each). The retest reliability coefficients for the separate memory tests ranged from .91 to .88 in the dementia sample.

The *verbal fluency* score was a composite of the number of words recalled in one minute for the letters F, A, and S (FAS; Benton & Hamsher, 1976), the one minute recall of names within the animal category (Goodglass & Kaplan, 1983), and the score from the initiation factor of the DRS (0–37 points). The retest coefficients for the individual tests ranged from .77 to .86. The Geriatric Coping Schedule (GCS; Quayhagen & Chiriboga, 1976) and the conceptualisation factor items (DRS) were used to measure *problem solving*. The score was the sum of alternative logical responses to the 12 short situations and the points (0–39) obtained on the conceptualisation factor. The retest coefficients for the two tests were .79 and .71 respectively. The intercoder reliability for the GCS ranged from .95 to .99. The 24-item Marital Needs Satisfaction Scale (Stinnett, Collins, & Montgomery, 1970) was used to assess the degree of satisfaction with *marital interaction* in the spousal relationship in six need fulfilment areas: love, respect, communication, personality fulfilment, life meaningfulness, and integration of life experiences, with a summed score obtained across items, giving a potential range from 24 to 120. This scale had an internal consistency alpha of .97 and factorial validity.

Results

Repeated measures multivariate procedures, using SPSS 8.0 for Windows (SPSS, 1998), were applied to the data to examine differences in groups over time. When violations of the assumption of compound symmetry occurred, the Huynh-Feldt epsilon correction was used. Pillai's criterion was applied when there was lack of homogeneity of dispersion matrices. All variables were examined for initial (pre-test) group differences that may have existed due to attrition effects over the three month period, and when differences were noted, appropriate covariate procedures were applied to the data. Significance was established at the .05 level of probability for all statistical procedures.

Results of the repeated measures multivariate procedures applied to the patient data revealed group by time interactions for immediate memory and for verbal fluency, $F(2, 53) = 4.18, p = .021; F(2, 53) = 6.54, p = .003$, respectively. Further examination of the interaction, using pairs of means, documented the source of the interaction and the directions of change as occurring between the cognitive stimulation (experimental) and the control groups. Specifically, there was a significant increase in both immediate memory and verbal fluency for the cognitive stimulation group as compared to the control group who demonstrated a decrease in these abilities, $F(1, 35) = 10.12, p = .003; F(1, 35) = 12.09, p = .001$, respectively. On the other hand, only a trend interaction $(p < .052)$ was noted between the cognitive stimulation group and the placebo, whereas no interaction was noted between the placebo and the control group.

To control for initial differences in the caregiver data, covariate procedures were applied to marital interaction and revealed only a trend for group differences, $F(2, 50) = 2.51, p = .092$, but Scheffe's multiple contrast documented significant decline in the control group post-treatment compared to the experimental group. In addition, improvement in the spousal interaction was documented by the experimental group caregivers who kept process log recordings as the intervention was being implemented. Table 1 displays means and standard errors for the outcome variables.

TABLE 1
Scores (mean + SE) for outcome variables in Study 1

Variables	Active cognitive stimulation (N = 20)	Passive stimulation (Placebo) (N = 19)	Control (N = 17)
Memory—Immediate			
Pre	34.15 ± 3.5	32.16 ± 2.7	32.12 ± 2.4
Post	38.95 ± 3.8	31.95 ± 3.0	30.12 ± 2.4
Memory—Delayed			
Pre	4.84 ± 2.3	4.00 ± 1.3	3.93 ± 1.2
Post	6.60 ± 2.8	4.21 ± 1.3	4.67 ± 1.4
Fluency			
Pre	57.05 ± 4.2	58.00 ± 4.0	58.71 ± 3.3
Post	63.55 ± 4.8	54.42 ± 4.2	51.65 ± 3.8
Problem solving			
Pre	55.65 ± 2.3	57.00 ± 2.1	55.35 ± 2.0
Post	59.80 ± 2.8	56.00 ± 1.6	53.18 ± 2.6
Marital interaction			
Pre	92.00 ± 3.6	83.95 ± 5.2	80.35 ± 4.3
Post	91.55 ± 3.5	85.05 ± 4.8	74.93 ± 5.5

Discussion

The above findings confirm cognitive improvement in the patients in immediate memory and verbal fluency. However, for delayed memory and problem solving skills the patients showed only a tendency toward improvement which did not reach a level of significance. Although improvement had been predicted, the experimental group maintained their level of marital interaction, while the control group declined as expected. One possible explanation for this finding of maintenance rather than improvement in marital interaction might be a ceiling effect in the responses, indicating need for a more sensitive measure. The pre-existing differences (for which a covariate analysis was used) in the caregiver outcome were attributed both to differential attrition within each group and to the fact that the participants were randomised by the cognitive functioning level of the patient rather than by caregiver similarities.

EXPERIMENTAL STUDY 2

Method

Design and participants

For comparing Study 2 with Study 1, the data analysis was limited to spousal caregiving units (patient and caregiver) who met the previously stated criteria, and who had been randomly assigned to either the active cognitive intervention or to a waiting list control group. The procedures for consent, assessment, and intervention were identical to those in Study 1. The 30 dementia diagnosed patients (19 men; 11 women) had an average age of 74.97 (SEM = 1.36) years, and education of 14.31 (SEM = 0.63) years, while their spousal caregivers (11 men; 19 women) had an average age of 72.57 (SEM = 1.51) years and education level of 14.31 (SEM = 0.52) years. Ninety percent were Caucasian, with the other 10% of Hispanic or African–American ethnic origin. The treatment and control groups did not differ on age or education, and ethnic participants were randomly distributed across groups.

Intervention

In this study, two major modifications were made in the experimental intervention of active cognitive stimulation. The length of the programme was shortened from 12 to 8 weeks. Further, each weekly focus included tasks and activities from all three of the intervention components (memory, verbal fluency, and problem solving), in contrast to the earlier study where only one component was addressed per week. As before, the tasks and activities represented a hierarchy of complexity to allow for varying levels of abilities. Also, the actual intervention continued to be one hour daily for five days each week of active cognitive stimulation, using the prescribed activities or tasks. As in the previous study, the research team provided one hour of instruction weekly to the family.

Measures

All assessment measures for the patients and the interaction (marital satisfaction) scale for the caregivers were identical to those used in the previous research.

Results

Using repeated measures multivariate procedures, a group by time interaction was found for both problem solving and verbal fluency, $F(1, 28) = 4.39$, $p = .045$; $F(1, 28) = 5.13$, $p = .031$, respectively. Specifically, the cognitive stimulation (experimental) group demonstrated a significant increase over time when compared to the control group which tended to decrease on both problem solving and fluency. Contrary to the previous study, memory differences were not found which may be attributed to the integrated focus across the three components in this latter study, and to a stronger focus on problem solving techniques. Even though marital interaction was not significant, in a qualitative evaluation of the intervention, 71% of the caregivers who received the cognitive stimulation program identified enhanced communication and interaction as a major benefit of the intervention. The means and standard errors for the outcome variables are displayed in Table 2.

TABLE 2
Scores (mean + SE) for outcome variables in Study 2

Variables	Cognitive stimulation (N = 18)	Control (N = 12)
Memory—Immediate		
Pre	41.00 ± 3.9	38.83 ± 4.4
Post	42.44 ± 4.9	38.50 ± 5.7
Memory—Delayed		
Pre	6.61 ± 2.2	6.92 ± 3.6
Post	9.56 ± 2.9	7.17 ± 3.9
Fluency		
Pre	60.44 ± 4.6	59.58 ± 6.1
Post	63.33 ± 5.3	54.00 ± 7.2
Problem solving		
Pre	64.52 ± 2.9	67.67 ± 5.7
Post	69.83 ± 3.8	65.08 ± 7.7
Marital interaction		
Pre	92.22 ± 3.5	95.25 ± 7.1
Post	91.06 ± 3.3	93.92 ± 8.6

Comparison of intervention effects between studies.   In this final analysis the intervention conditions from both Study 1 and Study 2 were compared for their effects on the outcomes, using the repeated measures multivariate procedure. There were no interaction or treatment main effects between the groups administered the longer versus the shorter version of the intervention. However, there were time main effects for immediate memory, verbal fluency, and problem solving, $F(1, 36) = 6.28$, $p = .017$; $F(1, 36) = 8.97$, $p = .005$; $F(1, 36) = 5.12$, $p = .030$, respectively, with both cognitive stimulation groups showing improvement regardless of the length of the intervention programme. An additional finding for this comparison was in delayed memory where another time main effect was noted with improvement in both groups, $F(1, 35) = 4.18$, $p = .048$. Given the similarities from these analyses, it appears that changes in the intervention program from one group to another were not substantial enough to make a difference, except when comparing the interventions with their respective control groups.

DISCUSSION

When comparing the results of Study 2 for the patients with dementia to those of the preceding experiment using Quayhagen et al. (1995) data, the results support a differential improvement in the cognitive components for the patients who participated in the home-based cognitive stimulation intervention even though it was shortened from 12 to 8 weeks, and modified in weekly focus. From the data, however, the memory component appeared stronger in the former study, as more aspects of memory skill were improved. A plausible explanation is that the memory component was more prominent in the longer protocol where seven of the weeks had a single focus on a specific aspect of memory. In contrast, in the latter study the problem solving component received greater emphasis and findings were stronger. Perhaps this result could be attributed to the weekly inclusion of the practical problem solving techniques, although the situations for solution varied.

The findings of cognitive improvement for patients, using the more specifically focused intervention of the initial study, were in accord with the results of Sandman (1993) and Camp et al. (1996). Also improvement in verbal fluency was not surprising since Bourgeois (1992) had similar results even with more debilitated patients. The qualitatively documented positive effect on interaction through joint completion of cognitive tasks was also similar to that found by Cavanaugh et al. (1989), Quayhagen and Quayhagen (1996), and Quayhagen et al. (in press). However, there were no significant correlations between marital interaction and level of cognitive function in either study.

Comparison of the two cognitive stimulation studies was only possible by imposing sampling, design, and measurement restrictions which allowed data analysis to be applicable to both projects. For example, since the second study was limited by the absence of longitudinal data, only the pre- and post-intervention assessments could be compared, even though the first study had included a nine month follow-up assessment. Knowing the longer-term effect of using a shorter form of the intervention would have been a valuable piece of information. In addition, the criterion of using only spousal caregivers and patients functioning at or above 100 on the DRS reduced the sample sizes from the larger studies from which the data were drawn. It is encouraging, however, that even with these limitations, significant improvement has been noted, although differentially, in the outcomes of interest. These findings support the value of including the spousal caregiver as an active participant in cognitive stimulation intervention. Further research is recommended into the use of meaningful, financially affordable stimuli for converting spousal interaction time into a cognitively challenging experience.

REFERENCES

Abrahams, J., & Camp, C. (1993). Maintenance and generalization of object naming training in anomia associated with degenerative dementia. *Clinical Gerontologist, 12,* 57-72.

Bäckman, L. (1992). Memory training and memory improvement in Alzheimer's disease: Rules and exceptions. *Acta Neurologica Scandinavica: Supplement, 139,* 84–89.

Benton, A.L., & Hamsher, K. deS. (1976). *Multilingual aphasia examination.* Iowa City: University of Iowa.

Bourgeois, M.S. (1992). Evaluating memory wallets in conversation with persons with dementia. *Journal of Speech and Hearing Research, 35,* 1344–1357.

Bourgeois, M.S., Burgio, L.D., Schulz, R., Beach, S., & Palmer, B. (1997). Modifying repetitive verbalizations of community-dwelling patients with AD. *Gerontologist, 37,* 30–39.

Butti, G., Buzzelli, S., Fiori, M., & Giaquinto, S. (1998). Observations on mentally impaired elderly patients treated with THINKable, a computerized cognitive remediation. *Archives of Gerontology and Geriatrics, (Suppl. 6),* 49–56.

Camp, C.J., Foss, J.W., O'Hanlon, A.M., & Stevens, A.B. (1996). Memory interventions for persons with dementia. *Applied Cognitive Psychology, 10,* 193–210.

Camp, C.J., Judge, K.S., Bye, C.A., Fox, K.M., Bowden, J., Bell, M., Valencic, K., & Mattern, J.M. (1997). An intergenerational program for persons with dementia using Montessori methods. *Gerontologist, 37,* 688–692.

Cavanaugh, J.C., Dunn, N.J., Mowery, D., Feller, C., Niederehe, G., Fruge, E., & Volpendesta, D. (1989). Problem-solving strategies in dementia patient–caregiver dyads. *Gerontologist, 29,* 156–158.

Cohn, M.D., Smyer, M.A., & Horgas, A.L. (1995). *The ABC's of behaviour change: Skills for working with behavior problems in nursing homes.* State College, PA: Venture Publishing.

Craik, F.I.M. (1977). Age differences in human memory. In J.E. Birren & K.W.Schaie (Eds.), *Handbook of the psychology of aging.* New York: Van Nostrand.

Dal Canto, P.G., Darnley, S., Jacob, T., & Gallagher-Thompson, D. (1997). An observational study of the relationship between distress in Alzheimer's disease caregivers and their interaction style. *Psychologists in Long Term Care Newsletter, 10,* 2–4.

D'Zurilla, T.J. (1986). *Problem solving therapy: A social competence approach to clinical intervention.* New York: Springer.

Feier, C.D., & Leight, G. (1981). A communication-cognition program for elderly nursing home residents. *Gerontologist, 21,* 408–416.

Friedman, R., & Tappen, R.M. (1991). The effect of planned walking on communication in Alzheimer's disease. *Journal of the American Geriatrics Society, 39,* 650–654.

Gerdner, L.A., Hall, G.R., & Buckwalter, K.C. (1996). Caregiver training for people with Alzheimer's based on a stress threshold model. *Image, 28,* 241–246.

Goodglass, H., & Kaplan, E. (1983). *The assessment of aphasia and related disorders.* Philadelphia: Lea & Febiger.

Hofmann, M., Hock, C., Kuhler, A., & Muller-Spahn, F. (1996). Interactive computer-based cognitive training in patients with Alzheimer's disease. *Journal of Psychiatric Research, 30,* 493–501.

Lawton, M.P. (1996). Behavioral problems and interventions in Alzheimer's disease: Research needs. *International Psychogeriatrics, 8,* 95–98.

Mattis, S. (1988). *Dementia Rating Scale: Professional manual.* Odessa, FL: Psychological Assessment Resources.

Montgomery, R.J.V. (1996). Advancing caregiver research: Weighing efficacy and feasibility of interventions. *Journal of Gerontology, 51B,* S109–S110.

Phillips, L.R., Morrison, E., Steffl, B., Chae, Y.M., Cromwell, S.L., & Russell, C.K. (1995). Effects of the situational context and interactional process on the quality of family caregiving. *Research in Nursing and Health, 18,* 205–216.

Quayhagen, M.P., & Chiriboga, D. (1976). Geriatric Coping Schedule. In D.J. Mangen & W.A. Peterson (Eds.), *Research instruments in social gerontology: Clinical and social psychology, Vol 1* (pp. 168–169, 182–183). Minneapolis: University of Minnesota Press.

Quayhagen, M.P., & Quayhagen, M. (1989). Differential effects of family-based strategies on Alzheimer's disease. *Gerontologist, 29,* 150–155.

Quayhagen, M.P., & Quayhagen, M. (1996). Discovering life quality in coping with dementia. *Western Journal of Nursing Research, 18,* 120–135.

Quayhagen, M.P., Quayhagen, M., Corbeil, R.R., Hendrix, R.C., Jackson, J.E., Snyder, L., & Bower, D. (2000). Coping with dementia: Evaluation of four non-pharmacologic interventions. *International Psychogeriatrics, 12,* 249–266.

Quayhagen, M.P., Quayhagen, M., Corbeil, R.R., Roth, P.A., & Rodgers, J.A. (1995). A dyadic remediation program for care recipients with dementia. *Nursing Research, 44,* 153–159.

Reisberg, B., Ferris, S.H., De Leon, M.J., & Crook, T. (1988). The Global Deterioration Scale (GDS). *Psychopharmacology Bulletin, 24,* 661–669.

Ripich, D.N., Vertes, D., Whitehouse, P., Fulton, S., & Ekelman, B. (1991). Turn-taking and speech act patterns in the discourse of senile dementia of the Alzheimer's type patients. *Brain and Language, 40,* 330–343.

Sandman, C.A. (1993). Memory rehabilitation in Alzheimer's disease: Preliminary findings. *Clinical Gerontologist, 13,* 19–33.

Spivack, G., Platt, J.J., & Shure, M.B. (1976). *The problem-solving approach to adjustment: A guide to research and intervention.* San Francisco: Jossey-Bass.

SPSS Inc. (1998). *SPSS 8.0 for Windows.* Chicago, IL: SPSS.

Stinnett, N., Collins, J., & Montgomery, J. (1970). Marital need satisfaction of older husbands and wives. *Journal of Marriage and the Family, 32,* 428–434.

Wechsler, D. (1987). *WMS-R (Wechsler Memory Scale—Revised).* San Antonio, TX: The Psychological Corporation.

Wilson, B.A. (1987). *Rehabilitation of memory.* New York: Guilford Press.

Woods, B. (1996). Cognitive approaches to the management of dementia. In R.G. Morris (Ed.). *The cognitive neuropsychology of Alzheimer-type dementia.* (pp. 310–326). Oxford, UK: Oxford University Press.

Woods, B. (1999). Promoting well-being and independence for people with dementia. *International Journal of Geriatric Psychiatry, 14,* 97–109.

Zanetti, O., Binetti, G., Magni, E., Rozzini, L., Bianchetti, A., & Trabucchi, M. (1997). Procedural memory stimulation in Alzheimer's disease: Impact of a training programme. *Acta Neurologica Scandinavica, 95,* 152–157.

Manuscript received May 1999
Revised manuscript received November 1999

Self-maintenance therapy in Alzheimer's disease

Barbara Romero[1,2] and Michael Wenz[1]

[1]*Alzheimer Therapiezentrum der Neurologischen Klinik Bad Aibling, Germany*
[2]*Klinik und Poliklinik für Psychiatrie und Psychotherapie der Technischen Universität München, Germany*

A short-term residential treatment programme designed to prepare patients with dementia and caregivers for life with a progressive disease was evaluated in a one group pretest–posttest design. The multicomponent programme included: (1) intensive rehabilitation for patients, based on the concept of Self-Maintenance Therapy, and (2) an intervention programme for caregivers. The results showed a consistent improvement in patients' depression and in other psychopathological symptoms, which can be seen as directly beneficial for patients. Following treatment, caregivers also felt less depressed, less mentally fatigued and restless, and more relaxed. Controlled studies are needed to support the preliminary results presented and to address hypotheses about factors responsible for benefits as well as for treatment resistance. The concept of Self-Maintenance Therapy allowed the prediction that experiences that are in accordance with patients' self-structures and processes support patients' well-being, reduce psychopathological symptoms, and facilitate social participation.

INTRODUCTION

Patients with dementia of Alzheimer type (AD) gradually lose their cognitive competence in the course of the disease. The lost and preserved competencies of patients are traditionally described in terms of neuropsychological functions and daily activities, such as "spatial orientation" or "naming" abilities. Rehabilitation programmes grounded on this traditional approach aim at facilitation of basic functions, for example, facilitation of memory performance or attention. However, interventions designed to improve basic

Correspondence should be sent to Barbara Romero, Alzheimer Therapiezentrum der Neurologischen Klinik Bad Aibling, Kolbermoorerstr. 72, D-83043 Bad Aibling, Germany. Email: romero@t-online.de.

The authors would like to thank L. Clare and R.T. Woods for providing helpful comments on a previous draft of this paper.

neuropsychological functions have not really proved beneficial for patients with AD. Neuropsychological research has revealed that the relevance of functional training for dementia patients has been limited (Bäckman, 1992; Heiss, Kessler, & Mielke, 1994; McKittrick, Camp, & Black, 1992).

We proposed a systemic approach for evaluating patients' psychosocial resources and for developing rehabilitation programmes (Romero, 1997; Romero & Eder, 1992; Romero & Wenz, 2000). There are two systems that should be stabilised and preserved in a rehabilitation programme for patients with dementia—the self as an intra-individual system, and the social network as an interpersonal support system.

Self-maintenance as a therapy goal in AD

Patients' abilities, cognitive functions, skills, and attitudes at each stage of the disease are organised in relation to the self system. The self mediates a sense of personal identity and continuity. The self mediates the way in which the patient understands and integrates new experiences, reacts and makes decisions. To maintain the feeling of continuous identity, the feeling of "I am still me" as well as the feeling of "I can understand what is going on" and "I can manage" is very important for the person's well-being and behaviour (Antonovsky, 1979, 1987; Greenwald & Pratkanis, 1984; Havens, 1968; Lyman, 1998; Romero, 1997; Romero & Eder, 1992).

The patient's self must cope with many changes in competence, social roles, and activities. According to Cohen and Eisdorfer (1986, p. 22): "Every few months I sense that another piece of me is missing. My life, my self, are falling apart. Most people expect to die some day, but who ever expected to lose their self first." When it is too difficult to integrate new experiences into prior self-structures, a patient reacts with shame, depression and/or aggression. Therefore, to reduce a patient's suffering, one has to support the patient's self.

The maintenance of the patient's self in its coherence and integrity is important not only for well-being. We can also expect that a patient can better make use of his or her cognitive competence and is less vulnerable to developing disturbed behaviour.

The following predictions can be made on the basis of psychological theories of the self concept:

1. The self is a cognitive schema, which actively encodes, processes and maintains information about the person and the environment. It enables a person to recognise situations, to make decisions, to develop attitudes and to orient to the environment (Epstein, 1979). Accordingly it can be predicted that Alzheimer patients will use their cognitive competence more effectively if self-structures are better integrated and self-processes are not overtaxed.

2. Experiences which violate self-based expectancies are likely to cause extremely negative emotions such as fear, shame, aggression or depression. Ronch (1993) calls this an inevitable feeling of hopelessness and despair. Accordingly it can be predicted that avoiding patients' self-violating experiences results in a reduction of strongly negative emotions. It must be emphasised that not all negative emotions can and should be avoided: Each patient can sometimes feel hopeless or angry and a caregiver should be able to validate these emotions.

3. In the course of Alzheimer's disease, behavioural disturbances like running away, aggressive outbursts, agitation, restlessness, and social withdrawal are very common. These symptoms are partly caused by incompatibility between patients' actual experiences on the one hand and patients' self-based expectations and preferences on the other. Accordingly, it can be predicted that increasing the number of experiences which fit the self-structures of patients (and reducing the number of contradictory experiences) results in a reduction of behavioural disturbances or psychopathological symptoms.

The self is a dynamic system that forms itself throughout the course of one's life. In planning interventions for self-maintenance it is important to take into account patients' personal goals and values, especially with regard to their present situation and to the experience of dementia. In this way, therapeutic interventions acquire more personal relevance.

Maintenance of the supporting social system

The other system that needs to be stabilised is an interpersonal one. Patients live in a social community, in most cases in a family, and they depend on social support to manage their daily lives. People providing social support themselves have to be supported. Caregivers in particular need help and integration within wider family networks as well as within other social structures. Psychosocial resources such as supporting coping strategies and a higher level of social support reduce physical health problems and depression in caregivers (Goode, Haley, Roth, & Ford, 1998). Caregivers receiving a multicomponent programme designed to provide counselling and social support were less depressed and more likely to care for dementia patients at home (Mittelman et al., 1996).

Self-Maintenance Therapy (SMT)

The primary aim of SMT is to maintain the sense of personal identity, continuity and coherence in patients with a progressive dementia for as long as possible. SMT incorporates procedures from existing, well-established methods like milieu therapy, validation, reminiscence therapy, and psychotherapy—modified in accordance with the primary aim of SMT (for a comparison of SMT and established methods, see Romero & Eder, 1992). There are four main components of SMT: psychotherapeutic support, self-knowledge training, facilitation of satisfying everyday activities, and validating communication in caregiving.

Psychotherapeutic support

In recent years support groups focusing on education and sharing of experiences about development of coping strategies as well as individual psychotherapeutic interventions have been recognised as valuable for persons in the early stage of dementia (Bauer, 1998; Hirsch, 1994; Petry, 1999; Radebold, 1994). In the Alzheimer Therapy Centre (ATC) programme, therapists aim to help patients to understand the disease and to maintain a sense of meaningfulness. It is helpful for the patients to be oriented towards those goals in life that do not yet have to be given up. Learning how to deal wisely with the disease offers opportunities for personal growth, despite the inevitable cognitive decline.

Self-related knowledge training

SMT includes a training programme to hold in memory some chosen components of self-knowledge for as long as possible. There are theoretical reasons (see Romero, 1997; Romero & Eder, 1992) which offer the rationale for the prediction that overlearning of chosen biographical knowledge mediates the sense of personal identity, continuity and well-being. The training consists of three steps:

Step one. Therapists assess which biographical memories are not yet forgotten and are currently available to the patient. At the same time therapists evaluate which of these maintained memories have personal relevance to the patient and are self-related. The established way to find out the central contents of self-related knowledge is to ask the patient to tell stories about him or herself. After some sessions it becomes clear which stories are repeated most often and touch the patient at an emotional level. In addition to free narration, therapists use personal photos from all life periods to assess patients' memories more systematically. As a result there is a set of stories, family photos, tapes with songs and music, all of which can stimulate and support the patient's sense of personal continuity and identity.

Step two. Therapists record this set of self-knowledge components in a form of external memory storage. It depends on the therapeutic setting which media can be used for this purpose. At the ATC, some very promising results have been obtained using computers, which offer many possibilities for external memory storage (Riederer, 1999). Therapists scanned and stored personal photos on disk and used a microphone to record stories and comments by the patient. Special software made it possible to identify and display desired elements of the stored knowledge, for example: "everything about the patient's mother" or "names of school friends and teachers the patient recalled in her school class photograph, with her comments". Computer-supported training in personal memories has also been reported by Hofmann and co-workers (Hofmann, Hock, Kuhler, & Müller-Spahn, 1996). In the future computers will undoubtedly be used more often as a kind of substitute for a patient's personal semantic memory. Currently, patients prefer more traditional media like a personal memory book for an individual patient. In a personal memory book selected family photos and other pictures (e.g., familiar landscapes) are kept as a book together with the patient's comments. Other media like tapes and video-tapes can also be used for external memory storage.

Step three. The patient reviews the chosen components of self-related knowledge, supported by the external memory records. Systematic reminiscence with these memories is at first practised with therapeutic assistance. The family is instructed to continue the reminiscence later on at home with the assistance of the caregiver. In this way the central contents of self-related knowledge can be continuously available for patients.

Satisfying everyday activities

Even more important than the special training in personal memories are daily activities and the way in which caregivers communicate with patients. Psychosocial stress as well as a low level of satisfying activities and experiences are indicated as risk factors for additional problems in the course of the disease (Bauer, 1994; Broe et al., 1990; Friedland et al., 1996; Motomura et al., 1996).The activities from which patients previously derived satisfaction often have to be replaced by other similar or perhaps different activities (Teri & Lodgson, 1991). Therefore persons with dementia are in need of special help as well as a supportive environment. For example, a keen amateur photographer was still able to choose a subject for his pictures, but was no longer able to handle the camera. When his wife took over the technical part, he was able to resume his hobby. The couple took pictures together: The husband looked for interesting subjects (with obvious engagement and enjoyment) and his wife "pushed the button". After the pictures were developed, he was able to remember some of the subjects and was very proud of his creative activity. Art therapy offers many possibilities to engage in creative activity, even for patients with apraxia (Urbas, 2000). Of course common everyday activities such as walking, housework, dancing, visiting a church or meeting with other people can be integrated in a satisfying routine. Studies show that intervention focusing on enrichment of the activity spectrum is supportive to both patients and their carers (Aldridge, 1994; Beatty, 1999; Palo-Bengtsson, Winblad, & Ekman, 1998).Therapists at the ATC work out individual programmes to stimulate patients' participation in daily life in the context of their individual resources.

Validating communication in caregiving

Therapists educate caregivers to understand better patients' changed behaviour and to handle patients' problems more competently. Caregivers learn that the patient's way of making sense of personal experience should always be validated and supported respectfully, because it is the only and the best way in which the patient can integrate his or her experiences.

THE ALZHEIMER THERAPY CENTRE (ATC)

The ATC was founded in 1999 as a part of the Neurological Hospital Bad Aibling in co-operation with the Clinic and Polyclinic of Psychiatry and Psychotherapy of the Technical University Munich. The therapy centre provides a 4-week residential treatment programme for patients with dementia and their caregivers. The dementia syndrome with multiple, progressive cognitive deficits requires interdisciplinary and integrative rehabilitation concepts, which take into account somatic, psychiatric, functional and psychosocial aspects of the disease. The importance of a short-term intensive treatment programme, like that provided at the ATC, lies in the interdisciplinary planned preparation of each individual family for life with the disease at home (Baier & Romero, 2000). The best place to provide a treatment programme of this kind is in a specialised centre setting. There is a need for out-patient, day and residential treatment programmes which complement each other. Short-term in-patient rehabilitation programmes for dementia patients are a new concept, and we report our preliminary experiences in this field. Also, caregivers have not been consistently involved in rehabilitation programmes in the past although early results were very promising. Brodaty, Gresham, and Luscombe (1997) demonstrated in a prospective, randomised controlled study with an 8-year follow-up that a structured memory retraining and activity programme for dementia patients delayed institutionalisation of these patients provided that caregivers also received an intensive residential caregiver training programme.

Treatment goals

The treatment programme was designed to prepare patients with dementia and caregivers for life with a chronic progressive disease. The aim was to reduce patients' loss of confidence in social interaction and withdrawal as well as to reduce patients' psychopathological symptoms like depression, apathy, agitation or aggression, and to facilitate their participation in daily life in a manner that fits their level of competence. Intervention with caregivers was designed to support their psychological well-being, to improve their competence in accompanying the patient, and to support their social integration.

Treatment groups

One group consisted of patients with Alzheimer's disease, vascular dementia, frontotemporal degeneration and other dementias. The diagnosis of a dementia syndrome is a criterion for participation in the treatment programme. Patients in different stages of dementia are treated unless they are unable to take part in the treatment programme (for example, bedridden or extremely agitated and uncooperative patients).

The other group consisted of caregiving relatives. Over 80% of patients with dementia are cared for by the family, in most cases by *one* close relative. These relatives need help and support to fulfil their role as caregiver and to maintain and stabilise their own psychological and physical well-being. Integration of caregivers lies at the heart of the treatment programme.

Treatment programme

Diagnosis and medical treatment. Reliable diagnosis and adequate medical treatment are an essential starting-point for developing an appropriate rehabilitation programme. At the ATC patients are diagnosed and medically treated for somatic, cognitive and psychopathological problems. All patients with AD who tolerate acetylcholinesterase inhibitors are treated with donezepil or rivastigmine, which have been shown to slow down the progression of cognitive decline (Corey-Bloom, Anand, & Veach, 1998; Rogers & Friedhoff, 1998). Psychopathological symptoms like agitation, hallucinations or depression are treated medically with antidepressants and/or neuroleptics.

Rehabilitation programme for patients. The intensive therapy programme (approximately 20 hours per week) adopts an interdisciplinary approach which is tailored to the individual in the light of the medical, neuropsychological, and psychosocial assessment. Group and individual sessions are included. In addition to the programme for patients, there is also a joint programme for patients and caregivers designed to allow transfer of the experiences from treatment in the ATC to daily living. The rehabilitation programme includes art therapy, gymnastics, massage, relaxation, self-related knowledge training, everyday activities like cooking and working in the garden, making music and singing as well as different cultural and social activities. Therapists observe what kind of activities the patients prefer (or reject) and what kind of support is necessary to compensate for lost competence. Some patients in the early stages of dementia receive psychotherapeutic support to cope with the progressive cognitive decline. For some of the patients with very early dementia certain external memory aids (for example, always putting keys in the same place, taking notes) can be helpful. In these cases the use of individually-tailored aids is taught to the patients. A number of studies have demonstrated improvement in everyday functioning of Alzheimer patients resulting from the introduction of external memory aids (Clare, 1999; Clare et al., 2000; Woods, 1996).

Physical care.   Some of the patients are not yet in need of physical care, but others need help with dressing, personal hygiene, or going to the toilet. The physical care required during treatment is usually carried out by the relatives. The ATC nurse provides physical care in some cases to relieve the caregiving relatives or to educate them.

Physiotherapy and physical treatment.   If required, patients and care-givers can receive massage, fango, lymph drainage, electrotherapy, and physiotherapy.

Caregiver intervention.   The treatment programme in the ATC aims to support the caring relatives and to stabilise the social system to which they belong. Caregivers can improve their competence in accompanying the patient in a way that is anticipated to have a positive effect on the self of the patient. Additionally, therapists provide psychotherapeutic and social support for the caregivers to stabilise their well-being and to prevent an early decompensation and loss of the caregiver's resources resulting from strain and the burden of caregiving. Caregiver interventions include an education programme in the form of individual and family sessions and support groups as well as psychotherapeutic support in individual sessions, art therapy, relaxation training, and social work consultation. The core programme runs for 8 hours per week, but varies due to individual needs. Caregivers also experience relief while at the ATC because they do not have to care for the patient alone, and do not have to carry out their usual household tasks such as cooking or cleaning.

Staff

The therapeutic team consists of five different professionals—a medical doctor, a social worker, a psychologist, an art therapist, and a nurse—and the ATC director who is a neuropsychologist. This small team is supported by *Zivildienstleistende* (young men completing the civilian alternative to national military service) and trainees.

With respect to medical supervision, diagnostic procedures, laboratory tests, and medical consultations, the facilities of the Neurological Hospital are used. In emergencies and other special situations medical and nursing support is obtained from the Neurological Hospital.

Location and establishment

In order to support the therapy goals through provision of a friendly, homely atmosphere, the ATC is located in a modern residential area, close to the Neurological Hospital. Up to 15 couples can be accommodated in 15 two-room apartments. The ATC has in addition a small kitchen for patients, a dining room, several group and therapy rooms, and offices for staff. A living room and garden facilitate contact between the families.

Costs

The total costs of the patients' treatment are covered by patients' health insurance in most of the treated cases. Decisions about reimbursement of costs are made on a case-by-case basis following application by the patient to the relevant insurance company. For the caregivers the stay at the ATC (inclusive of accommodation, meals, and psychoeducational treatment) is free; that is to say, the ATC covers the caregivers' costs.

SHORT-TERM EFFECTS OF THE ATC PROGRAMME

We report preliminary results of an in-patient treatment programme for AD patients and their caregivers. We predicted that immediately after the treatment programme there would be an improvement in patients' social behaviour and a reduction of patients psychopathological symptoms such as depression, apathy, agitation or aggression. Memory functions and everyday functional abilities were predicted to remain unchanged. Caregivers' depression and mood were predicted to improve.

   Pre-treatment assessments were completed at the start of the programme, and follow-up assessments at the end of the programme (approximately 3 weeks after admission and a few days before discharge).

Method

Design

The treatment programme evaluated here was established as a clinical service and not specially designed for the project. In the study a one group pretest–posttest design was used. In this preliminary study there were no resources available to support a more powerful design using a control group.

A further study with a control group of patients receiving standard treatment is in preparation.

Patients

In this preliminary analysis, results are included for all patients with a diagnosis of Alzheimer's disease or mixed dementia (Alzheimer's disease with cerebrovascular components) according to ICD-10 criteria, and their caregivers, who had completed the treatment programme at the ATC between May 1999 and April 2000. Patients with other forms of dementia and patients who completed a programme shorter than 3 weeks (the standard duration of treatment is 4 weeks) were excluded. This resulted in a sample of 43 patients and 43 caregivers. For some people, not all data were available, and consequently the number of participants varies for the reported measures.

The treated patients were relatively young: the median and the mean was 70 years (range 55–90 years). A fairly high percentage of the patients, 52%, developed dementia before the age of 65. The percentage of women was relatively low (35%). The stage of dementia was assessed with the Mini Mental State Examination (MMSE, Folstein, Folstein, & McHugh, 1975). Most of the patients demonstrated a moderate stage of dementia, but the sample included patients in the early and late stages. The median and the mean MMSE score was 14; one patient achieved the maximal score of 30 and the most disturbed patient a score of 1.

Medical treatment with acetylcholinesterase inhibitors is standard in Alzheimer's disease and 37 patients (86%) were receiving donezepil or rivastigmine at follow-up. Six patients were not receiving this medication because of side-effects. The course of treatment with acetylcholinesterase inhibitors differed for individual participants. Most of the patients had been treated with donezepil or rivastigmine for some months or years before entering the programme. After admission the dose was increased for some of these patients, while for others donezepil was changed to rivastigmine or vice versa, because of side-effects. Some patients received an acetylcholinesterase inhibitor after admission for the first time; sometimes this was soon after admission, but in other cases where additional diagnostic investigations were needed, the medication was introduced at a later stage.

About 40% of the patient group (17 patients) were being treated at follow-up with antidepressant and/or neuroleptic medication, because of special indications.

Caregivers

The caregivers were most often spouses: 28 (65%) wives and 12 (28%) husbands. Three patients were living alone and were supported by a daughter (one patient) or brothers (two patients), who also accompanied the patients during treatment. All but these three patients were living with their caregivers. The average age of the caregivers was 66, ranging from 50 to 80 years.

Outcome measures

Patients. All questionnaires were completed by caregivers, who gave their perceptions of patients' difficulties. Patients with Alzheimer dementia are able to give a valid report about their own psychopathological symptoms only to a limited extent.

Cornell Depression Scale (CDS): Depressive symptoms in the patients were assessed using the Cornell Depression Scale (Alexopoulos, Abrams, Young, & Shamoian, 1988). This instrument was developed especially for patients with dementia. Caregivers rated the affective state of the patient at admission and at follow-up in a semi-structured interview with a psychologist.

CERAD Behavior Rating Scale for Dementia (BRSD): The BRSD (Tariot et al., 1995) was administered to the caregiver in a semi-structured interview to assess behavioural disturbances and other psychopathological symptoms in the patients. Symptoms like depression, affective lability, apathy, irritability, agitation, aggression, psychotic features and other psychopathological symptoms were rated with this scale.

NOSGER: For global judgement of disturbances in activities relevant to everyday life we administered the Nurses Observation Scale for Geriatric Patients (NOSGER; Spiegel et al., 1991), an instrument which is often used in evaluation studies with dementia patients.

The scores of the 30 items are summarised into six subscales (Memory, Instrumental activities of daily living (IADL), Self-care, Mood, Social behaviour, Disturbing behaviour), all of which assess the degree of deterioration or disturbance.

Caregivers. Center for Epidemiological Studies-Depression Scale (CES-D), German version, was used to assess depression in the caregiver group (Radloff, 1977; German version: Hautzinger & Bailer, 1993).

Mehrdimensionaler Befindlichkeitsfragebogen (MDBF) (Steyer, Schwenkmezger, Notz, & Eid, 1997, Multidimensional Mood States Questionnaire). Mood components were assessed with this well-validated German questionnaire for the assessment of momentary mood states. The MDBF includes 24 bipolar items which can be summarized into three subscales (good vs. bad mood; alertness vs. tiredness; rest/calmness vs. restlessness). The items are adjectives like "tired" or "well" and subjects have to judge each adjective on a 5-point scale concerning how they are feeling at the moment.

Data were available for 27 participants on the CES-D and for 40 participants on the MDBF.

Statistical analysis

In all analyses non-parametric procedures were used. To compare the outcome measures at pre-treatment and at follow-up, as well as in the two subgroups of patients, Wilcoxon Signed Rank Tests were used. The difference between pre-and post-treatment scores was taken as an Improvement Index (II). Additionally the standard effect size measure was calculated as a difference between a pre-treatment score and follow-up score divided by the pre-treatment standard deviation. Correlations were calculated using Spearman rank correlations.

Results

Patients

As predicted the mean changes from pre-treatment to follow-up reached statistical significance on all outcome measures except the NOSGER Memory, ADL, and Self-care subscales. The Cornell Depression Scale shows significantly lower scores at follow-up (Table 1). Additional analyses indicated the clinical relevance of high depression scores at pre-treatment as well as of reduction of depression scores at follow-up. Suggested cut-off scores of the CDS are 8 for mild depression and 12 for moderate depression. At pre-treatment there were 26 (63%) patients with a score higher than 7, and 15 (36.5%) with a score higher than 11. At follow-up there were only 3 patients (7%) with a score of 12 or higher and 10 (24%) patients with a score of 8 or higher.

The BRSD showed a reduction of psychopathological symptoms at follow-up (Table 1).

Disturbances of social behaviour (NOSGER subscale Social Behaviour) and psychopathological symptoms (NOSGER subscale Disturbing Behaviour) were reduced at follow-up ($z = -2.442$, $p = .05$; $z = -3.350$, $p = .001$, respectively). Changes on the subscales Memory, ADL, and Self-care failed—as predicted—to reach significance.

In terms of effect size, Table 1 indicates that large treatment effects were observed for patients' depression (CDS), moderate to large effects for patients' behaviour (NOSGER disturbing behaviour, BRSD), small effects for memory, IADL, mood and social behaviour (NOSGER subscales), and no effect for self-care (NOSGER subscale).

To analyse how outcome measures relate to the age of patients and the stage of dementia, correlations were used. NOSGER subscale scores for Memory and Self-care as well as NOSGER global score correlated mildly ($r = -.3$ to $-.4$), as could be expected, with the MMSE score (Memory: $-.3$ and $-.4$, pre-and post-test respectively; Self-care: $-.4$, post-test; NOSGER—global score: $-.3$, pre-test). No other NOSGER score correlated with the MMSE. There was also no correlation between NOSGER scores and the age of patients. Cornell

TABLE 1
Pre- and post-treatment comparison of patient measures

	Pre-treatment	Follow-up	p*	Effect size
Cornell Scale (n = 41)				
Median (range)	10 (2–23)	5,5 (1–20)	< .001	1.2
Mean (SD)	9.8 (3.9)	5.1 (3.6)		
CERAD Behavior Rating Scale (n = 38)				
Median (range)	35 (14–78)	20 (5–60)	< .001	0.87
Mean (SD)	37.1 (16.3)	23 (12.7)		
NOSGER (n = 38)				
"Memory"				
Median (range)	16 (9–23)	14.5 (8–22)	n.s.	0.15
Mean (SD)	15.3 (3.9)	14.7 (3.9)		
IADL				
Median (range)	18 (9–24)	17 (10–23)	n.s.	0.15
Mean (SD)	17 (3.9)	16.4 (3.9)		
Self-Care				
Median (range)	8 (5–18)	8 (5–17)	n.s.	0
Mean (SD)	8.8 (3.4)	8.8 (2.8)		
Mood				
Median (range)	12 (5–18)	11 (5–20)	n.s.	0.21
Mean (SD)	11.7 (3.2)	11 (3.6)		
Social behaviour				
Median (range)	15 (8–24)	13 (5–21)	.01	0.27
Mean (SD)	14.8 (4.7)	13.5 (4.8)		
Disturbing behaviour				
Median (range)	9 (5–15)	8 (5–15)	.001	0.46
Mean (SD)	9.5 (2.6)	8.3 (2.6)		

* Wilcoxon Test. Higher values on the Cornell Scale (maximum 38) indicate more depressive symptoms. Higher values on the CERAD-Scale (maximum 160) indicate more psychopathological symptoms. Higher values on the NOSGER subscales (possible range: 5–25) indicate more disturbances in everyday life.

Scale scores and CERAD Behavior Rating Scale scores similarly showed no correlation with patients' age. The Cornell Scale score again showed no correlation with the MMSE score. CERAD follow-up score but not pre-treatment score correlated mildly ($r = -.4$) with the MMSE score.

To analyse the influence of medication with neuroleptics and antidepressants on general treatment effects we compared the psychopharmacologically treated (PT, $n = 17$) and non-psychopharmacologically-treated (PnT, $n = 26$) groups. In the PT group the mean MMSE score was significantly lower, and the BRSD score at pre-treatment and at follow-up was significantly higher. This suggests that the PT group included patients with more advanced dementia and with more affective and behavioural problems than did the PnT group.

NOSGER and CDS demonstrated no group differences. In both subgroups following treatment there were significant differences in the predicted direction on CDS (PT: $z = -3.417$, $p = .001$; PnT: $z = -4.294$, $p = .001$) and on BRSD (PT: $z = -2.667$, $p = .01$; PnT: $z = -3.637$, $p = .001$). NOSGER global score changed significantly at follow in the PnT group ($z = -2.421, p = .05$) but not in the PT group ($z = -1.227, p = .2$).

To analyse the influence of factors like the age of patients, stage of dementia and medical treatment on treatment effects we calculated an improvement index (II) as a difference between pre-treatment and follow-up scores on outcome measures. There was no correlation between II and either age or MMSE scores. There was no difference in II in the PT and PnT groups.

Caregivers

In the caregiver group a comparison between pre-treatment and follow-up showed the predicted effect on depression and mood state.

Lower CES-D scores at follow-up indicate a reduction of depressive symptoms in the caregiver group (Table 2). At admission 48% of the caregivers (13 individuals) showed scores above the critical cut-off point (for the German version: 23 points). At follow-up the number of participants above this cut-off fell to 15% (4 individuals).

Higher post-treatment scores on the subscales of the MDBF indicate better mood, lower mental fatigue and lower feelings of restlessness. Pre-post

TABLE 2
Pre- and post-treatment comparison of caregiver measures

	Pre-treatment	Follow-up	p*	Effect size
CES-D-Scale ($n = 27$)				
Median (range)	22 (2–40)	9 (0–39)	< .001	0.71
Mean (SD)	20.2 (11.2)	12.2 (9.9)		
MDBF ($n = 40$)				
Good vs. bad mood				
Median (range)	29.5 (10–40)	35 (10–40)	.01	0.43
Mean (SD)	28.8 (7.8)	32.2 (6.9)		
Alertness vs. tiredness				
Median (range)	25 (8–37)	31 (9–40)	.01	0.5
Mean (SD)	25.8 (7.8)	29.7 (8.3)		
Rest vs. restlessness				
Median (range)	27 (8–40)	32 (10–40)	.01	0.43
Mean (SD)	26.5 (8.3)	30.1 (7.7)		

*Wilcoxon Test. Higher values on the CES-D (maximum 63) indicate more depressive symptoms. Higher values on the MDBF-subscales (possible range: 8–40) indicate better mood states.

comparisons were statistically significant (Table 2; good vs. bad mood: $z = -3.005$, $p = .01$; alertness vs. mental fatigue: $z = -3.102$, $p = .01$; rest vs. restlessness: $z = -2.878$, $p = .01$).

With regard to effect size, Table 2 shows that large treatment effects were observed for caregivers' depression (CES-D) and moderate effects for mood, tiredness and restlessness (MDBF subscales).

Patients and caregivers

It could be expected that the well-being of caregivers depends to some degree on the affective and behavioural disturbances of the patients. On the other hand caregiver reports about patients' mood and behaviour can depend on caregivers' own well-being, and may be influenced by biases in perception. Correlations were used to analyse the relationship between caregivers' well-being and caregivers' reports of patients' symptoms.

At pre-treatment as well as at follow-up there were mild to moderate correlations between measures of caregivers' well-being (three MDBF subscales and CES-D) on the one hand and measures for patients disturbances (NOSGER global score and Cornell Depression Scale) on the other hand. Correlation quotients ranged from .3 to .7 in the expected direction. CERAD scores correlated only at post-treatment with CES-D scores. Additionally caregivers of patients who were treated psychopharmacologically (PT subgroup) showed significantly more depressive symptoms on CES-D than caregivers in the PnT subgroup at follow-up.

There were no correlations between caregivers' well-being at post-treatment and patients' improvement index.

DISCUSSION

We have reported an in-patient treatment programme for AD patients and their caregivers designed to reduce patients' loss of confidence in social interaction, withdrawal and isolation as well as to reduce patients' psychopathological symptoms such as depression, apathy, agitation, or aggression and to facilitate a means of participation in life which fits the level of the patient's competence. Caregiver intervention aimed to support their psychological well-being and to improve their competence to accompany the patient. In the present paper we report the basic concept of the therapy and preliminary results with a follow-up immediately after the treatment programme. Studies with follow-up intervals of some months and years are required to evaluate how enduring the results are in the home setting.

The results from this study showed—as predicted—a consistent improvement in patients' depression and in other psychopathological symptoms as assessed by caregivers reports on the questionnaire measures (Table 1).

The effect size indicators were moderate to large. Even small reductions in depression and in other psychopathological symptoms can be seen as beneficial for patients. In particular, the reduced number of patients with mild or moderate depression, as assessed by the Cornell Depression Scale, shows the clinical significance of the affective changes. At the same time a considerable proportion of patients (24%) show mild depressive symptoms also at follow-up (pre-treatment: 63%) and a few patients (7%) even moderate depression (pre-treatment: 36%). This demonstrates that the treatment was beneficial for many but not all patients and further studies are needed to understand more about the factors that influence outcome and how therapy methods can be improved. Psychopathological symptoms are common in a dementia population and their treatment is important because problematic behaviours are a major precipitating factor in the decision to institutionalise a dementia patient (Radebaugh, Buckholtz, & Khachaturian, 1996; Steele, Rovner, Chase, & Folstein, 1990; Swanwick, 1995), in long-term hospitalisation (Eastley & Mian, 1993; Shah, 1992) and in over-medication (Martin, McKenzie, & Ames, 1994; Shah, 1993).

The results also support the prediction that social behaviour improves, at least to a limited extent, following the rehabilitation programme. In further studies, social behaviour and patients' social participation should be evaluated in a more specific way. In the present study social behaviour was assessed with a subscale of the NOSGER, which is geared more towards a global assessment of patients' deficits.

Behavioural and affective symptoms (NOSGER, BRSD, CDS) as well as an improvement index for these measures showed no correlation with patients' age. This result suggests that even very elderly patients can benefit from the rehabilitation programme. The programme was tailored to the individual resources of patients and of their social networks. In this way the programme was adjusted to take account of age and one could expect effects which are not dependent on age. However, this result needs to be interpreted with caution because the proportion of patients aged 80 years and over was low, and the few "old old" participants are not likely to be representative for this age group. Further studies, including a larger sample of older patients, should address this practically important question. Unfortunately many medical doctors as well as non-professionals believe that positive treatment results can only be achieved, if at all, in younger patients. There is no evidence for these beliefs.

As could be expected, patients with lower MMSE scores were reported to have more memory problems on the NOSGER. There was also a slight tendency for patients with lower MMSE scores to have more psychopathological symptoms, as assessed by the BRSD. The incidence of behavioural symptoms is reported to be highest in moderate and severe dementia (Reisberg et al., 1989). Patients' depression (Cornell Scale) did not depend on the stage of dementia (MMSE).

The improvement index computed for the NOSGER, BRSD, and CDS did not correlate with the stage of dementia (MMSE). This result suggests that similar treatment effects can be reached in very mild, moderate, and severe dementia. Medical services often expect, that, if at all, only mild dementia patients can benefit from rehabilitation programmes. We have found, however, that even in the severe stages of dementia one can discover some possibilities by which to guide a patient to feel more like his or her usual self: with some dance steps, a favourite melody, or familiar landscape, depending on the patient's individual preferences, biography and remaining competence. In the later stages of dementia non-verbal forms of communication and experiences are of great importance. Additionally, the behaviour and affect of a patient depend to a considerable degree, even in the later stages of dementia, on the competence of the caregiver and can be influenced by support for the caregiver.

Patients with early dementia and caregivers are afraid that confrontation with the course of the disease, especially in a residential setting which includes patients with severe dementia, is more likely to increase than reduce the depression. Appropriate psychological help in coping with the progressive cognitive decline can however support the patient and integrate the confrontation experience into the coping strategies. Treatment programmes for patients in different dementia stages require further development.

The next question is the influence of medical treatment on the patients' improvement at follow-up. The subgroup of patients receiving antidepressant and/or neuroleptic medication (PT group) showed more advanced dementia (lower mean MMSE) and more affective and behavioural disturbances (higher CERAD scores) at both pre-treatment and follow-up. This last result is consistent with what might have been expected: Patients treated with antidepressant and/or neuroleptic medication have more psychopathological symptoms. An improvement (significantly lower NOSGER, CERAD, and CDS scores) could be demonstrated in both groups, which suggests that the therapy benefit was not likely to be caused only by psychopharmacological medication. The PT subgroup did not reach the level of the PnT group (higher CERAD scores at follow-up) which shows the limits of both medical treatment and rehabilitation programmes for patients with more severe affective and behavioural disturbances like fear or restlessness. Earlier studies have shown that pharmacological interventions can be effective in the treatment of psychiatric symptoms and disruptive behaviours in dementia patients but the improvement is often only modest (Cummings & Knopman, 1999; De Deyn et al., 1999; Defilippi & Crismon, 2000; Rabins, 1996). For optimal management of emotional and behavioural problems an integration of nonpharmacological approaches can help (Carlson, Fleming, Smith, & Evans, 1995; Forbes, 1998). Further studies are needed to determine what affective and behavioural symptoms are therapy-resistant and whether new therapy methods can help. It is interesting that in the

present study the differences between PT and PnT subgroups were evident on
the BRSD but not on the CDS. One explanation may be that the BRSD directly
assesses psychopathological ("psychiatric") symptoms, which may be more
therapy-resistant, whereas CDS evaluates depressive mood and depressive
reactions which may be easier to improve.

Medical treatment with acetylcholinesterase inhibitors varied according to
the needs of the particular patient. Most of the patients had already received
donezepil or rivastigmine for some months or years before admission, some
patients received this medication only after admission, and some (6 patients)
were not receiving acetylcholinesterase inhibitors because of side-effects. The
dose and the product were changed after admission in some patients. Given this
diversity, it is not possible to evaluate the influence of treatment with acetylcholinesterase inhibitors. The improvement demonstrated in our patients is
likely to be caused partly by medication with donezepil and rivastigmine.
A beneficial effect of cholinergic therapies has been demonstrated for cognitive and non-cognitive symptoms, although cognitive *improvement* has been
shown only in the initial phase of the therapy (Levy, Cummings, & Kahn-Rose,
1999).

In the present study the evaluation of patients' behaviour and affect was
based only on caregiver reports. It is important to consider whether changes in
caregivers' well-being influenced caregivers' perception of patients. We found
no correlation between changes in caregivers' self-reports (improvement index
for caregiver outcome measures) and reports about patients (improvement
index for patient outcome measures). No bias was identified in caregiver
reports, although this does not necessarily mean that none was present (see
below for discussion of placebo effects). In future research some additional
measures of patients' behaviour and well-being should be included, e.g., standardised behavioural observation.

Caregivers also reported an improvement in their own depression and mood.
After treatment, caregivers felt less depressed and restless, and more relaxed
(significantly lower scores on CES-D and higher scores on three MDBF
subscales; effect size indicators of 0.43 to –0.71, Table 2). In agreement with
other studies (Baumgarten et al., 1992; Clipp & George, 1990; Schneider,
Murray, Banerjee, & Mann, 1999; Wilz, Adler, Gunzelmann, & Brähler, 1999)
we found under pre-treatment conditions a large proportion (48%) of caregivers with critically high depression scores (CES-D), which were then significantly reduced (4 caregivers, 15%) at follow-up. The results also reveal a
relationship between patients' affective and behavioural symptoms and caregivers' well-being. Interestingly at follow-up (but not at pre-treatment) the
caregivers' well-being (especially the depression score) seemed to depend only
on patients' strictly psychopathological symptoms, as assessed with BRSD,
and not on depression and general decline as assessed with CDS and NOSGER.
Additionally, caregivers of the PT subgroup, with patients showing more

psychopathological symptoms in terms of BRSD both at pre-test and at follow-up, also demonstrated higher depression scores at follow-up than caregivers of PnT patients. This suggest that therapy-resistant caregiver depression can be induced by patients' therapy-resistant psychopathological symptoms.

The preliminary results reported here require replication in further controlled studies, but they do support the effectiveness of the treatment programme, which combines standard treatments with new methods, and a new therapeutic approach in a new setting.

The effectiveness of the programme will need to be proven in controlled studies. We do not claim that the programme is generally superior to standard methods, which are far less intensive and are delivered mainly in out-patient settings. What kind of help the family needs depends on the individual problems and resources of the family (Baier & Romero, 2000). We suggest, however, that a high proportion of patients and caregivers have psychological and/or psychiatric problems that can be treated effectively.

In the absence of a control group there are only limited possibilities to determine whether an observed improvement was a function of specific factors (e.g., specific therapeutic interventions like art therapy or psychological support for coping with the disease, stimulating social activities, and medication) or rather of factors such as statistical regression to the mean or placebo effects. Placebo effects could result from the caregivers' expectation for improvement, demand characteristics (i.e., the implicit pressure engendered by the situation for caregivers to behave in accordance with what is expected of them), therapists' enthusiasm and support, the therapist–caregiver alliance, and effort justification, i.e., the tendency to report positive changes in order to justify the effort exerted. However, in addition to self-rated distress, caregivers also reported patients' symptoms and a pattern of improvement which can be interpreted as meaningful. As could be expected from Alzheimer's disease patients, caregivers reported an improvement in patients' affect and behavioural disturbances but not in memory and everyday functional ability (significant pre- to post-treatment differences on all outcome measures except the NOSGER Memory, IADL and Self-Care subscales). Additionally, caregivers' perception of patients' memory problems as assessed with the NOSGER Memory subscale correlated with MMSE score, which is an objective measure of patients' cognitive decline (inclusive of memory). Finally, caregivers reported significantly more psychopathological symptoms in the patients who were treated with antidepressant and/or neuroleptic medication, which validates the caregivers' reports. Taken together these results suggest that specific factors outperformed placebo effects at least partially in the present study. Controlled studies are needed to support the preliminary results presented here and to address hypotheses about factors responsible for benefits as well as for therapy resistance. The concept of self-maintenance therapy allowed a prediction, that experiences which are in accordance with patients' self-structures and self-processes support patients' well-being, reduce psychopathological symptoms, and facilitate social participation.

REFERENCES

Aldridge, D. (1994). Alzheimer's disease: Rhythm, timing and music as therapy. *Biomedicine and Pharmacotherapy*, *48*, 275–281.

Alexopoulos, G.S., Abrams, R.C., Young, R.C., & Shamoian, C.A. (1988). Cornell scale for depression in dementia. *Biological Psychiatry*, *23*, 271–284.

Antonovsky, A. (1979). *Health, stress and coping: New perspectives on mental and physical well-being*. San Francisco, CA: Jossey-Bass.

Antonovsky, A. (1987). *Unravelling the mystery of health. How people manage stress and stay well*. San Francisco, CA: Jossey-Bass.

Bäckman, L. (1992). Memory training and memory improvement in Alzheimer's disease: Rules and exceptions. *Acta Neurologica Scandinavica, 85 (Suppl. 139)*, 84–89.

Baier, B., & Romero, B. (2000). Rehabilitationsprogramme und psychoedukative Ansätze für Demenzkranke und betreuende Angehörige. In H. Förstl (Ed.), *Demenzen in Theorie und Praxis* (pp. 385–404). Berlin: Springer-Verlag.

Bauer, J. (1994). *Die Alzheimer-Krankheit. Neurobiologie, Psychosomatik, Diagnostik und Therapie*. Stuttgart: Schattauer.

Bauer, J. (1998). Interpersonal psychotherapy in the early stages of Alzheimer's disease: A potential remedy for dysfunctional interpersonal relations and self-imposed mental de-activation. *European Archives of Psychiatry and Clinical Neuroscience, 248 (Suppl 1)*, 12–13, A.

Baumgarten, M., Battista, R.N., Infante-Rivard, C., Hanley, J.A., Becker, R., & Gauthier, S. (1992). The psychological and physical health of family members caring for an elderly person with dementia. *Journal of Clinical Epidemiology, 45*, 61–70.

Beatty, W.W. (1999). Preserved cognitive skills in dementia: Implications for geriatric medicine. *Journal of the Oklahoma State Medical Association, 92*, 10–12.

Brodaty, H., Gresham, M., & Luscombe, G. (1997). The Prince Henry Hospital dementia caregivers' training programme. *International Journal of Geriatric Psychiatry, 12*, 183–192.

Broe, G.A., Henderson, A.S., Creasey, H., McCusker, E., Korten, A.E., Jorm, A.F., Longley, W., & Anthony, J.C. (1990). A case-control study of Alzheimer's disease in Australia. *Neurology, 40*, 1698–1707.

Carlson, D.L., Fleming, K.C., Smith, G.L., & Evans, J.M. (1995). Management of dementia-related behavioral disturbances: A nonpharmacologic approach. *Mayo Clinic Proceedings, 70*, 1108–1115.

Clare, L. (1999). Memory rehabilitation in early dementia. *Journal of Dementia Care, 7(6)*, 33–38.

Clare, L., Wilson, B.A., Carter, G., Breen, K., Gosses, A., & Hodges, J.R. (2000). Intervening with everyday memory problems in dementia of Alzheimer type: An errorless learning approach. *Journal of Clinical and Experimental Neuropsychology, 22*, 132–146.

Clipp, E.C., & George, L. (1990). Psychotropic drug use among caregivers of patients with dementia. *Journal of the American Geriatrics Society, 38*, 227–235.

Cohen, D., & Eisdorfer, C. (1986). *The loss of self: A family resource for the care of Alzheimer's disease and related disorders*. New York: Norton.

Corey-Bloom, J., Anand, R., & Veach, J. for the ENA 713 B352 Study Group (1998). A randomized trial evaluating the efficacy and safety of ENA 713 (rivastigmine tartrate), a new acetylcholinesterase inhibitor, in patients with mild to moderately severe Alzheimer's disease. *International Journal of Geriatric Psychopharmacology, 1*, 55–65.

Cummings, J.L., & Knopman, D. (1999). Advances in the treatment of behavioral disturbances in Alzheimer's disease. *Neurology, 53*, 899–901.

De Deyn, P.P., Rabheru, K., Rasmussen, A., Bocksberger, J.P., Dautzenberg, P.I.J., Eriksson, S., & Lawlor, B.A. (1999). A randomized trial of risperidone, placebo, and haloperidol for behavioral symptoms of dementia. *Neurology*, *53*, 946–955

Defilippi, J.L., & Crismon, M.L. (2000). Antipsychotic agents in patients with dementia. *Pharmacotherapy*, *1*, 23–33.

Eastley, R.J., & Mian, I.H. (1993). Physical assaults by psychogeriatric patients. Patients characteristics and implications for placement. *International Journal of Geriatric Psychiatry*, *8*, 515–520.

Epstein, S. (1979). Entwurf einer integrativen Persönlichkeitstheorie. In S.H. Filipp (Ed.), *Selbstkonzeptforschung*. Stuttgart: Klett-Cotta.

Folstein, M.F., Folstein, S.E., & McHugh (1975). Mini Mental State. A practical method for grading the cognitive state of patients for the clinician. *Journal of Psychiatric Research*, *12*, 189–198.

Forbes, D.A. (1998). Strategies for managing behavioral symptomatology associated with dementia of the Alzheimer type: A systematic overview. *Canadian Journal of Nursing Research*, *30*, 67–86.

Friedland, R.P., Smyth, K., Esteban-Santillan, C., Koss, E., Cole, R., Lerner, A.J., Strauss, M.S., Whitehouse, P.J., Petot, G., Rowland, D.Y., & Debanne, S. (1996). Premorbid environmental complexity is reduced in patients with Alzheimer's disease (AD) as compared to age and sex matched controls: Results of a case-control study. *Neurobiology of Aging*, *17*, *Suppl*, 122, A.

Goode, K.T., Haley, W.E., Roth, D.L., & Ford, G.R. (1998). Predicting longitudinal changes in caregiver physical and mental health. A stress process model. *Health Psychology*, *17*, 190–198.

Greenwald, A.G., & Pratkanis, A.R. (1984). The Self. In R.S. Wyer & T.K. Srull (Eds.), *Handbook of social cognition*. Hillsdale, NJ: Lawrence Erlbaum Associates Inc.

Hautzinger, M., & Bailer, M. (1993). *Allgemeine-Depressions-Skala (ADS)*. Weinheim: Beltz Test.

Havens, B.J. (1968). An investigation of activity patterns and adjustment in an aging population. *Gerontologist*, *8*, 201–206.

Heiss, W.D., Kessler, J., & Mielke, R. (1994). Long-term effects of phosphatidylserine, pyritinol and cognitive training in Alzheimers disease. *Dementia*, *5*, 88–98.

Hirsch, R.D. (1994). *Psychotherapie bei Demenzen*. Darmstadt: Steinkopff.

Hofmann, M., Hock C., Kuhler A., & Müller-Spahn, F. (1996). Interactive computer-based cognitive training in patients with Alzheimer's disease. *Journal of Psychiatric Research*, *30*, 493–501.

Levy, M.L., Cummings, J.L., & Kahn-Rose, R. (1999). Neuropsychiatric symptoms and cholinergic therapy for Alzheimer's disease. *Gerontology*, *45 (Suppl 1)*, 15–22.

Lyman, K.A. (1998). Living with Alzheimer's disease: The creation of meaning among persons with dementia. *Journal of Clinical Ethics*, *9*, 49–57.

McKittrick, L.A., Camp J.C., & Black, F.W. (1992). Prospective memory intervention in Alzheimer's disease. *Journal of Gerontology*, *47*, 337–343.

Martin, C., McKenzie, S., & Ames, D. (1994). Disturbed behaviour in dementia sufferers: A comparison of three nursing home settings. *International Journal of Geriatric Psychiatry*, *9*, 393–398.

Mittelman, M.S., Ferris, S.H., Shulman, E., Steinberg, G., & Levin, B. (1996). A family intervention to delay nursing home placement of patients with Alzheimer disease. A randomised controlled trial. *JAMA*, *276*, 1725–1731.

Motomura, N., Ohkubo, F., Asano, A., Tomoda, Y., Akagi, H., & Seo, T. (1996). Premorbid behavioral characters in demented patients. *Neurobiology of Aging*, *17*, *(Suppl)*, 122, A.

Palo-Bengtsson, L., Winblad, B., & Ekman, S.L. (1998). Social dancing: A way to support intellectual, emotional and motor functions in persons with dementia. *Journal of Psychiatric and Mental Health Nursing*, *5*, 545–554.

354   ROMERO AND WENZ

Petry, H. (1999). Support groups for patients in the early stage of dementia—usefulness and experiences. *Therapeutische Umschau, 56,* 109–113.

Rabins, P.V. (1996). Developing treatment guidelines for Alzheimer's disease and other dementias. *Journal of Clinical Psychiatry, 57, Suppl 14,* 37–38.

Radebaugh, T.S., Buckholtz, N., & Khachaturian, Z. (1996). Behavioral approaches to the treatment of Alzheimer's disease: Research strategies. *International Psychogeriatrics, 8, Suppl 1,* 7–12.

Radebold, H. (1994). Das Konzept der Regression: Ein Zugang zu spezifischen, bei dementiellen Prozessen beobachtenden Phänomenen. In R.D. Hirsch (Ed.), *Psychotherapie bei Demenzen.* Darmstadt: Steinkopff.

Radloff, L.S. (1977). The CES-D scale: A self-report depression scale for research in the general population. *Applied Psychological Measurement, 3,* 385–401.

Reisberg, B., Franssen, E., Sclan, S.G., Kluger, A., & Ferris, S.H. (1989). Stage specific incidence of potentially remediable behavioral symptoms in aging and Alzheimer's disease. *Bulletin of Clinical Neurosciences, 54,* 95–112.

Riederer, E. (1999). *Explorative Entwicklung informationstechnischer Innovationen. Systemenetwürfe von Therapie- und Alltagshilfen für Menschen mit Demenz.* Aachen: Shaker Verlag.

Rogers, S.L., & Friedhoff, L.T. (1998). Long-term efficacy and safety of donepezil in the treatment of Alzheimer's disease: An interim analysis of the results of a US multicentre open label extension study. *European Neuropsychopharmacology, 8,* 67–75.

Romero B. (1997). Selbst-Erhaltungs-Therapie (SET): Betreuungsprinzipien, psychotherapeutische Interventionen und Bewahren des Selbstwissens bei Alzheimer-Kranken. In S. Weis & G. Weber (Eds.), *Handbuch Morbus Alzheimer. Neurobiologie, Diagnose und Therapie* (pp. 1209–1252). Weinheim: Beltz PVU.

Romero, B., & Eder, G. (1992). Selbst-Erhaltungs-Therapie (SET): Konzept einer neuropsychologischen Therapie bei Alzheimer-Kranken. *Zeitschrift für Gerontopsychologie und -psychiatrie, 5,* 267–282.

Romero, B., & Wenz, M. (2000): Wie kann das Beste erhalten bleiben: Vorbereitung auf das Leben mit fortschreitender Demenz sowie Behandlungskonzept im Alzheimer Therapiezentrum Bad Aibling. In Deutsche Alzheimer Gesellschaft (Ed.), *Fortschritte und Defizite im Problemfeld Demenz. Referate auf dem 2. Kongreß der Deutschen Alzheimer Gesellschaft, Berlin, 9.–11. September 1999* (pp. 111–121). Berlin: Deutsche Alzheimer Gesellschaft.

Ronch, J.L. (1993). *Alzheimer's disease. A practical guide for families and other caregivers.* New York: Crossroad.

Schneider, J., Murray, J., Banerjee, S., & Mann, A. (1999). Eurocare: A cross-national study of co-resident spouse carers for people with Alzheimer's disease: I—Factors associated with carer burden. *International Journal of Geriatric Psychiatry, 14,* 651–661.

Shah, A.K. (1992). Violence and psychogeriatric inpatients. *International Journal of Geriatric Psychiatry, 7,* 39–44

Shah, A.K. (1993). Aggressive behaviour among patients referred to a psychogeriatric service. *Medicine, Science and the Law, 33,* 144–150.

Spiegel, R., Brunner, C., Ermini-Fünfschilling, D., Monsch, A., Notter, M., Puxty, J., & Tremmel, L. (1991). A new behavioral assessment scale for geriatric out- and in-patients: The NOSGER (Nurses' Observation Scale for Geriatric Patients). *Journal of the American Geriatrics Society, 39,* 339–347.

Steele, C., Rovner, B., Chase, G.A., & Folstein, M. (1990). Psychiatric symptoms and nursing home placement of patients with Alzheimer's disease. *American Journal of Psychiatry, 147,* 1049–1051.

Steyer, R., Schwenkmezger, P., Notz, P., & Eid, M. (1997). *Der Mehrdimensionale Befindlichkeitsfragebogen (MDBF).* Göttingen: Hogrefe.

Swanwick, G.R.J. (1995). Nonpharmacological treatment of behavioral symptoms. In B.A. Lawlor (Ed.), *Behavioral complications in Alzheimer's disease. Clinical Practice*. Washington: American Psychiatric Press.

Tariot, P.N., Mack, J.L., Patterson, M.B., Edland, S.D., Weiner, M.F., Fillenbaum, G., Blazina, L., Teri, L., Rubin, E., Mortimer, J.A., & the CERAD Behavioral Pathology Committee (1995). The Behavior Rating Scale for Dementia of the Consortium to Establish a Registry for Alzheimer's Disease. *American Journal of Psychiatry, 152*, 1349–1357.

Teri, L., & Lodgson, R.G. (1991). Identifying pleasant activities for Alzheimer's disease patients: The Pleasant Events Schedule—AD. *Gerontologist, 31*, 124–127.

Urbas, S. (2000). Kunsttherapie mit Demenzkranken. In Deutsche Alzheimer Gesellschaft (Ed.), *Fortschritte und Defizite im Problemfeld Demenz. Referate auf dem 2. Kongreß der Deutschen Alzheimer Gesellschaft, Berlin, 9.–11. September 1999* (pp. 179–187). Berlin: Deutsche Alzheimer Gesellschaft.

Wilz, G., Adler, C., Gunzelmann, T., & Brähler, E. (1999). Auswirkungen chronischer Belastungen auf die physische und psychische Befindlichkeit—Eine Prozeßanalyse bei pflegenden Angehörigen von Demenzkranken. *Zeitschrift für Gerontologie und Geriatrie, 32*, 255–265.

Woods, R.T. (1996). Psychological "therapies" in dementia. In R.T. Woods (Ed.) *Handbook of Clinical Psychology of Ageing*. Chichester, UK: Wiley.

Manuscript received October 2000
Revised manuscript received January 2001

Behavioural difficulties and cued recall of adaptive behaviour in dementia: Experimental and clinical evidence

Michael Bird

Centre for Mental Health Research, Australian National University, Canberra, Australia

The remarkably widespread belief that people with dementia are incapable of new learning is manifestly false. Results are briefly reviewed of experimental list-learning findings, based on the levels of processing framework, which suggest ways to optimise a grossly impaired but still residual capacity to learn limited amounts of new information in mild to moderate dementia. Studies of a more clinical bent are dealt with in some detail, demonstrating that is possible to utilise the methods of *spaced retrieval* and *fading cues* to train persons with dementia to associate a behaviour with contextual cues, and retain the information over time. Two case studies are also presented to illustrate clinical application to serious behavioural problems in dementia. It is suggested that research such as this, at the problem-specific level, may be more relevant for cognitive and behavioural scientists at this stage of the research enterprise than attempts, so far unsuccessful, to produce generalised cognitive improvement of any practical value in dementia.

INTRODUCTION

Despite many years of effort, from the heyday of classroom reality orientation to the present, there is still no convincing evidence that exposing people with dementia to cognitive exercises presumed to stimulate or retrain cerebral processes has any effect on the manifold practical problems they daily

Correspondence should be sent to M. Bird, Centre for Mental Health Research, Australian National University, Canberra, ACT 0200, Australia.

Grateful acknowledgement is due to the Commonwealth Government Office for Older Australians for financial support, and the willing participation of all the people with dementia and their carers who contributed to experimental and clinical work undertaken by the author and described in this paper.

encounter—presumably the goal of rehabilitation. Gains, where they occur, are small, usually limited to one or two cognitive tests, rarely persist, and can often be attributed to artefacts of the training procedure (Bird, 2000; Bowlby, 1998; Godfrey & Knight, 1987; Pliskin, Cunningham, Remondet-Wall, & Cassisi, 1996). Few studies assess whether there is any generalisation to real-life problems, for example, anxious or depressed mood, activities of daily living, or frequency of behavioural problems (e.g., Beck et al., 1988), or do so and find no effect (e.g., Breuil et al., 1994; Zanetti et al., 1995). Quayhagen et al. (1995), who trained family carers to deliver regular cognitive exercises, did find a reduction in behaviour problems but there was an equal reduction in a "placebo" control group.

A few authors have suggested that the problem is insensitive instruments (e.g., Breuil et al., 1994; Zanetti et al., 1995). This still places the onus of proof on researchers whose definition of rehabilitation extends beyond adding a few points to the odd neuropsychological test. At present, the most parsimonious explanation seems to be that the multiple and interacting affective, cognitive, and behavioural problems caused by dementing illnesses are impervious to the small gains occasionally produced by efforts to provide generalised improvement by cognitive exercise.

The work reported here, which concentrated on memory in dementia, attempted not restitution of lost function but better use of what was left. That is, it was based, not on attempts to increase memory capacity in dementia, but on assisting clinicians to tap into the grossly damaged but still partially intact capacity for new learning which often remains until at least the middle stages of dementia.

BACKGROUND: LIST-LEARNING STUDIES

In the late 1970s, cognitive psychologists started applying the levels of processing framework (Craik & Lockhart, 1972) to memory in dementia, using predominantly persons suffering from Alzheimer's disease. This framework posits that entry of new information into memory and its subsequent use is a multi-stage process whose efficiency is heavily dependent upon context. Contextual variables include the nature of the to-be-learned material, the way it is presented, and information available at the time the material must be retrieved from memory (Jacoby & Craik, 1979; Mitchell, 1989). The model of learning used almost exclusively has been a simple three-stage process: initial *acquisition* of the material, *retention* in memory over time, and *retrieval* from memory (Figure 1). The usual paradigm has involved acquisition of lists of words, pictures, objects, or motor actions under various experimental conditions, and then requiring the subject to retrieve as much of the list as possible, also under various conditions.

In summary, the results of these studies show that persons with dementia are impervious to more subtle aspects of the material, but that there are a number of

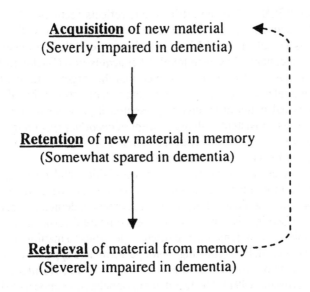

Acquisition of new material
(Severly impaired in dementia)

Retention of new material in memory
(Somewhat spared in dementia)

Retrieval of material from memory
(Severely impaired in dementia)

Figure 1.   Simple process model used in much dementia learning research.

contextual manipulations that can produce enhanced although still grossly impaired learning in at least mild to moderate dementia (for reviews, see Bäckman, 1992; Bäckman & Small, 1998). The most critical contextual variable for the purposes of this paper is the way the material is presented. It is essential for the experimenter or clinician actively to provide assistance at both acquisition and retrieval. There are profound deficits at both these stages of the learning process in the most common dementias (Bird & Luszcz, 1991; Diesfeldt, 1984; Tuokko & Crockett, 1989).

The usual assistance at acquisition has involved either multiple presentations or, more efficiently, presenting the material in a way that requires the subject to think beyond its face attributes. For example, assume that subjects with dementia are in the process of learning a list item, "elephant", by locating it in an array of pictures—thus ensuring attention. They are more likely later to be able to remember it if they are asked to find the "animal" and then to name it, rather than simply to find the "elephant" then name it (Bird & Luszcz, 1991; Diesfeldt, 1984). Forcing the subject to link the category—a contextual cue— with the target word during acquisition is consistent both with the notion of *cognitive effort* (Hasher & Zacks, 1979), and *elaborative processing* (Jacoby & Craik, 1979). Both are known to facilitate laying down accessible memory traces in normal subjects.

At retrieval, the assistance has been either forced choice recognition or, more commonly, the provision of cues to assist recall. An example might be a card showing "ELE ...". If the retrieval cue reflects features of the material highlighted at acquisition, successful recall is even more likely. For example, the efficacy as a recall cue of "ELE ..." will be greater if the written form of the target word, "elephant", has been involved at acquisition (Bäckman & Small, 1998; Bird & Luszcz, 1993). It is assumed that the target word and the high-lighted contextual material are encoded together in memory. When the same or similar contextual material is later re-presented it provides a more efficient recall cue. This is consistent with the concept of *encoding specificity* (Tulving, 1983); the more the context at retrieval resembles the context at initial acquisition, the greater the chance of successful recall.

The need for active assistance at both acquisition and retrieval, and the finding that the principles of elaborative processing, effortful processing, and encoding specificity appear to hold up to some extent in dementia, are central to the work described in this paper. One further contextual variable is of interest. Although subjects with dementia are often impervious to manipulations in the nature of the material, lists requiring motor performance appear easier for them to learn than lists of words (Bäckman & Nilsson, 1985; Herlitz, Adolfsson, Bäckman, & Nilsson, 1991). The fact that motor behaviour appears to be intrin-sically more memorable is of obvious importance in clinical application. It is behaviour that causes most problems in management of dementia (Donaldson, Tarrier, & Burns, 1997; Hagen & Sayers, 1995; MacPherson, Eastley, Richards, & Mian, 1994). In addition, there are a number of anecdotal accounts in the clinical literature that motor performance assists learning or re-learning of required tasks in dementia, for example, finding a location, or activities of daily living (e.g., Hanley, 1981; McEvoy & Patterson, 1986).

With regard to the middle stage of the model in Figure 1—retention of material in memory—most studies have tested retrieval only a few minutes after acquisition. Findings would therefore be of limited clinical utility unless there was evidence that subjects are able to retain new information from at least one day to the next. Fortunately, studies using forced choice recognition to assist retrieval several days after repeated trials to establish learning to criterion, have shown savings in persons with mild to moderate dementia (Hart, Kwentus, Taylor, & Harkin, 1987; Kopelman, 1985). That is, if sufficient acquisition support can be provided in the clinical setting, the material may be accessible in memory long enough to be of practical use, provided sufficient retrieval support is also available when the information is required.

SPACED RETRIEVAL AND FADING CUES

In the 1980s, Camp and associates began to experiment with the method of spaced retrieval to assist persons with dementia to acquire individual items of new information, rather than lists (for review, see Camp, Bird, & Cherry, 2000). Originally developed in the educational setting, the method capitalises on a well-established finding that learning trials where the information is simply repeated are less effective than learning trials that require subjects to remember the material for themselves (Bjork, 1988; Izawa, 1992). That is, the act of retrieval in itself is also an aid to acquisition. Each time information is successfully retrieved from memory it is, *de facto*, a fresh encoding of that material. Figure 1 is thus a circular and potentially continuous process, rather than a linear one. We may call this the *retrieval effect*. In addition, spacing trials as opposed to presenting them in rapid succession also has a mnemonic effect (Dempster, 1988). In both spacing and retrieval conditions, the less recognisable or accessible the material is on each trial, the better the effect, with cognitive effort posited by some authors as the causal mechanism in facilitating learning (Bjork & Bjork, 1992; Cuddy & Jacoby, 1982; Dellarosa & Bourne, 1985; Izawa, 1992).

The problem ingeniously overcome by Camp and associates in adapting spaced retrieval for dementia was that of ensuring, in a population partially defined by profound retrieval deficits, sufficient successful retrieval trials reliably to assist acquisition and consolidation of an accessible memory trace. The usual method is as follows. Subjects are presented with the material to be learned, for example: "Look at your calendar to help you remember what to do each day" (Camp, Foss, Stevens, & O'Hanlon, 1996). They are then immediately asked: "How will you remember what to do each day?" Assuming success, the next trial would be after about 20 seconds and the next after 40 seconds. Spacing between trials is thus progressively increased but with the process tailored to the subject's learning rate (See Figure 2). Where failure occurs (trials 5, 8, 9, and 10), the subject is reminded of the answer (e.g., "Go look at your calendar"), and spacing dropped back until the subject is again successful.

The process then continues based on the logic that, as each successful retrieval is a fresh and effective re-encoding of the material, the memory trace should be progressively strengthened until it is possible to build up to clinically significant intervals. Figure 2 shows 20 trials to consolidate the memory so that the subject can retain it unassisted for 4 minutes. Camp notes that, by this stage, the memory is often relatively secure, with savings apparent even after several days (Camp et al., 1996; 2000).

It is important to note that Camp and colleagues apply dementia-specific clinical realism to their work, and incorporate features somewhat removed from the tightly controlled laboratory conditions of much cognitive research. For example, with the study described above, the calendar was not abstract experimental information sprung on the subject at the time of testing. Each subject had already been made familiar with a large simplified one-day-a-page calendar and its location in the house. That is, the encoding context had been made as favourable as possible. The critical task, however, was to determine whether it was possible to induce persons with Alzheimer's disease to associate

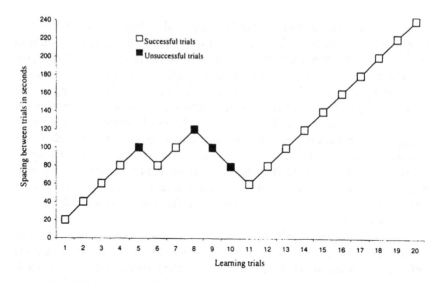

Figure 2. Representation of a spaced retrieval learning session for a subject with dementia. (After Camp et al., 1996.)

the desire to remember what to do with going to the calendar. The authors were successful with 75% of a sample of subjects with mild to moderate Alzheimer's disease in developing at least partial spontaneous calendar use, although spouses remained responsible for changing the page each day. More broadly, Camp and associates have repeatedly demonstrated the effectiveness of spaced retrieval as an acquisition aid in dementia (Camp et al., 2000). Foley (1996) has shown that both spacing and retrieval are necessary to the process.

Bird and Kinsella (1996) further developed this approach, both experimentally and clinically. In an explicit attempt to marry list-learning findings with direct clinical relevance, they trained subjects with Alzheimer's disease or vascular dementia to associate a tangible cue, for example, a beeper or a large word on a card, with a motor action, for example, opening a notebook. That is, acquisition of the task was explicitly contextual; the beeper or word became a contextual cue that was encoded together with the to-be-remembered task. Consistent with the principle of encoding specificity, the same contextual cue was to be the primary means to prompt later recall of the motor action.

The acquisition process consisted of repeated retrieval trials, but far fewer than in Figure 2, because spaced retrieval was supplemented with the method of fading cues (Moffat, 1992). This process is consistent with the concept of *errorless learning*. Learning support is manipulated to guarantee that the correct information, and only the correct material, is acquired on most trials (e.g., Clare, Wilson, Breen, & Hodges, 1999; Wilson, Baddeley, Evans, &

Shiel, 1994). Incorrect material generated by the patient tends to be rather salient and hard to shift (see Case 2 later).

Thus, in Bird and Kinsella (1996), when a subject failed to respond to the primary cue (e.g., the beeper) on any one trial or gave the wrong answer, it was assumed that it was a retrieval problem, not that the information was necessarily lost. Subjects were given supplementary elaborative cues, graded in the amount of help they provided, until they did remember the answer, for example: "Open the notebook". That is, elaborative contextual material was provided, but only the minimum required for successful retrieval, so the process was still assumed to be effortful. Only where subjects failed forced-choice recognition was it assumed that the information was lost; subjects were then given forced choice recognition with the correct answer heavily highlighted. With successful subjects, the number of supplementary cues required tended to diminish ("fade") as the memory consolidated, and retrieval became more automatic. To illustrate the process, Figure 3 shows the learning curves of two subjects being trained to open a notebook when a beeper sounded. Following initial successful trials AB, the less impaired subject as determined by a score of 19 on the Mini-Mental State Exam (MMSE; Folstein, Folstein, & McHugh, 1975), can be seen having difficulty after a delay of only one minute. The beeper sounded and she could not remember what it meant. The

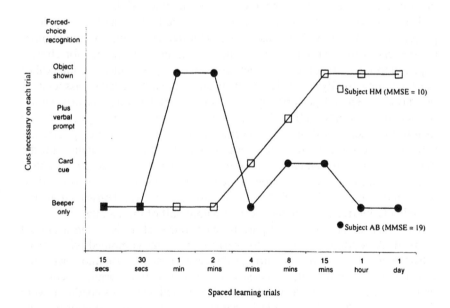

Figure 3. Progress of two subjects with dementia learning to associate a beeper with opening a notebook (Bird & Kinsella, 1996).

experimenter then raised a card showing NOTEBOOK but she still failed, and failed again when the experimenter said: "When you hear this beep you have to do something with a notebook." It was only when the subject was actually shown the notebook that she remembered the task. However, learning was still taking place. After the two-minute trial she had few problems, requiring the card prompt at most. One day later, she required only the beeper. By contrast, the much more impaired subject HM (MMSE = 10) got off to a good start, but thereafter needed more and more contextual cues until he levelled off at the 15-minute interval trial. One day later, he retained an accessible trace, but still needed to see the notebook before he could retrieve the task from memory.

Like subject AB, 12 out of 24 subjects taking part in this procedure could recall the task one day after the learning session requiring only the primary cue (e.g., the beeper). That is, although many could recall neither the learning process nor ever having seen the experimenter before, when the beeper sounded they remembered the task. Four required supplementary cues like subject HM, and eight had no retrievable memory of the task. Although higher functioning subjects were more likely to be successful after one day with the primary cue alone, some failed completely. Conversely, subjects with an MMSE score as low as 12 succeeded with the primary cue alone. One subject (MMSE = 12) failed on all experimental tasks, but proved responsive to clinical adaptation of the technique to ameliorate a severe behavioural problem, including violence (Bird, Alexopoulos, & Adamowicz, 1995).

Bird and Kinsella (1996) replicated these results with another sample of persons with Alzheimer's disease or vascular dementia, and examined other parameters of the learning process. The most important findings for clinical application were, first, that if subjects could work up to a retention interval of one hour, they usually still had a retrievable memory of the cue/task association one day later. Second, performing the task on each trial produced an effect independent of the retrieval effect. That is, retrieval was not necessary for subjects to link the beeper with the task, provided they were given the opportunity actually to perform it when the beeper sounded. This is consistent with the known sensitivity in dementia to the mnemonic advantage of task performance (Herlitz et al., 1991). Observation of the task only, without the opportunity to perform it, was much less effective in the absence of retrieval on each trial, and completely ineffective with the more impaired half of the sample.

However, even with motor performance, retrieval trials added a crucial element. A condition where motor performance was combined with verbal retrieval on each trial, thus requiring subjects to recall the task into consciousness before performing it, was easily the most effective learning method in practical terms. One day later, subjects who learned under this condition were far more likely to perform the task spontaneously on presentation of the cue. This would be a minimum requirement in the clinical setting; ability to remember an association is only of value if the subject also acts on that association. For this reason, in clinical work, it is important to induce the subject actually to perform the task on as many retrieval trials as practicable.

CLINICAL APPLICATION

It is impossible to open a book on management of dementia without seeing a lot about environmental cues. On the other hand, it is very rare to find mention of the fundamental point that a cue is utterly useless unless the person with dementia knows or can easily work out what it means. For example, in Australia it has become popular to paint toilet doors in special care units a different colour, a practice probably more therapeutic for interior designers than people with dementia. A red door is just a red door without the association in memory: "Red door = toilet". In now little cited but important studies two decades ago, Gilleard, Mitchell, and Riordan (1981) and Hanley (1981) showed that much more obvious cues were ineffective with confused patients unless they were trained, using motor performance, to use them.

The nature of the experimental tasks in Bird and Kinsella (1996) represented an explicit attempt to discover whether it was possible to assist persons with dementia to learn to associate a specific cue with a specific behaviour, and then retain the association over clinically significant intervals. Flexibly adapted by clinicians who are familiar with this population, the paradigm has proved to have fairly direct transfer to selected cases of severe behavioural problems in dementia. The cue becomes a retrieval prompt, not only for more adaptive behaviour to be recalled, but also for when it must be recalled.

Problems addressed have included obsessive toileting, incontinence, sexual assault, intrusive behaviour, and violence (Alexopoulos, 1994; Bird, 1998; Bird et al., 1995). In each case, patients with dementia have been taught, using the method of spaced retrieval and fading cues, to associate a cue with a behaviour or information affecting behaviour. Performance of the task on as many trials as possible has also been encouraged.

Based upon idiosyncratic requirements of the case profile, manipulation of the association, once learned, has usually permitted amelioration of the problem, with gains mostly maintained as long as the cue or cues remained available. This is consistent with the circular process illustrated in Figure 1. Because of the retrieval effect, each successful encounter with the cue acts as a new acquisition trial, helping to maintain the association between the cue and the behaviour. Two cases are presented here as illustration.

Case 1

An 83-year-old hostel resident with mild Alzheimer's disease (MMSE = 19) was referred for "paranoid delusions" and violence. The "delusions" related to a belief that staff had stolen her belongings and the violence occurred when, with increasing exasperation, they denied this. The language of psychosis was irrelevant although it could easily have led to use of antipsychotics, and usually does in dementia (Devanand & Levy, 1995; Elmståhl, Stenberg, Annerstedt, & Ingvad, 1998; Furniss, Lloyd Craig, & Burns, 1998). In fact this patient, a relatively new resident, was making a mistake because of cognitive impairment. She had lost memory for how she had disposed of her belongings, and found angry staff assertions that she had given most things away extremely implausible.

She was assisted to dimly recall the disposal process with the help of a trusted relative and multiple contextual cues (e.g., "Do you remember that rainy day we went to the Salvation Army to give them your sewing machine, and the struggle we had to get it out of the car?"). A list was then produced of where her most loved things had gone, which she signed. The next day, a poster-sized version was produced, embellished with a red smiley face as an extra contextual cue to assist the acquisition process. The goal was to assist her to acquire into memory the fact that the list was available to her every time she wondered about her belongings. The process is described in some detail later, to illustrate the clinical flexibility required within the basic paradigm.

The poster-sized list was first gone through and animatedly discussed in order to: (1) ensure that she still trusted it as a true document; (2) increase its familiarity; (3) help the patient herself arrive at the idea that the list would help her be less worried about where her belongings had gone; and (4) help her decide where to post it up in the room. This was done with some ceremony to make it more memorable.

Having made the context for learning as favourable as possible, including the establishment of collaborative rapport, she was then easily taught by the methods of spaced retrieval and fading cues to go to the poster each time she worried about or missed her belongings. Learning trials would be set off by questions such as: "What do you do when you worry about where your things have gone?", or, "What did you do with your sewing machine before you came in here?" If she could not answer, or answered incorrectly, for example, "I'll go and ask someone", she would be guided through a sequence of additional cues until she remembered the poster (see Table 1). On most trials she would then be encouraged, sometimes with difficulty, actually to go to the poster to increase the likelihood that the required behaviour would be undertaken as well as remembered post-training (Bird & Kinsella, 1996). This initial training phase took about 90 minutes, after which it was necessary to back off because the patient was becoming exasperated about repeatedly being asked to do such an "obvious" task. She was then re-visited after a delay of half an hour to ensure she still retained the association. A staff member with whom the patient had a good relationship, and who had observed some of the training, was deputed to administer further retrieval trials after delays of about one and four hours. The next day the association was still salient in memory.

TABLE 1
Methods used to introduce each Spaced Retrieval Trial in Cases 1 and 2, together with
Sequence of Subsidiary (Fading) Cues available when patient failed

Case 1. "Paranoid delusions" and violence	Case 2. Obsessive toileting
Introducing the retrieval trial: "What do you do when you wonder where your things have gone?"	*Introducing the retrieval trial:* Beeper sounded with no comment
Subsidiary prompts	*Subsidiary prompts*
1. "Is there somwhere you can go to find out?"	1. "Hear that?"
2. "Somewhere in this room?"	2. "What does it mean?"
3. "Isn't it something to do with a smiley face?"	3. (Beeper activated again) "That sound means you can go somewhere. Where?"
4. "Isn't there a poster somewhere with a smiley face?"	4. "It means you can go to the . . . ?"
5. "Isn't there a notice somewhere that looks like this?" (Blank poster with smiley face held up)	5. (Beeper activated again) "That sound means you can go somewhere beginning with T." Card held up showing "T" and, if he still failed: TOI. . . .
(The patient did not require contextual support beyond this level on any trial)	6. (Beeper activated again) "Does this beeper mean . . . ?" Card displayed showing: YOU *CAN* GO TO THE TOILET YOU *CAN'T* GO TO THE TOILET
Alternative introductions on some trials included:	7. As level 6, but with the correct message in larger print, and "CAN" additionally highlighted.
"Whatever happened to your sewing machine before you came in here?" "What's that poster with the smiley face for?"	Some alternative introductions were used as the memory consolidated. Appropriate fading cues were prepared but rarely needed by this stage.
	"What will remind you when it's time to go to the toilet?" "What's this thing for?" Pointing to beeper.

Only the minimum amount of contextual information required to retrieve the information was provided.

At a meeting with staff the same day, the issue of loss of possessions was discussed and they were encouraged to show empathy rather than exasperation. They were also shown how to use the sequence of fading cues illustrated in Table 1 to help her remember to go to the poster when she asked about the fate of her belongings. She soon stopped asking, the "paranoia" was cured, and staff stopped being angry and apprehensive of physical assault. (For outcome graph, see Bird, 1998.)

An important feature of Case 1, and also one with a more impaired subject who asked obsessively about medication (Bird et al., 1995), is that the poster was the means of allaying anxiety, not the primary cue prompting the behaviour. The primary cue was internal. It was an anxious thought and it was necessary during learning trials to induce it with questions such as: "By the way, whatever happened to your things?" This goes well beyond the experimental work, where only tangible cues were used, but is similar to the clinical work of Camp et al. (1996) with calendars. There the cue to go to the calendar was also internal—the desire to remember what to do.

Case 2

A 62-year-old man with hypoxic brain damage (MMSE = 18) obsessively toileted because of the interaction of fear of soiling himself with inability to remember whether or not he had visited the toilet. He was effectively house-bound because of this problem and his wife, accordingly, also semi-housebound and severely stressed. Anxiolytics were only minimally effective. He was taught to associate a beeper pinned to his shirt with going to the toilet, although there was initial difficulty. A powerfully salient message pressed on the subject for nearly two years, that he must not constantly visit the toilet, led him to learn: "The beeper means I mustn't go to the toilet." This false association had to be unlearned by using forced choice recognition on very closely spaced trials, with the correct message heavily highlighted, before we could proceed (see Table 1).

Thereafter, learning was relatively rapid. As in Case 1, motor performance was encouraged on as many trials as practicable in order to assist encoding but was easier to accomplish here because visiting the toilet was the patient's dearest wish. After the training session, which lasted about three hours because of having to unlearn the false association, his wife was instructed gradually to increase the intervals between signals, starting at 20 minutes. She used the sequence of supplementary cues employed in initial training where necessary (Table 1). It eventually proved possible to work him up to visiting the toilet only every two hours, although the interval could be manipulated as required to fit in with his wife's routine or that of the day care centre which he was now able to attend. His anxiety about soiling was apparent only when the beeper went off and he would rush to the toilet, or when he did not have the beeper on. Other-wise he was confident and calm, and able to take up more normal life. (For outcome graph see Bird et al., 1995.)

COMMENT ON CLINICAL APPLICATION

Although the basic paradigm rests on solid theoretical and experimental grounds, considerable flexibility is required to adapt it to the idiosyncrasies of the specific case profile. Rote application will inevitably fail; knowledge of cognitive science is not enough.

First, the spacing of trials in the research studies (Figure 3) was standardised for experimental consistency. This is not possible in the clinical situation, spacing as well as the level of cued support must be tailored to the patient's ability and progress in learning. Many individuals will require more trials than in Figure 3 with, in particular, a number of closely spaced trials early on. Case 2 is an obvious example and also an excellent example of the relationship of fading cues to errorless learning; the cues were manipulated until the error was corrected.

Second, the methods described here will usually only suit patients in the mild to moderate stages of dementia who retain some verbal skills, and it will only fit certain case profiles. For example, in an almost exactly similar situation to Case 2, training to associate a beeper with toilet visits was easily accomplished with a 79-year-old Alzheimer's disease patient. However, the technique proved inappropriate. Although, as in Case 2, the obsessive toileting was related to cognitive impairment (inability to remember whether or not he had been), it interacted not with fear of soiling himself but with a life-long belief that dire consequences ensue without a daily bowel movement. Failure to pass anything on a toilet visit greatly *increased* the patient's anxiety. The case was eventually ameliorated by supporting his wife and changing her responses (Bird et al., 1998). In Case 2, failure to pass anything reassured the subject that an accident was unlikely for a while.

Third, the contrasting solutions in the previous paragraph to what, on the face of it, was an identical problem illustrate a fundamental point. When planning use of the technique, it is essential not to become fixated on cognitive methods at the expense of the holistic clinical skills required to think any case through. This includes understanding the patient's viewpoint; the technique failed in the case here because this was not sufficiently considered. It also includes awareness of other potential factors that will affect outcome; few psychosocial interventions with difficult behaviour in dementia involve only one modality (Bird et al., in press). Although learning the association was critical, the beeper in Case 2 was also effective because of its reinforcing role as an anxiety reduction agent. The poster and learning it was there served a similar role in Case 1, but this intervention would have been ineffective if it had not also included counselling staff about responding with empathy, and why. The patient, a rather feisty person, would have been unlikely to respond to staff cueing to help her remember about the poster if interactions remained confrontational.

Finally, basic clinical skills are required. Tangible cues must be audible or visible—preferably in line of sight where the behaviour often occurs or, with auditory cues, carried around with the patient. Their suitability for the subject's sensory capacity is best tested before training begins, not afterwards. Although this falls more under the aegis of basic common sense, the frequency with which one sees supposed cues in nursing homes which are illegible or semi-visible even to the cognitively intact younger person suggests that common sense cannot be taken as a given.

Basic clinical skills also include the ability to establish and maintain rapport with cognitively impaired patients who may be difficult. Problems often arise in closely spaced early trials if this has not first been attended to. Once this stage is over, a particular advantage of spaced retrieval is that later trials can be slipped casually into general conversation, for example, in Case 1: "By the way, what's that smiley face poster for?" However, even here, this subject eventually became angry; it was necessary to know when to back off, and to utilise as co-therapist a member of staff with whom she had a close relationship.

CONCLUSION

There is a remarkably widespread belief, common even among health professionals, that persons with dementia are incapable of new learning. This belief is manifestly false, even on logical and observational grounds. Logically the idea of a categorical division—intact learning in normal aging versus no learning possible once dementia is diagnosed—is clearly absurd. Given the slow progress of many dementias, a gradual decline in learning ability is much more likely, from subtle problems very early on, through grossly disordered but still partially intact learning capacity in the middle stages to (perhaps) eventual complete loss. Even casual observation in nursing homes confirms this. Residents with dementia can be seen learning and acting on information unknown to them before admission, for example, the location of the garden, or the fact that there is a nursing home dog and, sometimes, the dog's name.

The work described in this paper backs up these conceptual and anecdotal arguments with unequivocal evidence. Persons with at least mild to moderate dementia can learn specific new information and act on it after clinically significant delays, if they are actively assisted to process that information both at initial acquisition and when it is necessary for them to retrieve it. There are now a few cases in the scientific literature where clinical application of the basic paradigm has been used to ameliorate serious problems associated with dementia.

The clinical cases, themselves, raise issues for further research, both experimental and clinical. For example, the rather surprising fact that, in several cases, it was possible to teach patients to associate a self-generated thought (e.g, "where are my belongings", "what am I supposed to do today") with a behavioural action merits further laboratory research. It is already known from the list-learning literature that that self-generated cues are more effective than experimenter-provided ones in dementia (Lipinska, Bäckman, Mäntalyä, & Viitanen, 1994). An example of the potential for clinical research would be to determine the kinds of problem for which cognitive strategies such as those described in this paper may be appropriate, and those where they are likely to be useless. At present, however, the clinical literature is minuscule. The suitability of these techniques can only be determined by scientist practitioners in the field who creatively use them with appropriate problems and then publish their case series in scientific journals, using objective evidence to report honestly success and failure. Such a body of literature would have the potential to generate a research agenda driven by specific identified clinical problems, and also by residual cognitive abilities of people identified from everyday clinical experience.

Generalised improvement following some kind of standard cognitive training is likely to remain superficially a very attractive idea, and the seam will certainly continue to be mined although at least 30 years of effort has yet to yield any coal. It sometimes appears to be based, implicitly or explicitly, on a fascinating idea that the brain is analogous to a muscle, but even more informed researchers are applying a standard cure or recovery model whose utility has still not been established in dementia (Woods & Bird, 1998; Woods & Britton, 1985). We simply do not know whether the quest for cognitive enhancement is a quest for a chimera.

The work described in this paper suggests that, in any case, a richer and more relevant although much messier seam for cognitive psychologists may be found directly at the clinical coalface. At this stage of the research enterprise, work at the micro-level is vital and there is a growing trend in this direction (Woods, 1999). The goal would be to identify specific severe clinical problems suffered by people with dementia and those who care for them, and then use or develop existing knowledge to devise scientifically validated ways to ameliorate those problems. It may help to minimise dissonance between cognitive science and clinical relevance. Much writing about psychosocial approaches to severe and confronting problems associated with dementia is poor science; the land of the unsupported assertion (Bird, 2000). Conversely, many cognitive texts, although good science, show minimal appreciation of the severe problems faced by people with dementia and those who care for them. One could be forgiven for believing that the worst problem likely to be suffered by someone with dementia is inability to remember appointments or someone's name.

Yet problems such as violence, sexual assault, resistance to personal care, suicide attempts, repetitive demands, screaming and yelling, and incontinence are common in dementia. They are usually the prime source of burden to home carers and the reason they surrender care to residential facilities, where similar but even more florid problems cause equivalent stress to nursing staff (Donaldson et al., 1997; Hagen & Sayers, 1995; Hallberg & Norberg, 1995; MacPherson et al., 1994; Morriss, Rovner, & German, 1996; Wijeratne, 1997). Currently these phenomena are, in the main, primitively managed, most commonly with antipsychotic medication, a practice whose limited efficacy and dangers have now been extensively documented (e.g., Aisen, Deluca, & Lawler, 1992; Devanand & Levy, 1995; Schneider, Pollock, & Lyness, 1990).

As in the two cases described earlier, which were causing severe distress to both the dementia sufferer and carers, the difficulty of making sense of the world because of cognitive impairment is commonly amongst the causal factors producing these behaviours. There is almost unlimited scope for cognitive and behavioural scientists willing to work at the clinical level to contribute to the range of tools, backed by solid experimental evidence, which can be used as alternatives or adjuncts to medication. For example, it is likely that few of the writers who confidently advocate use of differential reinforcement in management of problems in dementia have ever tried it. It is fiendishly difficult, especially in nursing homes, produces partial success at best (e.g., Bird et al., 1998), and there are few cases in the literature of the last 30 years where its successful use has been reported. References often cited in support (Pinkston & Linsk, 1984; Vaccaro, 1988) involved samples who were not dementing or mixed aged samples. Currently, the parameters of how to maximise the chances of persons with dementia associating a behaviour with a consequence, and then acting on that association, are simply not known because the basic experimental research has not been done.

Cued recall of behaviour is simply an example of a method, theoretically coherent, on which the basic experimental research has been done, and which has been developed by extending existing knowledge from the literature and marrying it to severe real-life problems. It will work with some patients in some situations some of the time, probably the best that can be hoped for with any one technique. In a recent large predominantly psychosocial intervention study, which produced a success rate of over 70% in alleviating difficult behaviour in dementia, cued recall of behaviour played only a minor role as opposed to changing the attitudes and practices of home carers or nursing home staff, adjusting the physical and sensory environment, or addressing remediable causes such as pain, depression, or infections (Bird et al., in press). Nevertheless, we are not so well endowed with techniques of proven experimental and clinical efficacy that we can afford to ignore it. At a minimum, the work reported in this paper demonstrates that clinicians who maintain the delusion that persons with dementia are incapable of new learning are working with an incomplete tool kit.

REFERENCES

Aisen, P.S., Deluca, T., & Lawler, B.A. (1992). Falls among geropsychiatry inpatients are associated with PRN medications for agitation. *International Journal of Geriatric Psychiatry, 7,* 709–712.
Alexopoulos, P. (1994). Management of sexually disinhibited behaviour by a demented patient. *Australian Journal on Ageing, 13,* 119.
Bäckman, L. (1992). Memory training and memory improvement in Alzheimer's disease: Rules and exceptions. *Acta Neurologica Scandinavica, Suppl. 139,* 84–89.

Bäckman, L., & Nilsson, L.-G. (1985). Prerequisites for lack of age differences in memory performance. *Experimental Aging Research, 11*, 67–73.

Bäckman, L., & Small, B. (1998). Influences of cognitive support on episodic remembering: Tracing the process of loss from normal aging to Alzheimer's disease. *Psychology and Aging, 13*, 267–276.

Beck, C., Heacock, P., Mercer, S., Thatcher, R.N., & Sparkman, C. (1988). The impact of cognitive skills retraining on persons with Alzheimer's disease or mixed dementia. *Journal of Geriatric Psychiatry, 21*, 73–88.

Bird, M. (1998). Clinical use of preserved learning capacity in dementia. *Australasian Journal on Ageing, 17*, 161–166.

Bird, M. (2000). Psychosocial rehabilitation for problems arising from cognitive deficits in dementia. In R. Hill, L. Bäckman, & A. Stigsdotter-Neely (Eds.), *Cognitive rehabilitation in old age*. Oxford: Oxford University Press.

Bird, M., Alexopoulos, P., & Adamowicz, J. (1995). Success and failure in five case studies: Use of cued recall to ameliorate behaviour problems in senile dementia. *International Journal of Geriatric Psychiatry, 10*, 5–11.

Bird, M., & Kinsella, G. (1996). Long-term cued recall of tasks in senile dementia. *Psychology and Ageing, 11*, 45–56.

Bird, M., Llewellyn-Jones, R., Smithers, H., Andrews, C., Cameron, I., Cottee, A. Hutson, C., Jenneke, B., & Kurrle, S. (1998). Challenging behaviours in dementia: A project at Hornsby/Ku-ring-gai Hospital. *Australasian Journal on Ageing, 17*, 10–15.

Bird, M., Llewellyn Jones, R., Smithers, H., Cohen, J., & Korten, A. (in press). *Challenging behaviour in dementia: A controlled trial of a predominantly psychosocial approach.* (Report to the Office for Older Australians, Commonwealth Department of Health and Family Services). Canberra: Centre for Mental Health Research, Australian National University.

Bird, M.J., & Luszcz, M.A. (1991). Encoding specificity, depth of processing, and cued recall in Alzheimer's disease. *Journal of Clinical and Experimental Neuropsychology, 13*, 508–520.

Bird, M.J., & Luszcz, M.A. (1993). Enhancing memory performance in Alzheimer's disease: Acquisition assistance and cue effectiveness. *Journal of Clinical and Experimental Neuropsychology, 15*, 921–932.

Bjork, R.A. (1988). Retrieval practice and the maintenance of knowledge. In M. Gruneberg, P. Morris, & R. Sykes (Eds.), *Practical aspects of memory: Current research and issues. Vol. 1: Memory in everyday life.* (pp. 396–401). Chichester, UK: Wiley.

Bjork, R.A., & Bjork, E.L. (1992). A new theory of disuse and an old theory of stimulus fluctuation. In A.F. Healy, S.M. Kosslyn, & R.M. Shiffrin (Eds.), *From learning processes to cognitive processes: Essays in honor of William K. Estes.* (Vol. 2, pp. 35–67). New Jersey: Erlbaum.

Bowlby, M. (1998). Reality orientation thirty years later: Are we still confused? *Canadian Journal of Occupational Therapy, 58*, 114–122.

Breuil, V., de Rotrou, J., Forette, F., Tortrat, D., Ganansia-Ganem, A., Frambourt, A., Moulin, F., & Boller, F. (1994). Cognitive stimulation of patients with dementia: Preliminary results. *International Journal of Geriatric Psychiatry, 9*, 211–217.

Camp, C., Bird, M., & Cherry, K. (2000). Retrieval strategies as a rehabilitation aid for cognitive loss in pathological aging. In R. Hill, L. Bäckman, & A. Stiggsdotter-Neely (Eds.), *Cognitive rehabilitation in old age*. Oxford: Oxford University Press.

Camp, C.J., Foss, J.W., Stevens, A.B., & O'Hanlon, A.M. (1996). Improving prospective memory task performance in persons with Alzheimer's disease. In M. Brandimonte, M. McDaniel, & G. Einstein (Eds.), *Prospective memory: Theory and applications.* (pp. 351–367). New Jersey: Erlbaum.

Clare, L., Wilson, B., Breen, K., & Hodges, J. (1999). Errorless learning of face–name associations in early Alzheimer's disease. *Neurocase, 5*, 37–46.

Craik, F., & Lockhart, R. (1972). Levels of processing: A framework for memory research. *Journal of Verbal Learning and Verbal Behaviour, 11*, 671–684.

Cuddy, L.L., & Jacoby, L L. (1982). When forgetting helps memory: An analysis of repetition effects. *Journal of Verbal Learning and Verbal Behaviour, 21*, 451–467.

Dellarosa, D., & Bourne, L.E. (1985). Surface form and the spacing effect. *Memory and Cognition, 13*, 529–537.

Dempster, F.N. (1988). The spacing effect: A case study in the failure to apply the results of psychological research. *American Psychologist, 8*, 627–634.

Devanand, D.P., & Levy, S.R. (1995). Neuroleptic treatment of agitation and psychosis in dementia. *Journal of Geriatric Psychiatry and Neurology, 8*, S18–S27.

Diesfeldt, H. F. A. (1984). The importance of encoding instructions and retrieval cues in the assessment of memory in senile dementia. *Archives of Gerontology and Geriatrics, 3*, 51–57.

Donaldson, C., Tarrier, N., & Burns, A. (1997). The impact of the symptoms of dementia on caregivers. *British Journal of Psychiatry, 170*, 62–68.

Elmståhl, S., Stenberg, I., Annerstedt, L., & Ingvad, B. (1998). Behavioural disturbances and pharmacological treatment of patients with dementia in family caregiving: A 2-year follow-up. *International Psychogeriatrics, 10*, 239–252.

Foley, L. (1996). *Spaced retrieval as a mnemonic in dementia: Its efficacy and the role of cognitive effort.* Unpublished Masters Thesis, Australian National University, Canberra.

Folstein, M.F., Folstein, S.E., & McHugh, P.R. (1975). Mini-mental state: A practical method for grading the cognitive state of patients for the clinician. *Journal of Psychiatric Research, 12*, 189–198.

Furniss, L., Lloyd Craig, S., & Burns, A. (1998). Medication use in nursing homes for elderly people. *International Journal of Geriatric Psychiatry, 13*, 433–439.

Gilleard, C., Mitchell, R.G., & Riordan, J. (1981). Ward orientation training with psychogeriatric patients. *Journal of Advanced Nursing, 6*, 95–98.

Godfrey, H.D.B., & Knight, R.G. (1987). Interventions for amnesia: A review. *British Journal of Clinical Psychology, 26*, 83–91.

Hagen, B., & Sayers, D. (1995). When caring leaves bruises: The effects of staff education on resident aggression. *Journal of Gerontological Nursing, 21*, 7–16.

Hallberg, I.R., & Norberg, A. (1995). Nurses' experiences of strain and their reactions in the care of severely demented patients. *International Journal of Geriatric Psychiatry, 10*, 757–766.

Hanley, I.G. (1981). The use of signposts and active training to modify ward disorientation in elderly patients. *Journal of Behavioural Therapy and Experimental Psychology, 12*, 241–247.

Hart, R.P., Kwentus, J.A., Taylor, J.R., & Harkin, S.W. (1987). Rate of forgetting in dementia and depression. *Journal of Consulting and Clinical Psychology, 55*, 101–105.

Hasher, L., & Zacks, R.T. (1979). Automatic and effortful processes in memory. *Journal of Experimental Psychology: General, 108*, 356–388.

Herlitz, A., Adolfsson, R., Bäckman, L., & Nilsson, L.-G. (1991). Cue utilization following different forms of encoding in mildly, moderately, and severely demented patients with Alzheimer's disease. *Brain and Cognition, 15*, 119–130.

Izawa, C. (1992). Test trials contributions to the optimization of learning processes: Study/test trials interactions. In A.F. Healy, S.M. Kosslyn, & R.M. Shiffrin (Eds.), *From learning processes to cognitive processes: Essays in honor of William K. Estes.* (Vol. 2, pp. 1–31). New York: Erlbaum.

Jacoby, L.L., & Craik, F.I.M. (1979). Processing at encoding and retrieval: Trace distinctiveness and recovery of initial context. In L.S. Cormack & F.I.M. Craik (Eds.), *Levels of processing in human memory.* (pp. 1–21). New Jersey: Erlbaum.

Kopelman, M.D. (1985). Rates of forgetting in Alzheimer-type dementia and Korsakoff's syndrome. *Neuropsychologia, 23*, 623–638.

Lipinska, B., Bäckman, L., Mäntalyä, T., & Viitanen, M. (1994). Effectiveness of self-generated cues in early Alzheimer's disease. *Journal of Clinical and Experimental Neuropsychology, 16*, 809–819.

MacPherson, R., Eastley, R.J., Richards, H., & Mian, I.H. (1994). Psychological distress among workers caring for the elderly. *International Journal of Geriatric Psychiatry, 9*, 381–386.

McEvoy, C., & Patterson, R. (1986). Behavioral treatment of deficit skills in dementia patients. *Gerontologist, 26*, 475–478.

Mitchell, D.B. (1989). How many memory systems? Evidence from aging. *Journal of Experimental Psychology: Learning, Memory, and Cognition, 15*, 31–49.

Moffat, N. (1992). Strategies of memory therapy. In B.A. Wilson & N. Moffat (Eds.), *Clinical management of memory problems.* (pp. 86–119). London: Chapman and Hall.

Morriss, R.K., Rovner, B.W., & German, P.S. (1996). Factors contributing to nursing home admission because of disruptive behaviour. *International Journal of Geriatric Psychiatry, 11*, 243–249.

Pinkston, E.M., & Linsk, N.L. (1984). Behavioural family interventions with the impaired elderly. *Gerontologist, 24*, 576–583.

Pliskin, N., Cunningham, J., Remondet-Wall, J., & Cassisi, J. (1996). Cognitive rehabilitation for cerebrovascular accidents and Alzheimer's disease. In P. Corrigan & S. Ydofsky (Eds.), *Cognitive rehabilitation for neuropsychiatric disorders.* (pp. 193–222). Washington DC: American Psychiatric Press.

Quayhagen, M.P., Quayhagen, M., Corbeil, R.R., Roth, P.A., & Rodgers, J.A. (1995). A dyadic remediation program for care recipients with dementia. *Nursing Research, 44*, 153–159.

Schneider, L., Pollock, V., & Lyness, S. (1990). A meta-analysis of controlled trials of neuroleptic treatment in dementia. *Journal of the American Geriatrics Society, 38*, 553–563.

Tulving, E. (1983). *Elements of episodic memory.* Oxford: Clarendon Press.

Tuokko, H., & Crockett, D. (1989). Cued recall and memory disorders in dementia. *Journal of Clinical and Experimental Neuropsychology, 11*, 278–294.

Vaccaro, F.J. (1988). Application of operant procedures in a group of institutionalized aggressive geriatric patients. *Psychology and Aging, 3*, 22–8.

Wijeratne, C. (1997). Pathways to morbidity in carers of dementia sufferers. *International Psychogeriatrics, 9*, 69–79.

Wilson, B., Baddeley, A., Evans, J., & Shiel, A. (1994). Errorless learning in the rehabilitation of memory impaired people. *Neuropsychological Rehabilitation, 4*, 307–326.

Woods, R. (1999). Promoting well-being and independence for people with dementia. *International Journal of Geriatric Psychiatry, 14*, 97–109.

Woods, B., & Bird, M. (1998). Non-pharmacological approaches to treatment. In G. Wilcock, R. Bucks, & K. Rockwood (Eds.), *Diagnosis and management of dementia: A manual for memory disorders teams.* Oxford: Oxford University Press.

Woods, R.T., & Britton, P.G. (1985). *Clinical psychology with the elderly.* London: Croom-Helm.

Zanetti, O., Frisoni, G., De Leo, D., Buono, M., Bianchetti, A., & Trabucchi, M. (1995). Reality orientation therapy in Alzheimer's disease: Useful or not? *Alzheimer's Disease and Associated Disorders, 9*, 132–138.

Manuscript received June 1999
Revised manuscript received February 2000

Can reality orientation be rehabilitated? Development and piloting of an evidence-based programme of cognition-based therapies for people with dementia

Aimee Spector, Martin Orrell
University College London, UK

Stephen Davies
Princess Alexandra Hospital, Harlow, Essex, UK

Bob Woods
University of Wales, Bangor, UK

This study describes the development and implementation of a programme of cognition-based therapies for dementia. The programme was designed by distilling the evidence of the effectiveness of Reality Orientation and related approaches, following a broad-based systematic review. The most beneficial elements identified from previous studies were extracted and incorporated into the programme, using the expertise of specialists in the field. The programme comprised of 15 45-min, twice weekly sessions. It ran in one day centre and three residential homes, involving 27 people with dementia (17 treatment and 10 control subjects). The results of the pilot study showed positive trends in cognition, and trends towards reduced depression and anxiety following treatment. No negative effects were identified. We discuss how the outcomes of the pilot study were used to modify the programme, which now has a stronger cognitive element. This refined programme is currently being tested as part of a large multicentre, randomised controlled trial.

Correspondence should be sent to Prof. B. Woods, Dementia Services Development Centre, Neuadd Ardudwy, University of Wales Bangor, Holyhead Road, Bangor, Gwynedd LL57 2PX

We would like to thank the National Health Service Executive North Thames for funding this project, as part of their research and development programme on the health of older people. We also thank Harry Cayton, Chief Executive of the Alzheimer's Society, for enabling this project to be carried out in partnership with the Society.

INTRODUCTION

Reality Orientation (RO) is the archetypal approach to cognitive rehabilitation in dementia (Holden & Woods, 1995). Taulbee and Folsom (1966) described RO as a technique to improve the quality of life of confused elderly people, although its origins lay in an attempt to rehabilitate patients with long-term mental health problems in Veterans' Administration hospitals (Ruskin & Talbott, 1993). RO operated through the presentation and repetition of orientation information, which was thought to provide the person with a greater understanding of their surroundings, possibly resulting in an improved sense of control and self-esteem. RO can be of a continuous 24 hour nature, whereby staff involve the patients in reality throughout the day, or of a "class-room" type, where groups of elderly people meet on a regular basis to engage in orientation-related activities (Brook, Degun, & Mather, 1975). Woods (1979) found that classroom RO led to some improvement in cognitive function, with no effect on behaviour, whereas Baines, Saxby, and Ehlert (1987) found significant positive effects on behaviour, with no significant changes in cognition. A programme of classroom and 24 hour RO together has demonstrated significant positive changes in orientation (Citrin & Dixon, 1977).

RO lost its initial popularity in the 1980s, largely due to criticism of it being applied in a rigid and insensitive manner. More modern strategies which aim to improve cognition in dementia frequently involve memory training and cognitive stimulation programmes. Zarit, Zarit, and Reever (1982) provided subjects with "didactic training" (forming mental images of words) and "problem solving" (practical steps to manage daily problems, e.g., notebooks and calendars). They reported small and short-lived changes in memory performance, but increased depression in caregivers. The use of external memory aids, such as diaries, calendars, large clocks and clear signposting are becoming increasingly common for people with dementia. More recent research is identifying ways of creating an optimal learning environment. For example, "errorless learning" involves encouraging people, when learning new information, only to respond when they are sure that they are correct; and "spaced-retrieval" involves learning and retaining information by actively recalling information over increasingly long periods of time (Camp, Foss, O'Hanlon, & Stevens, 1996; Clare, Wilson, Breen, & Hodges, 1999) .

Other therapies commonly described in dementia care include "Reminiscence Therapy" (RT), which typically involves weekly meetings that promote the discussion of past events, often assisted with aids such as photographs, music, archive recordings, videos and items with an historical connection; and "Validation Therapy" (VT), which aims to validate the feelings of people with dementia by concentrating on the underlying meaning of their behaviour, rather than correcting it.

There has been much interest in the various therapies and approaches to dementia care, yet there is a distinct lack of quality, up-to-date research and information available about how helpful the approaches are. Additionally, many care staff are uncertain about the best approaches to use, and of the scale of their potential impact. With more information on how care staff may positively contribute to dementia care, their level of satisfaction and morale may increase. This paper is in three parts; first, we report the use of a comprehensive analysis of the evidence in the literature to develop a cognition-based therapy programme; second, we report pilot data on the use of the programme in a day centre and three residential homes; finally, we discuss the modification of the programme based on the experience gained from the pilot work.

Our ultimate aim is to develop a group-based programme which staff in residential homes and day centres may learn to use with confidence as a means of enhancing and maintaining group members' level of function. This could form one component of a person's plan of care—we certainly do not envisage such an approach obviating the need for additional individualised interventions aimed at the whole range of the person's needs.

DESIGNING AN EVIDENCE-BASED PROGRAMME

Cochrane Reviews

In order to consolidate the existing evidence, the authors (Spector, Orrell, Davies, & Woods, 1998a,b) conducted two Cochrane Systematic Reviews on the effectiveness of RO and RT as psychological interventions for people with dementia, using evidence from randomised controlled trials (RCTs). Combining the results from six RCTs, the RO review showed that people receiving RO improved significantly more than controls in both cognition and behaviour. The RT review was inconclusive, due to only one RCT being included, and highlighted an enormous gap in research. An inconclusive systematic review of Validation Therapy (Neal & Briggs, 1999) is also available, and a review of memory training is planned.

Systematic literature evaluation

A comprehensive literature search was conducted, which included searching Medline, PsychLIT, Embase, BIDS (Science Citation Index and Social Science Citation Index), OMNI (Organising Medical Networked Information), Dissertation Abstracts International, the Cochrane Database of Systematic Reviews, and SIGLE (System for Information on Grey Literature). Once all the literature on the principal psychological interventions (RO, RT, VT and memory training) was gathered, trials which provided details of the content of the programme and activities used were considered further. The therapeutic content of each study, and subsequent outcomes, were tabulated (see Table 1).

TABLE 1

Details of studies (interventions incorporated into the programme are in italics)

Authors, intervention, quality/details	Description (treatment group)	Outcome following treatment
Breuil et al. (1994); RO RCT, blind. 56 Ss (CS = 29, C = 27)	*Copying pictures, associated words, naming and categorising objects.*	Significant improvement in cognition.
Wallis, Baldwin, & Higginbotham (1983); RO RCT, 33 Ss (RO = 18, C = 20)	Repetition of orientation information (e.g., time, place, weather). Charts, pictures, *touching objects and material.*	No change in cognition. Insignificant positive trend in behaviour.
Gerber et al. (1991); RO RCT, 24 Ss (RO = 8, SC = 8, C = 8)	Simple exercises, self-care, *food preparation,* orientation room with RO board, large clock, coloured illustrations.	Improved cognition in both RO and social interaction groups, especially in orientation and language (both significant)
Woods (1979); RO RCT, 14 Ss (RO = 5, ST = 5, C = 4)	Daily personal diary, group activities (dominoes, spelling, bingo). *Naming objects,* reading RO board.	Significant improvement in memory, learning, information and orientation in RO groups.
Hogstel (1979); RO RCT, 44 Ss (RO = 22, C = 22)	Introductions, reading RO board, tell time, discuss lunch menu. Patients had large clock and calendar in bedrooms. Additional input from staff outside RO class.	No significant differences. Observations: RO patients became more co-operative, and began communicating much more with each other.
Baines et al. (1987); RO RCT, 15 Ss (RO = 5, RT = 5, C = 5)	RO board, *old and current newspapers, personal and local photos, materials to stimulate all senses (e.g., cinnamon, silk, honey).*	Significant improvement in behaviour. No significant change in cognition. Positive effects reported by staff.
Goldstein et al. (1982); RO RCT, 14 Ss (RC = 7, C = 7)	Reading RO board, naming people, use of RO questionnaire (e.g., day, month, season, etc.).	Insignificant improvement in ADL.

Authors, intervention, quality/details	Description (treatment group)	Outcome following treatment
Hanley, McGuire, & Boyd (1981); RO RCT, 57 Ss (RO = 28, C = 29)	RO board, clocks, calendars, *maps* and posters. Room overlooked garden area to enable discussion.	Significant improvement in verbal orientation, in response to basic orientation items. No changes in behaviour.
Vockel (1978); RO RCT, 20 Ss (RO = 10, RT = 10). No statistics used.	Greeting, touching, RO board, calendars, clocks, antiques. Simple activities, e.g., identifying pictures.	No significant improvement in RO group, significant improvement in RT group.
Coen Micli et al. (1991); RO CT. No. of Ss and method of allocation unknown.	Space and *time orientation, memory prompting, naming objects* and body parts, training cognitive, semantic and phonetic abilities.	"Medium" overall improvement. Patients become less passive Increase in effort and ability to concentrate.
Zanetti et al. (1995); RO CT, 28 Ss (RO = 16, C = 12)	Early classes: personal, time and space orientation. Later: *historical events, famous people,* attention, memory and visuospatial exercises.	Significant improvement in verbal abilities. No changes in other cognitive functions or disability measures. No changes in self-rated depression scores.
Citrin & Dixon (1977); RO CT, 25 Ss (RO = 12, C = 13)	Personal and environmental information presented individually, 24 hr RO.	Significant improvement in RO information sheet. Geriatric Rating Scale was inconclusive.
Reeve & Ivison (1985); RO CT, 20 Ss (RO = 10, C = 10)	Classroom and 24 hour RO (environmental symbols, signposts, clocks and 2 RO boards).	Significant improvements in cognition and behaviour.
Gotestam (1987); RO ABA, 5 Ss	Time Orientation: diary, clock. *Person orientation: name games.* Room orientation: maps and nameplates on walls.	Significant improvements in time and room orientation, insignificant improvement in person orientation.
Cornbleth & Cornbleth (1979); RO ABA, 22 Ss	RO board, copying, telling time, *counting money.*	Significant improvement in orientation and ADL.
Barnes (1974); RO ABA, 6 Ss, No statistics	RO board, calendar, maps. Discussed names, lunch menu, etc.	Insignificant improvement (questionnaire).

TABLE 1 continued

Authors, intervention, quality/details	Description (treatment group)	Outcome following treatment
Greene, Nicol, & Jamieson (1979); RO ABA, 3 Ss, No statistics	"Personal Orientation Questionnaire" for each person. (Time, place, *current affairs, family, friends, history*.)	Increased orientation, generalising to other areas of behaviour (especially other items of information).
Goldwasser, Auerbach, & Harkins (1987), RT RCT, 30 Ss (RT = 10, SS = 10, C = 10)	Topics: food, family personal artefacts, jobs, songs, music, celebrations.	Increased depression. Insignificant improvement in cognition. No significant change in behaviour.
Baines et al. (1987): RT RCT, 15 Ss (RT = 5, RO = 5, C = 5)	*Old photos (local scenes, personal)*, books, *magazines, newspapers, domestic articles*.	Insignificant decrease in information/orientation after RT. Insignificant improvement in behaviour. Positive staff reports, e.g., got to know people better.
Orten, Allen, & Cook (1989); RT RCT, 56 Ss (RT = 28, C = 28)	Structured topics, covering life-span. Pictures and memorabilia discouraged.	Insignificant improvement in social behaviour. Group differences attributed to experience of leaders.
Kiernat (1979); RT ABA, 23 Ss	*Topics in chronological sequence. Multisensory materials*, e.g., popped corn to add sound and smell to circus discussion. *Pictures, recordings, historical items.*	Positive qualitative results, e.g., initially only responded to direct questions from staff. Later responded to other residents without prompting.
Gibson (1993); RT 5 individual case studies.	*Chronological events, family life and work*, major life crises, landmarks and transitions, place lived and visited.	"Staff became excited, intrigued and fascinated with the person's past." "Music especially evocative."
Zarit et al. (1982): Cognitive stimulation RCT, 35 Ss (and caretakers) in 3 groups (didactic training, problem solving, control)	Didactic training: Forming mental images of words, linking words with images. Problem-solving: Practical management of daily problems, e.g., notebooks, calendars.	Small and short-lived changes in memory performance. Increased depression in caregivers.

382

Authors, intervention, quality/details	Description (treatment group)	Outcome following treatment
Koh et al. (1994); "3R Mental Stimulation" CT, Quasi-randomised. 39 Ss (E = 15, C = 15)	Basic elements of RT, RO and remotivation. *Weekly discussion topics, e.g., money, hobbies, pets, fruit, and festivals. Stimulated all senses.*	Significant improvement in mental state score.
Quayhagen & Quayhagen (1989); Cognitive stimulation given on one-to-one basis by caregivers. Non-randomised.	*Communication exercises: Conversation skills, facts, opinion, etc.; memory-provoking techniques: verbal and non-verbal;* problem-solving exercises: planning/categorisation.	Qualitative findings reported by caregivers: improved emotional status of patients, maintenance over time in aspects of cognitive functioning. No improvement in carer well-being.
Bourgeois (1990); Memory training ABA, 3 Ss	Developed prosthetic memory aids: plastic wallets containing information of personal relevance (photos, daily schedule, etc.).	Content and quality of conversation doubled or tripled, but highly qualitative with Likert ratings.
Tosland et al. (1997); VT RCT, single blind, 88 Ss (VT = 31, SC = 29, C = 28)	Four segments. (1) Warm greetings, hold hands, sing songs. (2) Focus on topic of interest, reminisce. (3) Activity, e.g., poetry. (4) Refreshments, goodbyes. Used Feil's validation approach throughout.	Limited support for VT. Staff reported reduced physically and verbally aggressive behaviour (not reported by observers). No change in medication, physical restraint, or nursing time needed.
Bleathman & Morton (1992); VT Qualitative accounts, 20 groups	Welcoming, hand-shaking and holding, *singing,* discussion (on planned theme), closing song, thanking, refreshments. Roles given, e.g., song leader, welcomer, and hostess.	Individual observations, e.g., one person expressed empathic understanding, another expressed the desire to kill herself.

RCT = Randomised Controlled Trial, CT = Controlled Trial, ABA = Repeated measures (ABA) design, Ss = Subjects, RO = Reality Orientation group, RT = Reminiscence Therapy group, VT = Validation Therapy group, SC = Social Contact group, SS = Social Support group, ST = Social Therapy group, CS = Cognitive Stimulation group, Significant = $p < .05$, E = Experimental group.

Studies which did not include this information were excluded from these tables, as they provided little insight into which features of each intervention might be more or less beneficial. Studies with positive outcomes were drawn out from the tables, and the contents of the intervention examined. Through this process, potentially beneficial elements of each type of therapy were identified, and were incorporated into the design of the new programme. Priority was given to studies with stronger design methodology, such as RCTs. In Table 1, the studies and elements which contributed to the design of this programme are highlighted in italic type.

The most influential study in the design of this programme was that of Breuil and colleagues (1994). This was a single blind RCT, demonstrating the strongest improvements in cognition and memory of all the trials examined. Additionally, it weighted the results of the Cochrane review, being the largest study. The authors described their technique as "Cognitive Stimulation", although others (Holden & Woods, 1995) have compared it to RO. Subjects attended 10 hourly therapy sessions; activities included connecting dots to form pictures of common objects, drawing common objects from different perspectives, associated words, and naming and categorising objects.

Design of the package

The five "guiding principles" of the programme, developed from the literature search and the extensive clinical experience of the research team, were as follows:

1. Experiential learning involving the use of all five senses to promote cognitive stimulation and memory processes.
2. Focused psychological interventions which address the difficulties of everyday living.
3. Acknowledgment of the emotional lives and enhancment of the cognitive skills of people with dementia.
4. Implicit learning (familiarity and "intuition"), rather than explicit "teaching". Extensive rehearsal and consolidation of essential information about themselves and their world are thought to be most beneficial.
5. The reciprocal, psychological process (involving cognitive and emotional states) in which people with dementia and those who care for them learn more about each other's capabilities and vulnerabilities.

These principles were observed when designing and running the groups, and draw in part on the understanding of dementia set out by Kitwood (1990). Kitwood offered a deeper insight into dementia care, emphasising the importance of treating people with dementia as individual adults, with much to contribute when staff are able to recognise their "personhood" (Kitwood, 1997; Woods, 1999). These principles were vital in ensuring that the programme did not repeat the insensitivity and rigidity that became associated with some applications of RO (Dietch, Hewett, & Jones, 1989; Gubrium & Ksander, 1975).

A 15 session programme was designed with four phases; (1) The senses, (2) Remembering the past, (3) People and objects, (4) Everyday practical issues. Sessions were planned to last 45 min, commencing with a 10 min "introductory phase", where the group was to be welcomed, the "theme song" sung, and tea and biscuits consumed. The "intervention phase" was to be of 25 min duration, with sessions ending with a 10 min "consolidation phase", where the discussion and ideas were to be summarised, the theme song sung again, and farewells said.

Phase 1: The Senses

This phase involving sound, vision, smell/taste, and touch used multisensory stimulation, which has been used successfully in other programmes. Sensory elements were introduced, to be continued in all subsequent sessions ("theme tune", scented candle, unusual biscuits, lava lamp). This aimed to help identify the abilities of the group, create a sense of continuity, and to differentiate the sensory experience of these sessions from usual activities.

Phase 2: Remembering the past

This phase concerned growing up, work and home, and recent years. The RT review was inconclusive, but there was strong clinical support and evidence from other studies for the benefits of reminiscence; that people enjoy it, and that it increases interaction and engagement (Gibson, 1993; Woods & McKiernan, 1995). Hence these chronological reminiscence sessions were incorporated into the programme.

Phase 3: People and objects

This phase, recognising people from the past, recognising people in the group and staff members, recognising people in the family, familiar and modern objects, and using familiar objects, was based on Breuil et al.'s (1994) study, which placed great emphasis on the use of common objects, and naming and categorising objects. Naming objects was also used by Woods (1979), as part of an RO programme. Breuil et al.'s use of associated words was incorporated into the sessions on people.

Phase 4: Everyday practical issues

This was a general orientation phase, with a session on identifying and using money (also used by Koh et al., 1994), and a session on knowing your way around. The final session was designed as a summing up and consolidation session, ending with a tea party.

THE PILOT STUDY

Method

The programme was piloted in a day centre and three residential homes. The research team had existing clinical links with the day centre and one home, and Jewish Care put forward two of their homes to participate. Ethical approval was obtained through the appropriate NHS research ethics committee.

Inclusion criteria were as follows:

1. Diagnosis of dementia according to DSM IV criteria; the sub-type of dementia was not evaluated, as the programme was designed to be used with the typical residential and day-care population, where reliable information of this type is often not available, and many mixed dementias are found.
2. No severe hearing or visual impairments which might affect the participant's ability to co-operate in a group.
3. Some ability to communicate and understand communication (a score of 1 or 0 in questions 12 and 13 of the CAPE Behaviour Rating Scale; Pattie & Gilleard, 1979).
4. No serious health problems that could affect the ability to attend groups.
5. No challenging behaviour that could disrupt group activities (loud or constant talking, wandering about, etc.).

All participants were assessed in the week prior to the first group session, and the week following the final group session. Staff and carers completed the relevant assessment forms at the same times. Data collected included demographic details and a range of scales for subjects and carers. Thirty five participants completed the first assessment, 12 from the day centre and 23 from the three residential homes. Their mean age was 85.7 years (SD = 6.7), ranging from 71 to 95 years. The treatment group comprised six participants from the day centre, and five from each of the three homes. Four of the treatment group and four of the controls were not assessed at follow-up. Reasons for attrition included refusal (3), ill health (4), and the person moving away (1). Thus baseline and follow-up data are available for 10 participants in the control group and 17 in the experimental group. Ten family care givers of people attending the day centre took part, with staff completing the relevant assessments for the two day-centre attenders without carers and for participants in the residential homes. Participants were randomly allocated to treatment and control groups in each setting, by drawing names from a sealed container. Treatment groups were led by a member of the research team, with a staff member from the home/centre as co-facilitator, in a separate room. Participants in the control groups received usual care during the group sessions.

Instruments

1. *Mini-Mental State Examination* (MMSE; Folstein, Folstein, & McHugh, 1975): A brief test of cognitive function, with good reliability and validity. It is widely used in the evaluation of psychological therapies, enabling this study to be easily compared to others.

2. *Alzheimer's Disease Assessment Scale—Cognition* (ADAS-Cog; Rosen, Mohs, & Davis, 1984): A more sensitive scale measuring cognitive function, which includes additional items assessing short-term memory. It is frequently used in drug trials as the principal cognitive outcome measure.

3. *Holden Communication Scale* (Holden & Woods, 1995): Completed by staff, this covers the patient's social behaviour and communication, including conversation, awareness, pleasure, humour, and responsiveness.

4. *Clinical Dementia Rating* (CDR; Hughes et al., 1982): Completed by the researcher, this provides a global rating of dementia severity, including memory, orientation, judgement and problem solving, communication skills, domestic skills, and personal care.

5. *Cornell Scale for Depression in Dementia* (Alexopoulos, Abrams, Young, & Shamoian, 1988): This evaluates depression in dementia (mood-related signs, behavioural disturbance, physical signs, biological functions and ideational disturbance) using information from clinician's interviews with carers and patients.

6. *Rating Anxiety in Dementia* (RAID; Shankar, Walker, Frost, & Orrell, 1999): Rates anxiety from interviews with carers and patients. Categories are worry, apprehension and vigilance, motor tension, autonomic hypersensitivity, phobias, and panic attacks. It has good reliability and validity.

7. *Behaviour Rating Scale* (from the Clifton Assessment Procedures for the Elderly, CAPE; Pattie & Gilleard, 1979): Completed by the carer, this evaluates general behaviour, including personal care, behaviour towards others, and level of dependency.

8. *General Health Questionnaire* (GHQ-12; Goldberg, 1978): A standard self-report scale which has been frequently used to measure carer mental health, with demonstrated validity and reliability.

9. *Relative's Stress (RS) Scale.* (Greene, Smith, Gardiner, & Timbury, 1982): This evaluates carer stress arising specifically from care giving.

Results

An analysis of covariance was used to compare the follow-up score between groups in each test, with baseline score as the covariate (Table 2). The programme was associated with positive trends in cognition, demonstrated by the ADAS-Cog and MMSE. Anxiety (measured by the RAID) and depression (Cornell) both fell in the treatment group and rose for controls, the Cornell reaching significance. Behaviour (BRS) and communication (Holden) declined marginally in both groups. The severity of dementia (CDR) increased for controls, demonstrating an overall decline in this group. Two scales examined the effect of the programme on carers. Care-giving stress (RS) increased slightly in the treatment group and more substantially for controls. There was a significant improvement in carers' general psychological distress in the treatment group (GHQ), with little change for the controls.

REVIEW AND MODIFICATION
OF THE PROGRAMME

Phase 1: The senses

There were a number of difficulties encountered with this phase. It proved problematic to find particular smells, tastes or visual material which most people could identify and/or relate to. People appeared to enjoy feeling different textures in the tactile session, although the predominantly male group in one of the residential homes did question the "point" of this activity. On the positive side, these sessions generally focused on pleasant sensations, not high-lighting people's areas of deficit. They offered a gentle introduction to the programme, allowing the co-ordinators to judge how people responded and their potential limitations. However, it appeared that isolating the senses in this way was highly artificial, as most real-life experiences are multisensory. Asking a person with dementia, for whom sensory abilities are already impaired, to identify something when provided with information from only one sensory modality was evidently unrealistic. Accordingly, the senses phase, as such, was not included in the modified programme, but an attempt was made to introduce multisensory material implicitly throughout the programme.

Phase 2: Remembering the past

Sessions on childhood stirred clear memories, and were generally successful. As later life was discussed, memories tended to fade and discussion frequently reverted back to childhood. Introducing newspaper articles as prompts for discussion on different eras was unsuccessful. People had little memory for historical information where it held no personal meaning for them. Individuals varied enormously in their reactions to "old" objects from the "reminiscence

TABLE 2

Means (and standard deviations) for each group at baseline and follow-up, extent of changes on each scale, and test of between group difference at follow-up

Variable assessed	Test used	Baseline scores Treatment control	Follow-up scores Treatment control	Change (+: positive direction, −: negative)	Between group differences: Ancova
Cognition	MMSE	11.5 (4.4) *15.5 (4.4)*	14.6 (5.5) *15.5 (5.5)*	+3.1 *0*	t = −1.8 p = .08
	Adas − Cog	63.5 (11.9) *71.7 (14.5)*	67.8 (12.6) *70.7 (14.5)*	+4.3 *−1*	t = −0.9 p = .4
Anxiety	RAID	9.7 (10.2) *8.1 (3.2)*	6.6 (5.7) *11.3 (8.9)*	+3.1 *−3.2*	t = 1.7 p = .09
Depression	Cornell	8.1 (7.1) *7.3 (2.6)*	5.5 (3.8) *9.5 (6.7)*	+2.6 *−2.2*	t = 2.6 p = .02*
Communication	Holden	13.2 (7.2) *12.6 (6.8)*	13.9 (7.7) *13.1 (6.5)*	−0.7 *−0.5*	t = −0.2 p = .9
Behaviour	BRS	13.4 (4.2) *12.7 (5.1)*	14.5 (4.4) *13.3 (4.9)*	−1.1 *−0.6*	t = −0.5 p = .7
Global	CDR	2.1 (0.7) *0.9 (0.6)*	1.9 (0.5) *1.9 (0.7)*	+0.2 *−1*	t = 1.3 p = .2
Carer (N = 10)	RS	29.0 (4.6) *24.0 (18.8)*	30.0 (11.9) *33.0 (18.8)*	−1 *−9*	t = 1.1 p = .3
	GHQ	4.8 (2.8) *5.7 (3.1)*	1.0 (0.8) *6.0 (3.6)*	+3.8 *−0.3*	t = 2.8 p = .04*

Treatment group scores are in standard font, *control group scores are in italics.* * p < .05

box" with some often reverting back to the "old days", and others more interested in the here and now. Thus, for example, a "dolly peg" may not generate enthusiasm, as people are unlikely to have strong emotional memories of this object; indeed, a person with dementia may not be aware that this is even an unusual or old-fashioned item. On the other hand, showing people a mobile phone and demonstrating the different sounds it makes generated great enthusiasm in the pilot study. It is intended that the new programme provides scope for reminiscence as a natural component of the entire programme, in that all activities may create scope to reminisce; for many, talking about their past was an important way to contribute. A specific session on early memories has been retained.

Phase 3: People and objects

People enjoyed both taking and discussing pictures of themselves, the staff and their families. The pictures of famous faces were less successful, as people were sometimes only able to recognise very few faces, hence this session has been modified for the new programme. Attempting to "teach" each others' names through the use of name-badges and rehearsal was perceived as patronising, and created hostility, and so will not be retained. The session on using objects, which involved either making an apple crumble or changing a fuse, was an excellent way of enabling a number of people actively to engage in a collective task. Many appeared fascinated when demonstrated the use of various modern objects, such as a mobile phone and personal CD player.

Phase 4: Everyday practical issues

Guessing the prices of modern objects in the session on using money created laughter and debate. The orientation session involved collectively creating a plan of either the home, day centre or local town. This generated optimal input from all the groups. Constructing these sessions in a game-like way appeared to be enjoyable and non-threatening for the group. Using the day's newspapers, particularly those containing lots of pictures, was extremely evocative. The group responded better when given concrete material to discuss, such as the money quiz and the creation of the map of Britain, and in the modified programme, all discussion is accompanied by specific aids or activities.

Responding to different levels of ability

Based on the reactions of the four groups, it was clear that provision needed to be made for differing levels of ability. In the modified programme, most sessions are presented at two levels, depending on the ability of the group. Although for most groups, a combination of these two levels should be used, the more able groups might focus more on level 1 and the less able, on level 2. The modified programme is shown in the Appendix.

DISCUSSION

This study shows that it is feasible to develop a programme of psychological therapies, based on systematic evaluation of the literature and a careful appraisal of the evidence for effectiveness. The programme was popular and generally well tolerated. Positive trends in cognition, depression and anxiety were demonstrated. There were minimal changes in behaviour and communication. In the limited day-centre sample, relatives' stress increased in the control group, and there was an appreciable improvement in relatives' general psychological distress in the treatment group. If the findings in carers were to be supported by our larger study this would add further value to the programme and be the first replication of Greene, Timbury, Smith, and Gardiner's (1983) report of the impact of RO on relatives' stress in a day-hospital context.

The American Psychiatric Association, in their 1997 Practice Guideline on the treatment and management of dementia, suggest that the small gains associated with cognitive approaches such as RO do not justify the risk of negative effects. On the other hand, Gatz et al. (1998), using American Psychological Association criteria conclude that "reality orientation is probably efficacious in slowing cognitive decline". They point out, as we have acknowledged, that cognitive approaches can be implemented without sufficient sensitivity to the patient, leading to possible frustration and distress in the patient. So far, under the relatively controlled conditions of the pilot study, it appears that our efforts to develop a cognitive programme that is respectful and sensitive have borne fruit, in that participants' affect appeared to improve as well as cognition. Given that RO is the first psychosocial approach to dementia to find support from a Cochrane systematic review, we would argue that the effort to ensure any programme we develop is delivered appropriately is worth while.

Limitations

Problems in scheduling sessions were encountered in the day centre, as only around 10 clients attended each day, and activities tended to occur at all times. It was sometimes difficult to invite half those attending to the other room, essentially splitting them up from their friends and taking them away from whatever activity they might be engaged in. Additionally, the staff, who had received extensive training in dementia care, appeared slightly disappointed that parts of the programme involved elements found in their daily activities, perhaps expecting something "new and improved". These problems did not occur in the residential homes, as people were typically taken out of a lounge of up to 30 people, other activities seldom occurred, and staff did not have the unusually large amount of training found in the day centre. The context in which any intervention occurs has a great influence on it (see, for example, Woods, 1994, p. 441).

These early results must be interpreted with some caution. The population was small, and random allocation did not produce samples that were well matched, with the treatment group scoring lower in cognition and higher in anxiety and depression than controls at the outset. Although the analysis of covariance statistically adjusts for differences at baseline, these two slightly different populations could potentially have differed in their reaction to the programme. Additionally, there was the possibility of rater bias, as assessments were conducted by the group coordinator, staff and carers, all aware of group allocation. The treatment group inevitably received more attention than the control group, and an attention-placebo control would provide a stronger test of the specific efficacy of the procedures used. This may be especially the case for the residential homes, where there were relatively few alternate activities. Although numbers are too small for a comparative analysis, the results appeared more positive from the day centre than from the residential homes, despite the evident difference in existing stimulation and activity in the two contexts.

The results included here are presented as preliminary and in need of replication, although we have attempted to use a conservative statistical analysis to reduce the risk of overstating the current findings. We were not able to control for other factors that might have led to between-group differences, e.g., health changes, changes in medication, etc., although we have no reason to suspect that these were more likely in one group than the other.

Given the weight afforded by the Cochrane review to the cognitive stimulation work reported by Breuil et al. (1994) we have made a detailed comparison of our approach with the on-going programme of cognitive stimulation on which their report was based, led by Jocelyne de Rotrou, neuropsychologist at the Hospital Broca in Paris. There, people attend twice weekly sessions which are similar to traditional RO groups, with a large component of each session involving people engaging in a cognitive task, such as calculating the price of a shopping list. The Paris participants and our samples differed in the severity of dementia and their attitude to their cognitive difficulties. In Paris, people who had recently been diagnosed with dementia were attending groups with the aim of improving their cognition and allowing them to function independently. People in long-term residential care may have different attitudes towards their cognition, or indeed be less aware of its failings. For this reason, sessions in our programme are presented in a "game-like" manner, involving teams; so that cognitive stimulation is less overt, and individual failings are not so apparent. Explicit memory, as in learning the names of other people in the group, or seeking recall of specific historical events, led in our programme to participants potentially being exposed to the extent of their difficulty. The primary focus of the modified programme is on harnessing implicit memory, emphasising active engagement with materials and the plentiful provision of retrieval cues. This minimises conscious memorisation, with the danger of overt failure and promotes general cognitive stimulation and individual well-being.

Future plans

Using the modified programme, a large multi-centre, randomised controlled trial is now under way. This trial also includes a quality of life measure and an economic evaluation of the programme. The programme now divides sessions into "levels", to cater for groups of different abilities. A detailed manual to accompany the programme is being prepared (available from the authors) which should provide the group leader with both a choice of content for each session, and activities to suit a range of abilities.

This study has described the development, piloting and modification of an evidence-based package of cognitive-based therapies for people with dementia. Benefits in the pilot study include improved cognition, and reduced anxiety and depression following treatment. Perhaps just as important, there were no evident negative effects on the person with dementia or his/her relatives. This paper demonstrates that an evidence-based approach, tempered with the input of experienced clinicians, is feasible, but replication of these preliminary findings with a larger sample size and more rigorous methodology is needed before it can be claimed that they add to the evidence-base for the benefits of cognition-based psychological therapies for people with dementia.

REFERENCES

Alexopoulos, G.S., Abrams, R.C., Young, R.C., & Shamoian, C.A. (1988). Cornell Scale for Depression in Dementia. *Biological Psychiatry, 23,* 271–284.

American Psychiatric Association (1997). Practice guideline for the treatment of patients with Alzheimer's disease and other dementias of late life. *American Journal of Psychiatry, 154,* 1–39.

Baines, S., Saxby, P., & Ehlert, K. (1987). Reality orientation and reminiscence therapy: A controlled cross-over study of elderly confused people. *British Journal of Psychiatry, 151,* 222–231.

Barnes, J.A. (1974). Effects of reality orientation classroom on memory loss, confusion and disorientation in geriatric patients. *Gerontologist, 14,* 138–142.

Bleathman, C., & Morton, I. (1992). Validation therapy: Extracts from 20 groups with dementia sufferers. *Journal of Advanced Nursing, 17,* 658–666.

Bourgeois, M.S. (1990). Enhancing conversation skills in patients with Alzheimer's disease using a prosthetic memory aid. *Journal of Applied Behaviour Analysis, 23,* 29–42.

Breuil, V., Rotrou, J.D., Forette, F., Tortrat, D., Ganansia-Ganem, A., Frambourt, A., Moulin, F., & Boller, F. (1994). Cognitive stimulation of patients with dementia: Preliminary results. *International Journal of Geriatric Psychiatry, 9,* 211–217.

Brook, P., Degun, G., & Mather, M. (1975). Reality orientation, a therapy for psychogeriatric patients: A controlled study. *British Journal of Psychiatry, 127*, 42–45.

Camp, C.J., Foss, J.W., O'Hanlon, A.M., & Stevens, A.B. (1996). Memory interventions for persons with dementia. *Applied Cognitive Psychology, 10*, 193–210.

Citrin, R.S., & Dixon, D.N. (1977). Reality orientation: a milieu therapy used in an institution for the aged. *Gerontologist, 17*, 39–43.

Clare, L., Wilson, B.A., Breen, K., & Hodges, J.R. (1999). Errorless learning of face–name associations in early Alzheimer's disease. *Neurocase, 5*, 37–46.

Coen Mieli, D., Spizzichino, S., Zuccaro, S.M., Menasci, A., Calvetti, D., & Manor, M.M., (1991). Effect of modified Reality Orientation therapy in patients with severe cognitive disorder. *Archives of Gerontology & Geriatrics, 2*, 143–146.

Cornbleth, T., & Cornbleth, C. (1979). Evaluation of the effectiveness of Reality Orientation classes in a nursing home unit. *Journal of American Geriatrics Society, 27*, 522–524.

Dietch, J.T., Hewett, L.J., & Jones, S. (1989). Adverse effects of reality orientation. *Journal of American Geriatrics Society, 37*, 974–976.

Folstein, M.F., Folstein, S.E., & McHugh, P.R. (1975). Mini-mental state: A practical method for grading the cognitive state of patients for the clinician. *Journal of Psychiatric Research, 12*, 189–198.

Gatz, M., Fiske, A., Fox, L. S., Kaskie, B., Kasl-Godley, J.E., McCallum, T.J., & Wetherell, J.L. (1998). Empirically validated psychological treatments for older adults. *Journal of Mental Health & Aging, 4*, 9–46.

Gerber, G.J., Prince, P.N., Snider, H.G., Atchinson, K., Dubois, L., & Kilgour, J.A. (1991). Group activity and cognitive improvement among patients with Alzheimer's disease. *Hospital and Community Psychiatry, 42*, 843–846.

Gibson, F. (1993). What can reminiscence contribute to people with dementia? In J. Bornat (Ed.), *Reminiscence reviewed: Perspective, evaluations, achievements*. Milton Keynes, UK: Open University Press.

Goldberg, D.P. (1978). *Manual of the General Health Questionnaire*. Slough, UK: NFER/ Nelson.

Goldstein, G., Turner, S.M., Holzman, A., Kanagy, M., Elmore, S., & Barry, K., (1982). An evaluation of Reality Orientation therapy. *Journal of Behavioural Assessment, 4*, 165–178.

Goldwasser, N.A., Auerbach, S.M., & Harkins, S.W. (1987). Cognitive, affective and behavioural effects of reminiscence group therapy on demented elderly. *International Journal of Aging and Human Development, 25*, 209–222.

Gotestam, K.G. (1987). Learning versus environmental support for increasing reality orientation in senile demented patients. *European Journal of Psychiatry, 1*, 7–12.

Greene, J.G., Nicol, R., & Jamieson, H. (1979). Reality orientation with psychogeriatric patients: Case histories and shorter communications. *Behaviour Research & Therapy, 17*, 615–618.

Greene, J.G., Smith, R., Gardiner, M., & Timbury, G.C. (1982). Measuring behavioural disturbance of elderly demented patients in the community and its effect on relatives: A factor analytic study. *Age & Ageing, 11*, 121–126.

Greene, J.G., Timbury, G.C., Smith, R., & Gardiner, M. (1983). Reality orientation with elderly patients in the community: An empirical evaluation. *Age & Ageing, 12*, 38–43.

Gubrium, J.F., & Ksander, M. (1975). On multiple realities and reality orientation. *Gerontologist, 15*, 142–145.

Hanley, I.G., McGuire, R.J., & Boyd, W.D. (1981). Reality orientation and dementia: A controlled trial of two approaches. *British Journal of Psychiatry, 138*, 10–14.

Hogstel, M.O. (1979). Use of reality orientation with aging confused patients. *Nursing Research, 28*, 161–165.

Holden, U.P., & Woods, R.T. (1995). *Positive approaches to dementia care*. (3rd ed.). Edinburgh: Churchill Livingstone.

Hughes, C.P., Berg, L., Danziger, W.L., Coben, L.A., & Martin, R.L. (1982). A new clinical scale for the staging of dementia. *British Journal of Psychiatry, 140*, 566–572.

Kiernat, J.M. (1979). The use of life review activity with confused nursing home residents. *American Journal of Occupational Therapy, 33*, 306–310.

Kitwood, T. (1990). The dialectics of dementia: With particular reference to Alzheimer's disease. *Ageing and Society, 10*, 177–196.

Kitwood, T. (1997). *Dementia reconsidered: The person comes first*. Buckingham: Open University Press.

Koh, K., Ray, R., Lee, J., Nair, A., Ho, T., & Ang, P.C. (1994). Dementia in elderly patients: Can the 3R mental stimulation programme improve mental status? *Age and Ageing, 23*, 195–199.

Neal, M., & Briggs, M., (1999). *Validation therapy for dementia* (Cochrane Review). The Cochrane Library, Issue 2, Oxford: Update Software.

Orten, J.D., Allen, M., & Cook, J. (1989). Reminiscence groups with confused nursing centre residents: An experimental study. *Social Work in Health Care, 14*, 73–86.

Pattie, A.H., & Gilleard, C.T. (1979). *Clifton Assessment Procedures for the Elderly (CAPE)*. Sevenoaks, UK: Hodder & Stoughton.

Quayhagen, M.P., & Quayhagen, M. (1989). Differential effects of family-based strategies on Alzheimer's disease. *Gerontologist, 29*, 150–155.

Reeve, W., & Ivison, D. (1985). Use of environmental manipulation and classroom and modified reality orientation with institutionalised, confused elderly patients. *Age and Ageing, 14*, 119–121.

Rosen, W.G., Mohs, R.C., & Davis, K.L. (1984). A new rating scale for Alzheimer's disease. *American Journal of Psychiatry, 141*, 1356–1364.

Ruskin, P.E., & Talbott, J.A. (1993). *Aging and post-traumatic stress disorder*. Washington DC: American Psychiatric Association.

Shankar, K., Walker, M., Frost, D., & Orrell, M.W. (1999). The development of a valid and reliable scale for anxiety in dementia. *Aging and Mental Health, 3*, 39–49.

Spector, A., Orrell, M., Davies, S., & Woods, B. (1998a). *Reality orientation for dementia: A review of the evidence for its effectiveness*. The Cochrane Library, Issue 4, Oxford: Update Software.

Spector, A., Orrell, M., Davies, S., & Woods, B. (1998b). *Reminiscence therapy for dementia: A review of the evidence for its effectiveness*. The Cochrane Library, Issue 4, Oxford: Update Software.

Taulbee, L.R., & Folsom, J.C. (1966) Reality orientation for geriatric patients. *Hospital and Community Psychiatry, 17*, 133–5.

Toseland, R.W., Diehl, M., Freeman, K., Manzanares, T., Naleppa, M., & McCallion, P. (1997). The impact of validation group therapy on nursing home residents with dementia. *Journal of Applied Gerontology, 16*, 31–50.

Update Software (1996). *RevMan*. Version 3.0 for Windows. Oxford: Update Software.

Voekel, D. (1978). A study of reality orientation and resocialisation groups with confused elderly. *Journal of Gerontological Nursing, 4*, 13–18.

Wallis, G.G., Baldwin, M. & Higgenbotham, P. (1983) Reality orientation therapy: A controlled trial. *British Journal of Medical Psychology, 56*, 271–277.

Woods, R.T. (1979). Reality orientation and staff attention: A controlled study. *British Journal of Psychiatry, 134*: 502–507.

Woods, R.T. (1994). Problems in the elderly: Treatment. In S.J.E. Lindesay & G.E. Powell (Eds.), *The handbook of clinical adult psychology* (Second ed., pp. 438–458). London: Routledge.

Woods, B. (1999). The person in dementia care. *Generations, 23*, 35–39.

Woods, R.T., & McKiernan, F. (1995). Evaluating the impact of reminiscence on older people with dementia. In B.K. Haight & J. Webster (Eds.), *The art and science of reminiscing: Theory, research, methods and applications* (pp. 233–242). Washington DC: Taylor & Francis.

Zanetti, O., Frisoni, G.B., De Leo, D., Buono, M.D., Bianchetti, A., & Trabucci, M. (1995). Reality orientation therapy in Alzheimer's disease: Useful or not? A controlled study. *Alzheimer's Disease and Associated Disorders*, *9*, 132–138.

Zarit, S.H., Zarit, J.M., & Reever, K.E. (1982) Memory training for severe memory loss: Effects on senile dementia patients and their families. *Gerontologist*, *22*, 373–377.

APPENDIX 1

At beginning of each session:

1. Five minute warm-up, such as soft ball game. When throwing the ball, people may either state their own name or (for the more able) the name of the person they are throwing the ball to.
2. Discuss the day, month, year, season, time, name and address of home.
3. Short-term memory prompts, such as asking people what they had for breakfast/lunch, what they thought of yesterday's weather.
4. Discuss something that is currently in the news.

Sessions

1. Physical game, such as rollaball or indoor boules, which involves teamwork. This should be a relatively relaxed activity for the first session, incorporating movement, touch and score calculations.
2. Sound: Sound effects tapes, which include different categories, such as "indoor sounds" and "outdoor sounds", to be matched with the correct picture. This provides people with both visual and auditory stimulation, making the task easier. Percussion instruments given to each person in the group, to be played with music (such as popular 1940s music).
3. Childhood: Activities include people filling out a sheet asking their name, father's name, mother's name, schools attended, etc.; construction of their childhood bedroom or house on a board; and demonstrating the use of old-fashioned childhood toys.
4. Food: Using miniature grocery replicas which have been priced, give people a budget and a scenario, e.g., dinner for four. Alternatively, categorise these objects, e.g., different mealtimes, special occasions, savoury foods. Additionally, eat food with reminiscent or personal meaning, and brainstorm food categories on the whiteboard.
5. Current affairs: Discuss issues from a selection of the day's national and local newspapers, and picture magazines. Use cue cards to evoke conversation on news, views, attitudes, dreams and aspirations.
6. Faces/scenes: To reduce the attentional problem of only one person being able to look at each picture at a time, multiple sets of the famous faces cards (added to more modern pictures) have been created. Give people four cards. Ask them to identify named person/scene. Ask opinions, e.g., most beautiful, oldest. Attempt to use opinions to generate memories for names.
7. Associated words/discussion: Sentence completion task. Includes amounts (e.g., a cup of . . .), famous couples (e.g., Laurel and . . .), famous places (e.g., Westminster . . .). Use "Golden Expression" cards to stimulate discussion, e.g., "What do you think of medicine today?".
8. Using objects: Creative session, such as cookery. Multiple tasks enable all to participate (e.g., greasing bowl, mixing ingredients, making crumble mixture, peeling and slicing apples).
9. Categorising objects: People think of words beginning with a particular letter (picked from a card) in a particular category (picked from a card). Alternatively, brainstorm categories on board.

10. Orientation: Construct map of England, local area or home on whiteboard. Fill in the "map" by asking the group to suggest different places or landmarks, such as the post office, and draw them in the appropriate position.

11. Using money: Use laminated cut-outs of common objects from a catalogue, with prices on the back. Tasks could involve guessing the prices, adding prices (how much will the bill be?), or matching the pricetag with the object.

12. Number game: involving the recognition and use of numbers.

13. Word identification game ("Hangman"): involving the recognition and use of letters and words. Draw a number of dashes for each letter of a word, and ask the group to guess the letters. Incorrect letters contribute to the drawing of a "hangman" and losing the game. The group is required to guess the word.

14. Team games: divide the group into two teams, ask them to choose a team name, and play trivia quiz. Give prizes to all the group, and say farewells.

Manuscript received August 2000
Revised manuscript received October 2000

Effects of memory aids on conversations between nursing home residents with dementia and nursing assistants

Laura Hoerster

Healthsouth Harmarville Rehabilitation Hospital, Pittsburgh, PA, USA

Ellen M. Hickey, and Michelle S. Bourgeois

Department of Communication Disorders, The Florida State University, Tallahassee, FL, USA

The effects of personalised memory books on the conversations between four residents with dementia and three nursing assistants (NAs) were evaluated using an experimental, single-subject design. Most residents increased their production of factual utterances, NAs decreased their use of non-facilitative conversational behaviours, and conversational turn-taking became more equitable when residents used their books. The addition of NA instruction resulted in further reduction of non-facilitative NA behaviour. The effects of the intervention were somewhat weaker with residents with greater dementia severity. Social validity measures suggested that this intervention may hold promise for improving conversations between NAs and residents with dementia.

Nursing home residents' communicative interactions are influenced by the institutional environment of the setting, wherein the quality of communication between nursing staff and residents is often observed to be less than optimal (Baltes & Reisenzein, 1986; Bohling, 1991; Burgio & Bourgeois, 1992;

Correspondence should be sent to Michelle S. Bourgeois, Department of Communication Disorders, 304 Regional Rehabilitation Center, Tallahassee, FL 32306-1200, USA. Tel: (850) 644-6639, email: mbourgeo@garnet.acns.fsu.edu.

This research was supported by grants from the National Institute on Aging to the University of Pittsburgh (R01 AG 09291) and the Florida State University (R01 AG 13008). The authors thank Connie Tompkins, Ph.D., and the residents and staff of Marion Manor Nursing Home for their contributions to this research.

Caporael & Culbertson, 1986; Grainger, 1995; Kaakinen, 1992; Liukkonen, 1995; Lubinski, 1995; Nussbaum, Robinson, & Grew, 1985; Seers, 1986; Sigman, 1985). Among the factors detrimental to communication in long-term care settings are limited communication partners for the residents, interactions restricted to social amenities, trivial and short interchanges, and administrative philosophies placing little emphasis on communication (Lubinski, 1978). Nursing home staff perceive themselves as too busy to talk with residents, and that little staff–resident interaction occurs apart from giving and receiving nursing care (Lubinski, 1978). Most of the interactions between staff and residents are task-oriented rather than relational (Bowers & Becker, 1992; Grainger, 1995; Jacelon, 1995). When staff members have the opportunity to talk, they more frequently talk to each other than to the residents (Sigman, 1985). Staff are noted to have low expectations for residents, especially those with cognitive or communicative disabilities, leading to low levels of social interaction.

Residents also perceive staff as too busy to engage in conversation, and feel that they should not bother the staff unnecessarily (Jacelon, 1995; Kaakinen, 1992; Liukkonen, 1995; Sigman, 1985). Residents have complained of the restriction of caregiver conversational topics to health and the perception that staff members resent residents (Lubinski, Morrison, & Rigrodsky, 1981). Other implicit rules reported by residents regarding communication include not talking too much, and not talking to those who are thought to be senile (Kaakinen, 1992). Physical and cognitive impairments are positively correlated with decreased engagement, conflict, and distress in nursing home residents (Mor et al., 1995; Schroll et al., 1997). Disabled residents' efforts at social integration are often met with rejection because of this conflict and distress, propagating low levels of interaction.

The negative climate for staff–resident communication is compounded by the high proportion of nursing home residents with dementia (up to 74%) (Burgio & Bourgeois, 1992). Long-term care staff are required to deal with the problem behaviours of residents with dementia, including communication deficits, often without specific training. Among the negative behaviours common in this population are verbal and physical agitation, inability to follow directions, and wandering (Burgio & Bourgeois, 1992). Behaviour problems are sometimes attributed to limited communication abilities (Bartol, 1979; Bourgeois et al., 1997). Communication impairment in individuals with dementia is characterised by word-finding difficulties and production of off-topic and meaningless sentences, and production of fewer utterances per turn than normally ageing individuals (Bayles & Tomoeda, 1991; Hutchinson & Jenson, 1981). Individuals with dementia also have decreasing conciseness and increasing ideational repetitions as the dementia progresses (Ripich, Carpenter, & Ziol, 1997; Tomoeda et al., 1996). The inability to sustain a conversation is one postulated result of these deficits (Bayles & Tomoeda,

1991), as language use is more significantly impacted than specific linguistic abilities (Fromm & Holland, 1989; Ripich & Terrell, 1988).

Burgio, Butler, and Engel (1988) reported that nursing staff expressed concern about the severe behaviour problems in residents with dementia, but felt that they had not received sufficient training to manage these problems. A physically and emotionally demanding job with few rewards, residents with severe behaviour deficits related to dementia, and lack of training to manage problematic resident behaviour result in non-facilitative behaviours on the part of the nursing assistants (NAs). NAs find ways to increase their efficiency, including anticipating the needs of the residents (Grainger, 1995), and cutting corners (Bowers & Becker, 1992), further reducing the interaction with the residents. Other strategies NAs use to deal with residents' problematic issues include ignoring or contradicting the residents, referring the resident to a higher authority (e.g., nurse or doctor), and making light of the residents' troubles (Grainger, 1995).

Several investigators have provided descriptive data regarding types of communicative behaviours observed in caregivers. Baltes, Kinderman, Reisenzein, and Schmid (1987) discovered that institutional staff conversing with elderly residents produced a high frequency of requests and commands. The use of excessive questioning by caregivers has been identified as a behaviour that is non-facilitative when dealing with individuals with dementia (Bourgeois, 1992; Ostuni & Santo-Pietro, 1986). The questioning style adopted by caregivers is paradoxical. Although caregivers feel a need to ask questions to obtain verbal communication from residents with dementia, a common result of extensive questioning is to increase residents' frustration and decrease their desire to communicate (Bourgeois, 1992). Other studies (Macleod-Clark, 1981; Nussbaum et al., 1985; Seers, 1986) have classified the conversational content of nursing staff in terms of topic matter (e.g., task, medical, personal, social). Few of these descriptive studies have specifically addressed caregiver communication with residents who have dementia. One such study (Bohling, 1991) investigated listening patterns of adult day care workers conversing with individuals who had dementia. Bohling's (1991) results suggested that by listening sensitively and adopting a person's frame of reference, caregivers could prevent high levels of anxiety from building in their residents with dementia.

Changing the communicative behaviour of nursing staff could have a strong, positive impact on residents (Grainger, 1995). For example, NAs who discussed the topics of "old times", "religion", and "hobbies of the resident" reported higher levels of affinity for the resident with whom they conversed than NAs who discussed topics such as the resident's health, the NA's personal problems, and the NA's job (Nussbaum et al., 1985). Macleod-Clark (1981) also emphasised the importance of addressing the emotional and communication needs of residents as a significant component of total care.

Although individual differences exist in the personalities and communication styles of nursing staff, it is necessary to improve the communication skills of less competent staff members through direct training (Macleod-Clark, 1981).

Two areas of intervention can be developed in response to the existing communication problems in the nursing home, training NAs and treating residents with dementia. Direct training of NAs may help to curb their negative and non-facilitative responses to residents with dementia. In addition, direct interventions for residents with dementia are needed to modify the wide range of problematic behaviours that are frequently antecedent to negative staff responses and perpetuate the negative communication setting in the nursing home. However, there have been limited scientific investigations of these types of interventions.

One promising approach designed to maintain conversation skills in individuals with dementia addresses the semantic deficits underlying conversational breakdown (Bourgeois, 1990). Bourgeois (1990) evaluated the performance of individuals with Alzheimer's disease (AD) using prosthetic memory aids, known as "memory wallets", in conversations with spouses and familiar partners. When using memory wallets, individuals with moderate dementia increased the number of factual statements made (both on-topic and elaborated) and decreased the number of ambiguous, error, perseverative, and unintelligible statements made in 5-min conversations. In this initial study, naïve judges rated the conversational performance of individuals with AD as significantly improved when memory wallets were utilised (Bourgeois, 1990). This memory aid approach has been investigated further in a variety of settings and with a variety of conversational partners. Bourgeois (1992) demonstrated improvements in conversations of individuals with moderate dementia using wallets in an adult day care setting with experimenters and members of the adult daycare staff. Familiar trainers noted positive changes in the conversational behaviours of individuals with AD including increased elaboration of topics, decreased repetitiveness, increased initiation, and decreased memory loss (Bourgeois, 1992). In a nursing home setting, members of conversational dyads in which both participants had moderate to severe dementia evidenced similar improvements in semantic aspects of conversation (Bourgeois, 1993). Additionally, equity of conversational turn-taking improved when a memory aid was used, even for a resident who was functioning at a low cognitive level. Unfamiliar judges rated dyad members using memory aids as being better at maintaining topics, introducing novel information, turn-taking, and responding to partners than members of dyads conversing without memory aids (Bourgeois, 1993).

Using a memory aid to enhance the semantic content of residents has the potential to improve interactions between NAs and residents with dementia. Bourgeois (1990, 1992, 1993) found the most significant changes in residents with moderate dementia; the few severely cognitively impaired residents (Bourgeois, 1993) showed less robust effects of the memory aid intervention. More research is needed to determine the usefulness of memory aid treatments with lower functioning individuals with AD, especially residents in nursing homes, whose difficulty maintaining communication skills may be exacerbated by the limitations of the nursing home environment. If lower functioning residents are able to benefit from the treatment, and NAs perceive improvements in the communication skills of the residents, NAs may alter their communicative behaviours while interacting with the residents. These changes in communicative interactions may result in a more stimulating and satisfying communication environment for both NAs and residents with dementia.

This study examined conversational interactions between NAs and nursing home residents with dementia using prosthetic memory aids containing personal information about the residents. Changes in the conversational content produced by residents with severe dementia using a memory aid, and conversational behaviours of NAs were evaluated during 5-min timed conversations throughout baseline and treatment phases. Clinical significance was measured using two social validation techniques, the ratings of naïve judges, and reports of NAs' satisfaction. The following specific research questions were addressed:

1. Do residents with dementia conversing with NAs in a nursing home setting produce more on-topic statements of fact, and fewer off-topic statements in conversations with NAs when personal memory aids are used as compared to unaided conversational situations?
2. Does NA production of non-facilitative communicative behaviours (e.g., requests and assertions) change in conversations with residents with dementia when the residents use memory aids?
3. Does the equity of conversational turn-taking improve when the residents use memory aids?
4. Are the changes clinically significant, as judged by naive listeners and by reports of NAs' satisfaction?

METHOD

Participants

Residents with dementia. Four female residents with dementia (RD1–RD4) participated. Each resident had a primary diagnosis of one of the following types of dementia: Alzheimer's disease (AD), multi-infarct dementia (MID), or organic brain syndrome (OBS), established by a board-certified physician. Information about residents with dementia was obtained via chart review, and by interviews with nursing staff, residents, and families of residents. Table 1 summarises the characteristics of the residents with dementia.

Residents with dementia were sampled from those identified to be "verbal communicators" by nursing supervisors, using the following criteria: (1) makes spontaneous attempts to vocalise, (2) has intelligible speech at least 50% of the time, and (3) uses verbalisation as her primary mode of communication. In addition, participants had to have involved family members who could provide the information and photographs needed to complete the residents' memory books. All participants were observed to initiate conversations with staff, peers, and family members during activities of daily living and social visits.

Table 1 also displays the results of cognitive and language testing. The Bourgeois Reading Screening (Bourgeois, 1992) was administered to assess reading ability and to determine which size print (0.25" or 0.5") each resident could read best in her memory book. All residents exceeded the 70% criteria (maximum number of errors = 3/25) for reading both sizes, and all residents stated a preference for the 0.5" print. The presence and extent of deficits in naming ability and informativeness of connected speech were assessed by measuring the number of content units (CUs) produced while describing the "Cookie Theft" picture (Goodglass & Kaplan, 1972). Residents had to score in the moderate to severe range (5–15 content units) on this task (Yorkston & Beukelman, 1980). A minimum of five CUs was considered sufficient to ensure adequate verbal output in the timed conversational probes (Nicholas, Obler, Albert, & Helm-Estabrooks, 1985; Yorkston & Beukelman, 1980). The poor performance (two CUs) of RD3 on the day of formal testing differed from a prior informal assessment using the same instrument, and was not thought to reflect her optimal ability.

Nursing assistants. Four female full-time NAs volunteered for participation in this study. These four NAs were recommended by the Director of Nursing and their unit supervisors based on the appraisal of their skills as representative of the "average" NA at the home and their availability for participation in the study. All NAs had been employed on the daylight shift and had worked on the same unit of the nursing home for a minimum of 1 month. Three of the four had completed a Nursing Assistant training course approved by the State of Pennsylvania, and the fourth was enrolled in such a course at the time of the study. Additionally, all NAs had received on-the-job training from an NA from the Pennsylvania Nurse Aide Registry, Division of Long-Term Care. For this study, NAs were paired with residents who were on their assigned floor but not on their regular care caseload. Therefore, NAs were casually familiar with the residents, but had minimal personal knowledge of them. All NAs were native speakers of English. Table 2 summarises demographic characteristics of the four NAs.

TABLE 1
Characteristics of residents with dementia (RDs)

	RD1	RD2	RD3	RD4
Primary diagnosis	MID	AD	OBS	AD
Co-occurring neurological or psychological diagnoses	–	Early PD, right CVA with cerebellar ataxia	MID, right CVA with slight left hemiparesis	Depression
Age (years)	90	88	89	83
Education (years)	14	12	14	16
MMSE	12	9	8	8
Content units	6	8*	2	6
Oral reading errors	0*	1*	1*	2*
	0**	0**	0**	1**
Length of residence at nursing home (months)	17	16	14	19
Total length of institutionalisation (months)	17	40	44	19

MID, Multi-Infarct Dementia; AD, Alzheimer's disease; OBS, organic brain syndrome; CVA, cerebrovascular accident; PD, Parkinson's disease. MMSE, Mini-Mental Status Exam score, 30 total. Content units: number of information units generated on picture discription subtest of the Boston Diagnostic Aphasia Examination. Oral reading errors: out of 25 possible on the Bourgeois Reading Screening.
* print size 0.25"; ** print size 0.5".

TABLE 2
Characteristics of nursing assistants (NAs)

	NA1	NA2	NA3	NA4
Age (years)	20	20	29	22
Education (years)	13	12	13	13
Length of employment at nursing home (months)	1	24	1	1
Total length of NA employment (months)	1	48	8	1

In addition, each NA who had been identified as a good candidate for the study was asked to have a 5-min conversation with a resident with dementia who was not a study participant. NA target behaviours were observed in order to verify high levels of the target non-facilitative behaviours (i.e., requests and assertions). The NA was instructed to find out as much about the resident as she could. No additional prompts were given to NAs or residents. As shown in Table 3, all three NAs produced a high frequency of requests. Assertions were relatively few in number, but remained target behaviours because the residents did not have an opportunity to respond to these utterances or to initiate topics. Additionally, two NAs dominated the conversation by producing more utterances per conversation than residents.

Setting and apparatus

This study was conducted on one mixed-population wing with two floors in a non-profit Catholic nursing home. Each of the floors in this section of the building housed 26 of the 212 residents in the nursing home. The level of care required by residents on each floor varied from total independence (resident performed all activities of daily living independently) to total care (resident required assistance with all activities of daily living). All conversational probes occurred in the residents' rooms. NAs and residents sat in chairs facing each other. All sessions were audio-taped and timed using a digital countdown timer with electronic alarm. Background noise was eliminated to maximise hearing conditions and to decrease distractions for residents.

TABLE 3
Prebaseline results: Frequency of NA behaviours in 5-min conversation with non-experimental residents with dementia

	NA1	NA2	NA3
Requests	52	29	51
Assertions	6	4	2
Directives	1	0	0
Responses	38	20	26
Other	7	6	2
Total utterances—NA	106	59	81
(RD)	(76)	(65)	(71)
Utterances/turn—NA	1.49	1.11	1.25
(RD)	(1.04)	(1.23)	(1.09)

NA4 did not participate in this phase of the study because she was recruited later.

Stimuli

A memory book containing 25 pages of picture and sentence stimuli (Bourgeois, 1990) was constructed for each resident with dementia. Each memory book included facts related to the resident's memory failures for personally relevant information, as reported by family members on a question-naire. Facts that were of particular significance to the resident, and availability of corresponding photographs to accompany them, were also criteria for choosing memory book stimuli (Bourgeois, 1993). Sentences were developed based on this personal information, and were printed in 0.5" block letters with upper and lower case on the bottom of sheets of 8.5" × 11" unlined white paper. Corresponding picture stimuli were then mounted on each page. Pages were inserted into clear plastic protective sleeves then placed in a ring binder.

Memory book training

Following the baseline phase and prior to treatment, the experimenter trained each resident with dementia to use her memory book in conversation. The resident was given her memory book and instructed: "This book is for you. It has a picture and a sentence on each page to help you remember things about your life, your family and friends, and things you like to do. Let's look at it together. Open your book. We'll look at each page. Look at the picture and read the sentence on each page aloud." Residents were praised for spontaneously reading a sentence correctly and for elaborating on the sentences. The experi-menter allowed at least 5 s for the resident to read the next sentence or to elabo-rate on a sentence. If the resident did not read a sentence spontaneously, the experimenter prompted her to do so by pointing to the sentence, then, if neces-sary, by saying, "Read the sentence aloud". If the resident did not produce a spontaneous elaboration within 30 s of reading a sentence, the experimenter said, "Tell me more about that". Training continued until the resident read each sentence at least once and elaborated on 30% of the sentences in one session.

Data collection and procedures

Nursing assistants were asked to have a 5-min conversation with their resident with dementia once a week. The experimenter sat across the room from the dyad in an inconspicuous place. Instructions to the dyad are described below for each condition. The conversations were audio-taped for later scoring.

Scoring. All probe conversations with the RDs were transcribed verbatim by the experimenter, using standard punctuation and adding contextual notes. Each transcript contained the utterances for both the NA and the RD, numbered sequentially, and identified for speaker. All scoring was done using the transcripts and supplemented by the audio recordings when necessary.

Operational definitions of the five RD and five NA behaviours are provided below.

RD Behaviours:

1. *On-topic statements* were self-initiated intelligible and unambiguous information contained in the memory book, or other statements of fact that contributed additional personally relevant information (e.g., "My children are Mary and John" and "I was a teacher for 30 years").

2. *Off-topic statements* contained ambiguous, perseverative, or error information, including misread memory book statements (e.g., Memory book open to picture of son: "That's my nephew" and "I want to go home, I want to go").

3. *RD other statements* functioned as questions, placeholders, organisational devices, or social conventions, or did not meet the criteria for on-topic or off-topic statements. RD other statements included laughter and factual statements about the physical environment (e.g., "Let me see" and "It's all right.").

4. *RD responses* were intelligible and unambiguous requests for clarification, answers to questions, or repetitions of preceding partner utterances that served to acknowledge or clarify (e.g., after NA asks where the RD lived: "Where did I live?" or "I don't know", or "Well, let me see").

5. *Unintelligible statements* included neologisms, literal, verbal, semantic, and phonological paraphasias, sentence fragments, non-English phrases, and multiple joined sentence fragments (e.g., "My brother's uh...").

NA Behaviours:

1. *Requests* were used to elicit information from the RD, and were usually used to initiate a conversation, and included giving additional cues or parts to a question (e.g., "What is your daughter's name?" and "How long were you married?"). Requests were not necessarily in response to an RD utterance.

2. *Assertions* were meant to identify, describe, or explain observable events, and were not in response to an RD utterance. Assertions included statements of fact unrelated to the RD ("Your son is handsome" and "This is your book").

3. *Directives* were intended to command/direct the patient to do some action, and may have served a possible teaching function, including modelling, or labelling of objects (e.g., "Turn the page" or "Look at the picture").

4. *Responses* served to acknowledge previously presented information and to maintain a conversation, to affirm or repeat a preceding RD comment, to answer an RD's question, or to request clarification without soliciting new information (e.g., after RD tells NA she had three children "You

sure did" or "What nice children"). Responses also included those that appeared to be related to probable nonverbal communicative gestures (e.g., nodding) of the RD.

5. *NA Other statements* either did not meet the criteria of the above utterances, or functioned as social conventions, placeholders, or responses to the RD's physical rather than communicative actions (e.g., "Let me see" or "Are you having trouble sitting still today?"). NA other statements could also be attempts to gain the RD's attention (e.g., "Hey, Jane").

Experimental design

A multiple baseline design across subjects was used to assess changes in the conversational interactions of NA–RD dyads as a function of the presence of a memory book. Experimental control was demonstrated by beginning baseline concurrently for the first three NA–RD dyads, then introducing the memory book treatment sequentially to each dyad while the others remained in baseline. Dyad 4 began baseline at Session 4 because RD4 was recruited into the study later as a backup when RD3 was hospitalised temporarily. Baseline probes continued until the primary target behaviour remained at a stable and high level for each NA. Movement between experimental phases was made after visual inspection of line graphs indicated a stable or increasing trend in baseline or a stable or decreasing trend in treatment for the target behaviours. It was expected that the number of requests made by each NA would decrease in the treatment phase as a function of the resident using her memory book. If visual inspection of a minimum of three data points revealed that questioning still occurred at a high level during this treatment phase, or if the experimenter judged that the level of change was not clinically significant, a second treatment phase was implemented. Treatment sessions (Treatment 1 and Treatment 2) continued until a minimum of 5 and a maximum of 10 data points were collected across both treatment phases.

Baseline. Each nursing assistant participated in 5-min conversational interactions once a week with their resident with dementia. Memory books were not available during baseline conversations. The NAs were instructed as follows: "I would like you to have a conversation with (Resident) now. Talk with her about her life, her family, and things she likes to do." The residents with dementia were instructed as follows: "I would like you to have a 5-minute conversation with (NA). You could tell her about your life, your family, and things you like to do. I'll tell you when the 5 minutes are over. You can begin now." A tape recorder was turned on, and the countdown timer was started. The experimenter sat in an inconspicuous place in the room where the NA and the resident remained observable. If 30 s elapsed with no conversation from either participant, the experimenter interjected a general prompt, "Tell her more about that" or "Talk about (*Resident's*) family now".

Treatment 1. Memory books were introduced to the NA during the first treatment conversation with the instructions: "This is a book with pictures and sentences to help (*Resident*) remember things about her life, her family and friends, and things she likes to do. Let her use her book to help her have a conversation with you." Residents were then instructed: "Tell (*NA*) about the pictures in your book. You can begin now."

Treatment 2. To counteract the NA questioning behaviour, the following instruction was added: "When you look at (*Resident's*) memory book with her, try to let her talk more. She may need extra time to think of what she wants to say. Pointing to the sentence on the page may help her. When she does read a sentence, you can say, 'Tell me more about that before moving on'."

Reliability

Throughout the experiment, an independent observer (a graduate student in speech–language pathology) was given tapes and transcripts that were randomly selected from each dyad to obtain word-by-word reliability on at least one baseline and one treatment session for each dyad. She indicated transcription disagreements on 11 out of 43 conversations by marking an "X" above the word in question on the transcripts. Overall word-by-word agreement was 98.4%. The independent observer also indicated agreements and disagreements for utterance per turn for 10 out of 43 transcripts. Agreement on the number of utterances per turn was 100%. Conversational behaviours were coded by the independent observer for 33% of all transcripts (at least one transcript per dyad for each of the three phases) throughout the study. The mean point-to-point agreement per probe session for coding the dependent variables for Dyads 1, 2, 3, and 4 was 89.2% (range 85.2–92.8%), 91.9% (range 87.5–96.1%), 87.8% (range 85–90%), and 87.8% (range 83–90.5%), respectively.

Social validation measures

Unfamiliar judges. A social validation procedure was implemented following the study to assess whether unfamiliar listeners could detect changes in the conversations of the dyads over time (Bond & Lader, 1974; Guyatt, Berman, Townsend, & Taylor, 1985). One baseline and one treatment probe was randomly selected for each of the four dyads for social validity rating. The audiotapes from these sessions were dubbed onto a master tape in random order for each dyad, with baseline and treatment sessions for each dyad dubbed consecutively.

Ten unfamiliar judges who were all college graduates ranging in age from 24 to 31 used a 5.8 cm visual analogue scale to rate one baseline and one treatment session along six dimensions (Bourgeois, 1993). The dimensions included (a) comfortable vs. awkward, (b) ambiguous vs. unambiguous information provided, (c) novel content, (d) topic maintenance, (e) equity of turn taking, and (f) responsiveness to the partner's prior turn. Judges listened to the audio-tapes of each session played on a stereo cassette player. The tape was stopped after each segment so they could mark a vertical pencil line along the continuum for each dimension. The first two dimensions were rated on scales of 100% comfortable to 100% awkward, and 100% ambiguous to 100% unambiguous. The topic maintenance, new information, equity of turn taking, and responsiveness dimensions were rated on scales from 0% to 100% of the time for that dimension. Once judges had marked their forms, the next segment was played, until all eight conversations were rated. The mean rating for each dyad was calculated by measuring the distance from the end of each scale to the judge's mark using a centimetre ruler. The mean distance for all 10 ratings in each segment for each dimension was calculated and divided by 5.8, then multiplied by 100 for the total percentage rating.

NA satisfaction. An informal post-treatment interview comprised of seven questions was used to assess NA satisfaction with the memory aid treatment. The experimenter posed questions that addressed general communicative style with nursing home residents and specific changes in conversations effected by the memory aid. Each interview was taperecorded and transcribed by the experimenter.

RESULTS

Memory book training

Training session data are displayed in Table 4. RD1 and RD 2 met the training criteria of oral reading of sentences with elaboration of 30% of sentences within two sessions. RD3 and RD4 required multiple training sessions due to fatigue and/or agitation. Within three sessions, RD3 met the reading, but not the elaboration criteria. Although RD4 failed to meet criteria for reading within four sessions due to limited attention, she elaborated on 28% of the sentences in the fourth trial.

Effects of memory aids on NA–RD conversations

Changes in residents' conversational content. The frequency of on-topic (total of memory aid and elaborated statements) and off-topic utterances produced by each resident in the 5-min conversations are shown in Figure 1. In

TABLE 4
Memory book training data for residents with dementia

	RD1	RD2	RD3	RD4
Number of training sessions	2	1	3	3
Number of trials to criterion	2	1	3	4*
Mean correct per trial	19.5	25	17.33	11.25
Mean elaborations per trial	12	20	4	5.25

* Did not reach criterion after four training sessions.

baseline sessions, all residents produced a low and stable level of on-topic utterances. RD2, RD3, and RD4 produced a comparatively high level of off-topic statements, while RD1 produced few of either type of targeted behaviours. Three nontargeted behaviours (responsive, unintelligible, and other) were also measured. Mean frequencies per condition are presented in Table 5. Unintelligible and other behaviours remained stable at low levels, while responses remained stable at high levels for all four residents throughout baseline.

All residents demonstrated an increase in on-topic statements with use of a memory aid in Treatment 1. RD2 showed the most dramatic increase in on-topic utterances, with a concomitant decrease in off-topic utterances, during the first treatment phase. RD4 also showed a dramatic increase in on-topic utterances, but with less of a decrease in off-topic utterances with use of a memory

TABLE 5
Mean number (and standard deviations) of nontargeted RD conversational
behaviours across experiment phases

	RD1	RD2	RD3	RD4
Responses				
Baseline	30.50 (10.14)	21.60 (7.06)	31.00 (5.60)	12.67 (7.85)
Treatment 1	41.67 (4.64)	11.25 (7.66)	12.00 (1.41)	13.67 (7.36)
Treatment 2	22.50 (2.69)	6.00 (1.00)	19.00 (5.89)	11.67 (4.64)
Unintelligible				
Baseline	0.25 (0.43)	11.40 (6.65)	1.17 (0.37)	4.00 (2.83)
Treatment 1	0.33 (0.47)	2.50 (1.19)	1.00 (0.82)	2.00 (1.63)
Treatment 2	0 (0)	2.50 (1.50)	0.67 (0.47)	3.67 (1.70)
Other				
Baseline	7.00 (1.00)	15.4 (6.5)	1.83 (1.07)	6.00 (2.83)
Treatment 1	6.67 (1.70)	4.75 (2.17)	2.00 (0)	9.33 (0.47)
Treatment 2	3.75 (1.48)	5.5 (0.5)	1.00 (1.41)	5.33 (1.25)

Memory aid; Treatment 2, memory aid + NA instructions.

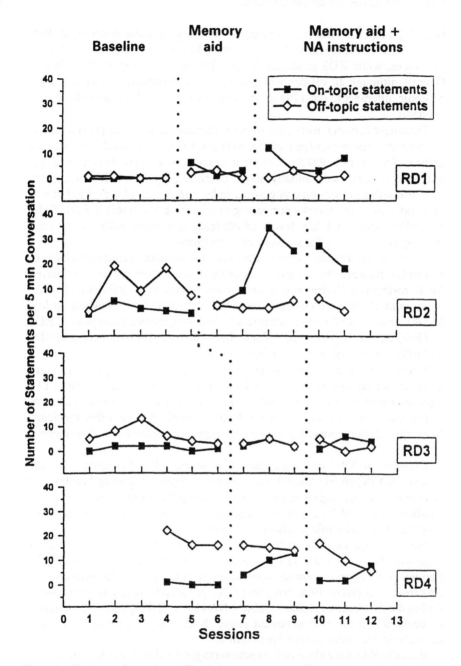

Figure 1. Frequency of on-topic and off-topic statements across residents with dementia (RD1, RD2, RD3, RD4) and experimental phases (Baseline, Memory aid, Memory aid with NA instructions). Filled squares represent on-topic statements and open diamonds represent off-topic statements.

book. RD1 and RD3 had similar effects of memory book use for on-topic utterances, but at lower levels. RD1 maintained a low and stable level of off-topic utterances, while RD3 produced fewer off-topic utterances in Treatment 1. Overall, although all residents increased on-topic utterances, and decreased off-topic utterances, the effects of Treatment 1 varied in quantity across residents.

Treatment 2, direct instruction of NAs, resulted in further improvements in the quantity of on-topic utterances for RD1 and RD3, who had achieved smaller gains in Treatment 1. RD2's on-topic utterances declined in Treatment 2, but remained at levels substantially above baseline frequencies. RD4 produced similar numbers of on-topic utterances in both treatment phases, but her off-topic utterances continued a decreasing trend during Treatment 2. RD1, RD2, and RD3 maintained low levels of off-topic utterances with use of their memory books during the second treatment phase.

Additionally, treatment effects were seen for the nontargeted behaviours of residents with dementia. Overall, a decrease in responsive utterances occurred for all residents with dementia in the treatment conditions. RD2, who had the most unintelligible utterances at baseline, decreased this behaviour to low levels that were similar to the other residents during the treatment phases. RD1 and RD2 decreased production of other behaviours during treatment, and RD3 and RD4 maintained other behaviours at low levels.

In summary, three of the four residents demonstrated the expected changes in target behaviours, with increased on-topic utterances and decreased off-topic utterances when using memory aids. The fourth resident showed changes in the expected direction, but at much lower levels than the other residents. Nontargeted behaviours also showed the expected decrease for all residents.

Changes in NAs' conversational behaviours. The frequencies for the primary NA dependent variables are shown in Figure 2. During baseline, all NAs demonstrated high levels of requests during the 5-min conversations. In addition, NA1 and NA2 produced high levels of assertions. NA3 and NA4 produced low and stable levels of assertions.

For all NAs, a reduction in the frequency of one or both dependent variables occurred when a memory aid was present during conversations. For NA1, the frequency of requests showed little change overall between baseline and the first treatment phase. Both NA2 and NA3 produced slightly fewer requests during the first treatment phase. Subject NA4 showed the greatest reduction in requests during the first treatment phase. NA1 and NA2 exhibited a large decrease in assertions during Treatment 1.

Because NAs were observed to continue to give residents inadequate time to initiate conversation in Treatment 1, and the levels of change in NA behaviour did not appear to be clinically significant, Treatment 2 was implemented. When this expanded instruction condition was provided, NA1 and NA4 further

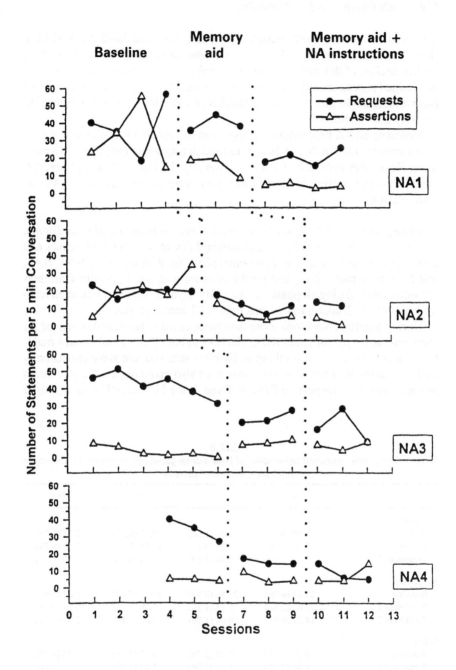

Figure 2. Frequency of requests and assertions across nursing assistants (NA1, NA2, NA3, NA4) and experimental phases (Baseline, Memory aid, Memory aid with instructions). Filled circles represent requests and open triangles represent assertions.

improved in limiting their requests, although NA2 and NA3 showed little change. Additionally, for NA1 and NA2, who had high levels of assertions, further decline of this non-facilitative behaviour was demonstrated. NA3 had maintained approximately the same level of assertions across all phases. NA4 had variable slight increases in the number of assertions that she produced in memory aid conditions.

Nontargeted NA behaviours are displayed in Table 6. Overall, three of four NAs increased the number of directives used during treatment phase conversations. Responses decreased for all four NAs by the last treatment phase. NA other behaviours were at low levels during baseline, and decreased across treatment phases.

Changes in social discourse behaviours of residents and nursing assistants. Table 7 shows the mean number and standard deviation of total utterances and utterances per turn for each experimental phase for RDs and NAs. NA1, NA3, and NA4 took more turns, and produced more utterances per turn than their respective RDs during all phases of the study. Dyad 2 had more balanced turn-taking, with RD2 taking more turns than NA2 across phases.

During baseline, NA1 took more than twice as many turns, and produced far more utterances per turn than RD1. The NAs in both Dyad 3 and Dyad 4 maintained stable levels of turn-taking in baseline sessions that were consistently higher than those of the RDs. NA3 and NA4 also maintained more utterances per turn than their respective RDs. In Dyad 2, the NA and RD took a similar

TABLE 6
Mean number (and standard deviations) of NAs' nontargeted conversational behaviours across experimental phases

	NA1	NA2	NA3	NA4
Directives				
Baseline	1.00 (0)	2.50 (1.50)	0.17 (0.37)	3.33 (1.70)
Treatment 1	7.00 (3.00)	0.25 (0.43)	18.33 (7.04)	27.33 (8.73)
Treatment 2	9.25 (4.32)	2.00 (1.00)	22.33 (6.55)	22.33 (7.41)
Responses				
Baseline	20.75 (6.98)	20.80 (8.98)	16.17 (7.40)	18.67 (5.91)
Treatment 1	22.67 (2.62)	5.75 (1.30)	9.00 (4.08)	17.33 (3.68)
Treatment 2	14.50 (4.56)	6.00 (1.00)	3.00 (3.86)	5.33 (2.05)
Other				
Baseline	5.75 (3.56)	7.20 (5.38)	6.67 (4.19)	8.33 (1.25)
Treatment 1	4.00 (2.16)	1.25 (1.09)	2.67 (1.70)	5.33 (3.40)
Treatment 2	3.25 (1.79)	1.00 (0)	1.67 (0.94)	4.33 (1.25)

Baseline, no memory aid; Treatment 1, memory aid; Treatment 2, memory aid + instructions.

TABLE 7

Mean number (and standard deviations) of total number of utterances
and utterances per turn for each Dyad during each experimental phase

| | Experimental phase | | | | | |
| | Baseline | | Treatment 1 | | Treatment 2 | |
	T	U/T	T	U/T	T	U/T
Dyad 1						
NA	96.00 (9.42)	2.86 (0.85)	91.00 (6.08)	1.77 (0.34)	50.50 (9.43)	1.59 (0.33)
RD	38.50 (13.10)	1.04 (0.03)	53.67 (5.51)	1.03 (0.04)	34.00 (6.58)	1.07 (0.17)
Dyad 2						
NA	68.2 (18.51)	1.41 (0.24)	28.5 (15.42)	1.37 (0.29)	23.00 (7.07)	1.06 (0.08)
RD	61 (21.67)	1.24 (0.13)	39.25 (8.88)	2.03 (0.96)	40.50 (10.61)	1.88 (0.06)
Dyad 3						
NA	68.17 (20.97)	1.83 (0.26)	61.00 (5.20)	3.07 (0.17)	54.33 (7.23)	2.18 (0.51)
RD	41.83 (7.14)	1.14 (0.07)	21.33 (4.04)	1.06 (0.07)	26.67 (6.51)	1.05 (0.11)
Dyad 4						
NA	69 (13.45)	1.55 (0.13)	70.33 (12.10)	1.64 (0.06)	47.67 (11.93)	1.60 (0.16)
RD	50 (13.45)	1.10 (0.02)	49.00 (6.00)	1.15 (0.04)	29.33 (3.79)	1.06 (0.40)

T, total number of utterances; U/T, utterances per turn. Baseline, no memory aid; Treatment 1,
memory aid; Treatment 2, memory aid + NA instructions.

number of turns in the baseline phase, with the NA exceeding the resident for
only one data point. However, NA2 produced slightly more utterances per turn
than RD2 in baseline.

The effects of Treatment 1 on turn-taking were varied. In the case of Dyad 1,
the memory aid treatment resulted in the length of the partners' conversational
turns becoming more similar, while the RD took many more turns and the NA's
number of turns remained the same. When given direct instruction in the
second treatment phase, NA1 markedly reduced her number of turns, although
the RD reduced her turns to baseline levels. In Treatment 2, number of utterances per turn remained similar for NA1 and RD1. During both treatment
phases, RD2 actually took more turns and contributed more utterances per turn
than her NA, despite producing fewer turns in treatment phases than in
baseline. In Dyad 3, the NA and the RD produced fewer turns in treatment
phases than baseline, with the NA continuing to dominate the conversations
with more utterances per turn as well. Both members of Dyad 4 showed
stability in number of turns and utterances per turn across baseline and
Treatment 1. However, in Treatment 2, both members of Dyad 4 took fewer
turns than in the previous phases, but utterances per turn remained unaffected
by the treatment.

418   HOERSTER, HICKEY, BOURGEOIS

Social validity

Unfamiliar judges.   Ten unfamiliar judges used a 5.8 cm visual analogue scale (VAS) to rate one baseline and one treatment session along six dimensions. Table 8 shows the mean ratings and standard deviations obtained on each conversational dimension for baseline and treatment samples. Results revealed that judges rated one of four dyads as about the same and two of four dyads as improved when the residents used their memory books for the domains of topic maintenance, new information conveyed, unambiguous, and equity of turn-taking. Overall ratings for comfort vs. awkwardness decreased for three dyads when a memory aid was used. One dyad was judged to improve on responsiveness to prior turn.

Dyad 1 received the highest ratings overall, but Dyad 3 was judged to improve in the most categories, with the exception of comfort, when RD3 used her memory book. Judges rated Dyad 1 as improving on three categories, and declining on one category. Dyad 2 was judged to improve only for new information conveyed. Dyad 4 was not judged to improve on any dimension, and received equitable scores only for topic maintenance.

Nursing assistants.   In the post-treatment interview, all NAs stated that the memory aids affected the residents positively. NA1 stated that RD1's memory book refreshed her memory, and made it easier for her to talk about herself. In addition, NA1 thought she knew the resident better after introduction of the memory book. Positive changes in both the communication and behaviour of RD2 were reported by NA2, who reported that her resident talked about herself more easily and behaved less suspiciously during treatment conversations. For NA3, the memory aid made it easier for her to talk about topics of interest to the resident, despite RD3's minimal improvement in initiation of on-topic utterances. Also, NA3 stated that she was able to understand RD3 better by associating the resident's utterances with the memory book stimuli. NA4 stated that the memory book helped RD4 to converse about people she had not mentioned in the baseline condition. Additionally, NA4 thought that the resident did not discuss all of the memories that the prosthetic aid may have triggered (e.g., NA4 reported that RD4's facial expressions indicated recognition of her sister, but she did not seem to want to talk about her and turned the page).

Three of the four NAs perceived positive changes in their own communicative styles when memory aids were used during conversation. Only NA1 reported that aided conversations were more difficult for her. NA2 was aware of a decrease in the frequency of requests she produced during aided conversations, and perceived this as a positive change. In addition, she was relieved to not feel the need to evade the resident's suspicious questions. Both NA3 and NA4, who were paired with the residents who made the smallest treatment gains, reported feeling more at ease during the aided conversations. Although

TABLE 8
Results of social validation assessment:
Mean (and standard deviation) of perceived changes in resident behaviour

	Dyad 1		Dyad 2		Dyad 3		Dyad 4	
	B	Tx	B	Tx	B	Tx	B	Tx
Topic maintenance	61.38 (1.53)	73.45 (0.71)	38.45 (1.59)	33.62 (1.54)	43.10 (1.50)	72.24 (0.77)	22.76 (1.05)	21.90 (1.01)
New information	55.52 (1.38)	57.24 (1.38)	21.38 (0.77)	38.45 (1.63)	29.66 (1.28)	56.07 (1.39)	32.24 (1.69)	20.69 (0.91)
Unambiguous vs. ambiguous	45.69 (1.44)	54.48 (1.32)	26.03 (1.08)	23.97 (1.04)	27.07 (1.38)	48.97 (1.11)	24.14 (1.26)	21.21 (1.05)
Equity of turn-taking	33.45 (1.08)	44.66 (1.24)	36.90 (1.11)	36.72 (1.20)	37.59 (0.92)	51.03 (1.18)	44.31 (1.04)	26.38 (0.68)
Responsiveness	51.72 (1.31)	54.66 (1.44)	40.17 (1.58)	30.86 (1.43)	37.41 (1.39)	57.41 (1.25)	44.31 (1.04)	29.48 (1.18)
Comfort vs. awkward	65.52 (1.75)	59.83 (1.33)	49.48 (1.71)	39.14 (1.69)	45.34 (1.63)	47.59 (1.39)	52.07 (1.62)	30.69 (1.36)

Percentage ratings (and standard deviations): 0–100% of the time, calculated from 5.8 cm Visual Analogue Scales.

both of these NAs still felt the need to lead the conversations due to poor performance by their residents, they felt that the contents of the memory aid provided the means to do this with more sensitivity to resident knowledge and interest.

DISCUSSION

This study evaluated the impact of a communication intervention on the conversational behaviours of four residents with dementia and their nursing assistants. When residents had access to a memory book during conversations, the frequency of on-topic resident behaviours increased and non-facilitative staff behaviours decreased in all four dyads.

Resident effects

All four residents with dementia improved somewhat in their ability to initiate meaningful conversation when they used a memory aid. These results extend those of Bourgeois (1990, 1992, 1993) in validating the memory aid treatment for improving communicative abilities of individuals with dementia. The gains made by residents with dementia in this study were similar, but of a smaller magnitude, to results described by Bourgeois, in which individuals with dementia made more statements of fact and used fewer ambiguous utterances when using memory aids in conversations with familiar partners at home, in adult day care, and nursing home settings (Bourgeois 1990, 1992, 1993). Institutionalised residents who were functioning at a lower cognitive level than the individuals in Bourgeois' earlier studies were successful in producing more statements of fact when conversing with nursing home staff when using a prosthetic memory aid than in the non-aided condition.

The residents in this study had varied diagnoses and responded to treatment differently. RD2 and RD4 were initially the most verbal residents. However, many of their verbalisations were off-topic statements. Both residents responded to treatment with fewer off-topic statements. RD2 had the largest increase in on-topic statements; other residents' on-topic statements increased, but to a lesser extent. Qualitative aspects of the residents' on-topic statements, not captured in the quantitative data, also reflected improvements. The residents responded with more detailed statements and more novel statements when using memory aids. In addition, nonverbal behaviours showed less agitation and suspicion, and more pleasure in interactions in some residents (e.g., RD2, RD4). Some residents (i.e., RD3) needed more response time in order to use their memory aids effectively, as demonstrated by further increases in Treatment 2. Lethargy and other medical complications impacted the ability of some residents to respond to treatment (RD3, RD4).

Unfamiliar judges' ability to rate changes in residents' conversational behaviour was variable. Positive changes in topic maintenance, decreased ambiguity, and equity of turn-taking for RD1 reflect improved conversational abilities when using a memory aid and given more time to respond in Treatment 2. RD2's increases in on-topic statements were noted by improved new information ratings only. Similarly, RD3's use of more frequent and longer on-topic utterances is reflected in the social validity data where the treatment conversation was rated improved on five of the six dimensions. In contrast, RD4's modest improvements in reducing off-topic and increasing on-topic statements were not observed by the unfamiliar judges who rated her lower on most conversational dimensions post-treatment. These results are not surprising in light of the fact that this resident had the most severe cognitive deficits and the poorest training performance. In addition, her distractibility in conversations necessitated frequent prompting to use her memory book.

NA effects

Although the four NAs varied in their pre-treatment communicative styles, they all tended to produce a high frequency of requests. NA1 and NA2 tended to talk about themselves or other topics unrelated to the residents during baseline conversations. NA3 and NA4 produced many requests in attempts to increase their residents' verbalisations. As expected, all four NAs used fewer non-facilitative behaviours (requests, assertions) as a result of Treatment 1. But these effects were not as robust as desired; NAs continued asking many questions. For example, rather than allowing time for the resident to talk, NA1 would interrogate the resident about the pictures in the memory aid. Treatment 2 resulted in further decreases in requests for NAs 1 and 4. NA3's rate of questioning remained high throughout both treatment phases, possibly due to her resident's lethargy and relatively low level of initiation. Effects of the second treatment phase on NA2 are inconclusive due to the shortage of data points.

The immediate positive effect of the memory aids was to focus conversations on the residents. All NAs reported approaching interactions with the residents more positively after training. The training allowed them to view the residents as more knowledgeable and capable of participating in conversations. The NAs thought that the memory aid conversations were less effortful and more satisfying. Even when the residents continued to produce low levels of verbalisations, the NAs found the memory aids to be helpful, as the memory book provided a guideline for discussing topics that were relevant to the resident. The fact that all NAs reported positive changes in resident behaviour when the memory aid was used during conversations extends the results of Bourgeois (1990) by providing a validation from conversational partners. Bourgeois (1990) reported that familiar conversational partners and spouses did not judge improvements in the conversations of individuals with dementia following memory aid treatment. The contrast between the satisfaction ratings

of spouses in Bourgeois (1990) and the NAs in the present study may be attributed to the fact that the NAs did not serve the function of trainer. Conversations
in this study were purely social in nature, and NAs were not expected to learn to
implement a training regimen. In addition, Bourgeois (1990) postulated that
partners in this study were lifelong friends who were better able to interpret
ambiguous statements than were unfamiliar judges. In the present study, the
NA conversational partners did not have extensive knowledge of the residents'
history. To NAs, treatment effects might have been more obvious due to their
inability to interpret vague or confusing utterances of the residents prior to
treatment.

   The NAs' positive opinions of the use of memory books contrasted with the
judges' ratings of the comfort of the conversations. In the dimension of comfort
vs. awkwardness, three of the four dyads were rated significantly lower by the
judges. Dyad 3 was rated unchanged on this domain. The ratings for this dimension are consistent with those of Bourgeois (1993), in that the conversations of
four dyads consisting of partners with dementia were rated by unfamiliar
judges to be more awkward when a memory aid was used. The perceived artifi-
ciality of the residents reading from their books and the NAs frequently
adopting didactic roles may account for the consistently low comfort rating.

Turn-taking

The number of utterances per turn taken by the members of each dyad was
calculated as an indicator of length of conversational turns. Previous research
(Hutchinson & Jenson, 1981) has suggested that residents with dementia
generally produce fewer utterances per turn than individuals functioning at a
normal cognitive level. Bourgeois (1993) investigated the effects of memory
aid use on this social behaviour and found that three of four residents with
dementia increased their number of utterances per turn when using a memory
aid. In the present study, the effects of the memory aid on turn-taking had mixed
results. For Dyad 1, the treatment had the effect of equalising the number of
utterances per turn in both partners. Dyad 2's conversation was equitable in
baseline, but after treatment, the resident exceeded the NAs' turns and utterances per turn. The effects of the treatment on turn-taking for Dyads 1 and 2 was
consistent with Bourgeois' (1993) findings. In contrast, Dyad 3's utterances
per turn became less equitable as the NA produced more directives to the
resident to prompt her to talk about her memory aid and Dyad 4 maintained the
balance of turn-taking but with different types of statements produced by both
partners. The difficulties encountered by the NAs in these two dyads in getting
these residents to use their memory aids may explain these results. As stated
above, these two residents were more cognitively impaired and had medical
complications during the study.

Limitations of the study

Several factors inherent in the nursing home environment and the population being studied may have influenced the outcomes of this study. The unpredict-ability of fluctuations in resident status, combined with complicating staff variables, resulted in a less than optimal number of conversational sessions being conducted across all phases of the study. Such variables impacted the experimental design. For example, the steadily declining trends for both resident (off-topic) and NA (requests) dependent variables, as shown in Figures 1 and 2, were influenced by the rush to collect these data points after RD3 was hospitalised. Ideally, stability at each phase should have been more evident before moving on to consecutive treatment phases, but RD4's unpredictable medical fluctuations necessitated expediency.

Other limits of this study warrant discussion. First of all, the results of a small study with so few participants have limited generalisation to other residents. In addition, resident factors such as varied and co-occurring diag-noses, psychoactive medications, variable medical status throughout the study, and differences and deficiencies in hearing status are probable sources of uncontrolled variability that confound the internal validity of the results obtained here. All residents in this study were functioning at a low cognitive level. In the case of RD3 and RD4, their abilities were further impaired by co-occurring diagnoses and behaviour problems that were erratic and at times severe. The fact that results were highly variable for the residents within this study raises questions related to determining candidacy for the memory aid treatment.

In addition to environmental and resident factors, limitations in the experi-mental protocol affected outcomes further. Training of residents to use their memory books was extremely limited in this study. Although Bourgeois (1990) has demonstrated that residents with dementia require little training to use a memory aid, the residents in this study were functioning at very low cognitive levels. Ideally, all residents should have been trained to the original criteria for reading all 25 of their memory book sentences and for elaborating on 30% of them before treatment probes with the NAs began.

The necessity of a second treatment condition to effect a clinically signifi-cant reduction in NA non-facilitative behaviours raises questions about the extent of caregiver training needed for optimal treatment success. Bourgeois (1990) reported that spouses who were trained to implement a memory aid treatment protocol did so successfully, but expressed limited satisfaction with the treatment outcomes. Too much or too little training of caregivers might interfere with the overall impact of the treatment on communicative interactions.

An additional limitation of the study may be reflected in the inconsistency between quantitative data on dependent variables and qualitative ratings of improvements. Although RD2, for example, improved her on-topic statements following treatment, unfamiliar judges only rated the treatment conversation as improved on one dimension. Several questions about the differences in pre- and post-treatment behaviours and the overall impact of the treatment on the quality of communication must be addressed. A limitation of the social validity procedure itself was that NA and resident behaviour changes were assessed together, even on domains that specifically addressed one participant more than the other. The presentation of dyadic interactions may have confounded the ability of the unfamiliar listeners to detect changes in the behaviour of individual subjects. All residents made positive, but relatively small treatment gains. The results of the social validity procedure in this study differ from those of Bourgeois (1990), where unfamiliar judges consistently gave higher ratings to aided conversations. Further research is needed to determine whether more and/or more rigorous memory aid training in this lower functioning population would result in improvements that would be noticed by unfamiliar judges.

A final limitation of this study deals with maintenance and generalisation issues. It is not clear to what extent this protocol would be useful in other settings. It is realistic to expect that problems encountered throughout this study, such as variable resident health and busy nursing staff, will be encountered in any geriatric long-term care setting. Generalisation of resident memory aid skills in conversations with other staff members, residents, and family members, or in other settings (e.g., activity room) was not assessed in this study. In addition, generalisation of improved NA conversational skills to conversations with other nursing home residents was not examined in this study. The maintenance of memory aid skills in residents with dementia was an important area not addressed by this study. The amount of intervention in the form of booster sessions or feedback needed to maintain resident skills has not been determined yet. In addition, maintenance of improved NA conversational skills was not assessed. The amount and type of reinforcement necessary to maintain improved NA behaviours is an important area that needs more attention.

Future research

The findings of this study suggest several possible avenues of future research. Overall, the results suggest that a relatively simple treatment implemented with little formal training improved some of the communicative behaviours of some low-functioning institutionalised residents with dementia and nursing assistants. Future studies should consider more rigorous subject controls and training procedures. The optimal amount of training for caregivers in various settings to participate in conversations with residents who have dementia warrants further study.

Further validation of the memory aid treatment for a similar population is necessary. This study substantiates Bourgeois' (1993) contention that cognitive status and successful memory aid use may be related. The development of better assessment protocols to determine candidacy of institutionalised residents with dementia for the memory aid treatment is needed. The complicated medical and social variables common in this population have the potential to affect treatment outcomes. The influence of co-occurring neurological deficits, medications, and sensory deficits on successful use of a prosthetic memory aid during conversations also warrants further investigation.

Within this study, several anecdotal or incidental behaviours were noted that might warrant investigation as dependent variables in future studies. For example, the resident-oriented vs. self-oriented content of NA conversations may be worthwhile to investigate and manipulate when studying NA behaviour. Resident variables that deserve attention in future studies include new information conveyed, elaborated responses, and increased mean length of utterance in memory aid conversations.

Finally, interventions aimed more directly at changing and maintaining improved staff behaviours when dealing with institutionalised residents should be considered. Further classification of NA communicative behaviours across residents and settings within nursing homes is recommended to identify variables for which intervention would be most beneficial. Although a few studies have indicated that direct training of nursing assistants can improve interactions with residents (e.g., Cohn, Horgas, & Marsiske,1990; Koury & Lubinski, 1991), more specific direction of these efforts toward changing communication behaviours, and measurement of effects of NA communication training for staff and residents are also essential. Providing in-service training and direct instruction for NAs regarding the effects of NA behaviour on resident behaviour may be needed to increase the robustness of treatment effects in this setting. Replication of the protocol of this study with stronger effects is necessary to verify that the instructions to the NAs were responsible for the apparent effects exhibited by some NAs in Treatment 2.

REFERENCES

Baltes, M.M., Kindermann, T., Reisenzein, R., & Schmid, U. (1987). Further observational data on the behavioral and social world of institutions for the aged. *Psychology and Aging, 2,* 390–403.

Baltes, M.M., & Reisenzein, R. (1986). The social world in long-term care institutions: psychosocial control toward dependency. In M.M. Baltes & P.B. Baltes (Eds.), *The psychology of control and aging* (pp. 315–343). London: Lawrence Erlbaum Associates.

Bartol, M.A. (1979). Nonverbal communication in patients with Alzheimer's disease. *Journal of American Nursing, 5,* 21–31.

Bayles, K.A., & Tomoeda, C.K. (1991). Caregiver report of prevalence and appearance order of linguistic symptoms in Alzheimer's residents. *The Gerontologist, 31,* 210–216.

Bohling, H.R. (1991). Communication with Alzheimer's residents: An analysis of caregiver listening patterns. *International Journal of Aging and Human Development, 33*, 249–267.

Bond, A., & Lader, M. (1974). The use of analogue scales in rating subjective feelings. *British Journal of Medical Psychology, 47*, 211–218.

Bourgeois, M.S. (1990). Enhancing conversation skills in residents with Alzheimer's Disease using a prosthetic memory aid. *Journal of Applied Behavior Analysis, 23*, 29–42.

Bourgeois, M.S. (1992). Evaluating memory wallets in conversations with persons with dementia. *Journal of Speech and Hearing Research, 35*, 1344–1357.

Bourgeois, M.S. (1993). Effects of memory aids on the dyadic conversations of individuals with dementia. *Journal of Applied Behavior Analysis, 26*, 77–87.

Bourgeois, M.S., Burgio, L.D., Schulz, R., Beach, S., & Palmer, B. (1997). Modifying repetitive verbalisations of communityd-welling patients with AD. *The Gerontologist, 37*, 30–39.

Bowers, B. & Becker, M. (1992). Nurse's aides in nursing homes: the relationship between organization and quality. *The Gerontologist, 32*, 360–366.

Burgio, L.D., & Bourgeois, M.S. (1992). Treating severe behavioral disorders in geriatric residential settings. *Behavioral Residential Treatment, 7*, 145–168.

Burgio, L.D., Butler, F., & Engel, B. (1988). Nurses' attitudes towards geriatric behavior problems in long-term care settings. *Clinical Gerontologist, 7*, 23–34.

Caporael, L.R., & Culbertson, G.H. (1986). Verbal response modes of baby talk and other speech at institutions for the aged. *Language and Communication, 6*, 99–112.

Cohn, M.D., Horgas, A.L., & Marsiske, M. (1990). Behavior management training for nurse aides: Is it effective? *Journal of Gerontological Nursing, 16*, 21–25.

Folstein, M., Folstein, S., & McHugh, P. (1975). Mini-mental state. *Journal of Psychiatric Research, 12*, 189–198.

Fromm, D., & Holland, A.L. (1989). Functional communication in Alzheimer's disease. *Journal of Speech and Hearing Disorders, 54*, 535–540.

Goodglass, H., & Kaplan, E., (1972). *Boston Diagnostic Aphasia Examination*, Philadelphia: Lea and Febiger.

Grainger, K. (1995). Communication and the institutionalized elderly. In J.F. Nussbaum & J. Coupland (Eds.), *Handbook of communication and aging research* (pp. 417–436). Mahwah, NJ: Lawrence Erlbaum Associates.

Guyatt, G.H., Berman, L.B., Townsend, M., & Taylor, D.W. (1985). Should study subjects see their previous responses? *Journal of Chronic Diseases, 38*, 1003–1007.

Hutchinson, J.M., & Jensen, M. (1981). A pragmatic evaluation of discourse communication in normal and senile elderly in a nursing home. In L. Obler & M. Albert (Eds.), *Language and communication in the elderly* (pp. 59–73). Lexington, MA: Heath.

Jacelon, C.S. (1995). The effect of living in a nursing home on socialization in elderly people. *Journal of Advanced Nursing, 22*, 539–546.

Kaakinen, J.R. (1992). Living with silence. *The Gerontologist, 32*, 258–264.

Koury, L.N., & Lubinski, R. (1991). Effective in-service training for staff working with communication-impaired residents. In R. Lubinski (Ed.), *Dementia and communication* (pp. 279–289). Philadelphia: B.C. Decker.

Liukkonen, A. (1995). Life in a nursing home for the frail elderly: daily routines. *Clinical Nursing Research, 4*, 358–370.

Lubinski, R.B. (1978). Why so little interest whether or not old people talk: A review of recent research on verbal communication among the elderly. *International Journal of Aging and Human Development, 9*, 237–245.

Lubinksi, R. (1995). State-of-the-art perspectives on communication in nursing homes. *Topics in Language Disorders, 15*, 1–19.

Lubinski, R., Morrison, E.B., & Rigrodsky, S. (1981). Perception of spoken communication by elderly chronically ill residents in an institutional setting. *Journal of Speech and Hearing Disorders, 46*, 405–412.

Macleod-Clark, J. (1981). Communication in nursing. *Nursing Times, Jan 1*, 12–18.

Mor, V., Branco, K., Fleishman, J., Hawes, C., Phillips, C., Morris, J., & Fries, B. (1995). The structure of social engagement among nursing home resident. *Journal of Gerontology: Psychological Sciences, 50B*, 1:P1–P8.

Nicholas, M., Obler, L.K., Albert, M.L., & Helm-Estabrooks, N. (1985). Empty speech in Alzheimer's disease and fluent aphasia. *Journal of Speech and Hearing Research, 28*, 405–410.

Nussbaum, J.F., Robinson, J.D., & Grew, D.J. (1985). Communicative behavior of the long-term care employee: Implications for the elderly resident. *Communication Research Reports, 2*, 16–22.

Ostuni, E., & Santo Pietro, M.J. (1986). *Getting through: Communicating when someone you care for has Alzheimer's disease.* Plainsboro, NJ: The Speech Bin.

Ripich, D.N., Carpenter, B.D., & Ziol, E.W. (1997). Procedural discourse of men and women with Alzheimer's disease: A longitudinal study with clinical implications. *American Journal of Alzheimer's Disease, 12*, 258–271.

Ripich, D.N., & Terrell, B.Y. (1988). Patterns of discourse cohesion and coherence in Alzheimer's disease. *Journal of Speech and Hearing Disorders, 53*, 8–15.

Schroll, M., Jonsson, P.V., Mor, V., Berg, K., & Sherwood, S. (1997). An international study of social engagement among nursing home residents. *Age and Aging, 26* (S2), 55–59.

Seers, C. (1986). Talking to the elderly and its relevance to care. *Nursing Times, 82*, 51–54.

Sigman, S. (1985). Conversational behavior in two health care institutions for the elderly. *Institutional Journal of Aging and Human Development, 21*, 147–163.

Tomoeda, C.K., Bayles, K.A., Trosset, M.W., Azuma, T., & McGeagh, A. (1996). Cross-Sectional Analysis of Alzheimer Disease Effects on Oral Discourse in a Picture Description Task. *Alzheimer Disease and Related Disorders, 10*, 204–215.

Yorkston, K.M., & Beukelman, D.R. (1980). An analysis of connected speech samples of aphasic and normal speakers. *Journal of Speech and Hearing Disorders, 65*, 16–26.

Manuscript received June 1999
Revised manuscript received September 2000

Can repeated exposure to "forgotten" vocabulary help alleviate word-finding difficulties in semantic dementia? An illustrative case study

Kim S. Graham[1], Karalyn Patterson[1], Katherine H. Pratt[1,2], and John R. Hodges[1,2]

[1]MRC Cognition and Brain Sciences Unit, Cambridge, UK
[2]University Neurology Unit, Addenbrooke's Hospital, Cambridge, UK

The predominant, and most socially isolating, symptom typically seen in semantic dementia is anomia—word-finding difficulties—in conjunction with a deteriorating central semantic system. In this paper, we demonstrate that repeated rehearsal of the names of concepts paired with pictures of them and/or real items resulted in a dramatic improvement in the ability of a patient (DM) with semantic dementia to produce previously "difficult-to-retrieve" words on tests of word production. Although the substantial improvement shown by DM suggests that home rehearsal with pictorial and verbal stimuli could be a useful rehabilitative strategy for word-finding difficulties in semantic dementia, the experiment also revealed that constant exposure to items was necessary in order to prevent the observed decline in performance once DM's daily drill was stopped. The results are discussed with respect to the underlying neuroanatomical structures thought to be important for the acquisition and storage of long-term memory, and to techniques for facilitating word-finding in patients with aphasia.

THE NEUROPSYCHOLOGICAL PROFILE OF SEMANTIC DEMENTIA

More than a century ago, Pick (1892) drew attention to the fact that patients with neurodegenerative conditions could present with relatively focal symptoms, such as impaired language function. Following these initial reports,

Correspondence should be addressed to Kim S. Graham, MRC Cognition and Brain Sciences Unit, 15 Chaucer Road, Cambridge, CB2 2EF. Tel.: 44 (0)1223 355294 ext. 790; Fax: 44 (0)1223 359062; Email: kim.graham@mrc-cbu.cam.ac.uk

We would like to thank DM and his wife for helping us with the relearning experiments we describe in this paper.

there was little interest in these cases until Mesulam (1982; see also Schwartz, Marin, & Saffran, 1979; Warrington, 1975) described a number of patients with "slowly progressive aphasia without generalised dementia". Over 100 cases of progressive aphasia have now been described, and it is clear that there are at least two main variants of the disorder: progressive *fluent* aphasia and progressive *nonfluent* aphasia. Whereas patients with progressive nonfluent aphasia are impaired in the phonological and syntactic aspects of language, cases with the fluent variety show a progressive loss of semantic information about people, objects, facts, and concepts which disrupts the patient's ability to produce words in spontaneous speech and, as the disease advances, to comprehend word meaning. The diagnostic label semantic dementia has been applied to this latter disorder (Breedin, Saffran, & Coslett, 1994; Hodges, Patterson, Oxbury, & Funnell, 1992; Snowden, Goulding, & Neary, 1989; Snowden, Neary, & Mann, 1996b) in order to capture the primary deficit in the syndrome.

On neuropsychological tests, patients with semantic dementia perform poorly on any task which requires conceptual knowledge, including picture naming, naming an item when given a description (e.g., "a jar or ornament in which we keep flowers"), category fluency (producing multiple exemplars from a specified category), word–picture matching (pointing to the picture of an "elephant" amongst an array of pictures), sorting (grouping pictures or words on the basis of various conceptual distinctions), defining concepts in response to their names or pictures, and answering semantic probe questions (Hodges et al., 1992). Patients are also impaired on nonverbal tests of semantic memory, such as selecting the appropriate colour for a black and white line drawing [e.g., grey for an "elephant" and white for a "snowman" (Breedin et al., 1994; Graham, 1995) and drawing animals or objects from memory (Graham, 1995; Lambon Ralph, Howard, Nightingale, & Ellis, 1998; Srinivas, Breedin, Coslett, & Saffran, 1997)]. In striking contrast to their semantic deficits, these patients achieve near or completely normal scores on tests of visuoperceptual and spatial ability, nonverbal problem-solving, phonology, syntax, and working memory (Breedin et al., 1994; Hodges et al., 1992; Hodges & Patterson, 1996; Snowden et al., 1996b).

Neuroradiological studies of semantic dementia reveal focal atrophy of the inferolateral temporal neocortex on one or both sides, with sparing (at least early in the disease) of the hippocampi, parahippocampal gyri, and subiculum (Breedin et al., 1994; Graham & Hodges, 1997; Harasty, Halliday, Code, & Brooks, 1996; Hodges, Garrard, & Patterson, 1998; Hodges & Patterson, 1996). Although evidence regarding the neuropathological basis of semantic dementia is still limited, a meta-analysis of published and unpublished information for 13 cases seen in Cambridge revealed that all patients had either Pick bodies or nonspecific histological changes without Alzheimer's or Pick's pathology (Hodges et al., 1998).

New learning in semantic dementia

Until recently, there was surprisingly little empirical evidence on the status of episodic memory in semantic dementia, despite the fact that one of the five characteristics of the disorder is considered to be "relatively preserved autobiographical and day-to-day (episodic) memory" (Hodges et al., 1992, p. 1785). This statement was based mainly on clinical observations that patients with semantic dementia are well-oriented in time and place, rarely get lost in familiar surroundings and remember appointments (Breedin et al., 1994; Diesfeldt, 1992; Graham & Hodges, 1997; Graham, Patterson, & Hodges, 1999b; Hodges et al., 1992; Snowden, Griffiths, & Neary, 1994, 1995, 1996a).

Recent studies of episodic memory in semantic dementia have partially confirmed this view. Graham and Hodges (1997; see also Snowden et al., 1996a) demonstrated a reverse temporal gradient on tests of autobiographical memory: Six patients with semantic dementia were better at producing memories from the recent time period compared with childhood and early adulthood on the Autobiographical Memory Interview (Kopelman, Wilson, & Baddeley, 1989). By contrast, a group of amnesic patients with presumed early Alzheimer's disease showed the more typical temporal gradient, in which recent memories were more impaired than those from the distant past (Graham & Hodges, 1997). A similar effect of time has been noted on tests of semantic memory, such as identification of famous people: Patients with semantic dementia recalled more semantic information about recent personalities than those that have been famous in the distant past (Hodges & Graham, 1998; see also Graham, Pratt, & Hodges, 1998). New learning, as measured by tests of recognition memory, is also relatively normal early in the disease (Graham, Becker, & Hodges, 1997; Graham et al., 2000), and Funnell (1995) reported that a patient with semantic dementia was able to reacquire the names of six vegetables (names that she would easily have produced premorbidly but had now forgotten) when the patient practised with their names and some written descriptions.

Graham and Hodges (1997; Graham et al., 1999b) explained these results by suggesting that the hippocampal complex and the temporal neocortex play separate, but interactive, roles in the acquisition and maintenance of autobiographical and semantic knowledge (see Alvarez & Squire, 1994; Graham, Murre, & Hodges, 1999a; Hodges & Graham, 1998; McClelland, McNaughton, & O'Reilly, 1995; Murre, 1996; Squire, 1992 for more details). The proponents of this view differ on some specific details; but almost all agree that although ultimately our long-term memories are represented in neocortical regions, the hippocampus and related structures play a vital role in an initial phase of memory representation. The hippocampus is seen as crucial for the retrieval of a recently experienced event. As memory consolidates, the involvement of the hippocampus gradually diminishes, until eventually the memory is represented permanently in the neocortex. This consolidation theory provides an explanation for the selective preservation in semantic dementia of recent autobiographical and semantic memories, and the strikingly normal performance seen on some tests of new learning.

On a practical level, the profound word-finding (and comprehension) difficulties experienced by the patients, in particular the inability to remember the names of people, diminishes their social confidence, often leading to isolation for both patient and spouse. Given that new learning is possible early in semantic dementia, episodic memory might provide a suitable mechanism for developing strategies which arrest or at least delay the deterioration of vocabulary and semantic knowledge typically seen in the disease, as suggested by the results of Funnell's (1995) study. For example, relearning the names of regular partners in sport or card games, or the names of newspapers and magazines, would avoid embarrassment over failure to produce these names and might thereby encourage more social interaction (e.g., playing golf and visiting the local newsagent). Although this strategy can only be successful for a limited time in a degenerative condition like semantic dementia, it may nevertheless be of genuine benefit, and would be even more appropriate for patients with non-progressive damage to lateral temporal lobe structures with sparing of the hippocampi.

The purpose of this study was to determine whether a patient with semantic dementia would benefit from repeated practice of words which he frequently failed to produce in spontaneous speech or under test conditions. Furthermore, we wished to explore the extent and the longevity of the benefit obtained from such practice, and to try to understand something about the mechanisms underlying any observed effects. Therefore, the first part of this article, Experiment 1, briefly describes an experiment reported in Graham, Patterson, Pratt, and Hodges (1999c) in which relearning of vocabulary was investigated in a patient with semantic dementia, DM. In the second part, Experiment 2, we describe new longitudinal data from DM which confirms some of the hypotheses discussed in the earlier paper.

CASE REPORT: DM

DM (born 1936), an ex-surgeon, presented in April 1995 with a two-year history of word-finding difficulties. DM had first noticed his anomic problems at work: During operations he had experienced increasing difficulty in producing the names of surgical instruments. Following his (early) retirement, he and his wife reported that his anomia had become worse and that, more recently, it had been accompanied by comprehension problems. For example, DM commented in July 1996 that he sometimes experienced problems reading long sentences in his daily newspaper, *The Times*, and in

August 1997 that he was finding it increasingly difficult to follow television programmes.

DM's insight into his condition was excellent and in an attempt to counteract his anomia, he started recording his "lost" words in a notebook from which he attempted to relearn words and phrases that he could not reliably retrieve (see Figure 1). In response to our testing of DM's ability to produce information about celebrities (from faces and/or names), he also produced a book of famous faces, collated from newspaper photographs (see Figure 2). DM also regularly used the *Oxford English Picture Dictionary* (Parnwell, 1977), which consists of pages of coloured drawings organised by category (e.g., the kitchen, the seaside, clothes, sports, etc.) which contain numbered items. For example, the "kitchen" drawing includes a cooker, bread-bin, tea-towel, sink, etc. Below the drawing is a list of the names of the numbered items. DM would cover the answers and attempt to name all the items in each drawing, uncovering the list to retrieve any failed name (see Figure 3). DM practised with these word and picture books regularly and was convinced that he would have much greater word-finding and comprehension difficulties without continual practice.

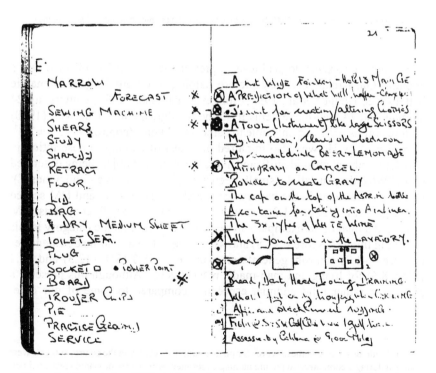

Figure 1.   Example from DM's notebook of words which he could no longer reliably produce.

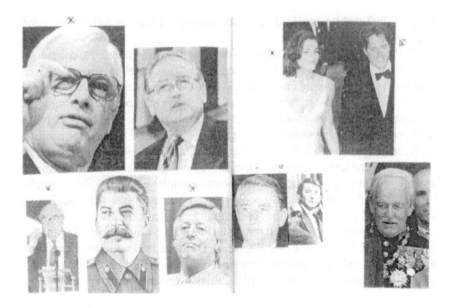

Figure 2. Example from DM's book of faces (contains people he could no longer name).

Formal neuropsychological tests at presentation in 1995 confirmed DM's anomia: On a relatively easy picture naming test from Hodges' semantic battery (see Hodges et al., 1992; Hodges & Patterson, 1995) comprising 24 animals and 24 man-made items from the Snodgrass and Vanderwart (1980) picture corpus, DM was only able to name 34/48 items (controls = 43.6 ± 2.3[1]; z score = −4.2). He was also impaired on a test of naming to description in which the subject must identify and name the animal or object being described (e.g., "What do you call the small green animal which leaps around ponds?"); half of the 48 items in the battery are tested in this fashion, and DM scored 15/24 (controls = 22.4 ± 1.3; z score = −5.7). On category fluency tests, DM produced a total of 36 exemplars in response to four semantic category labels for living things (z score = −1.8) and 41 for a set of four man-made categories (z score = −1.7; controls generate an average of 58.3 (SD = 12.3) and 55.4 (SD = 8.6) for living and man-made, respectively). Although this presents a picture of rather mild anomia, especially compared to some of our other

---

[1] It should be noted that these scores for picture naming accuracy in the control subjects were obtained during a computerised picture naming experiment which also measured reaction times. Control subjects achieve a higher average score if given unlimited time to name the pictures.

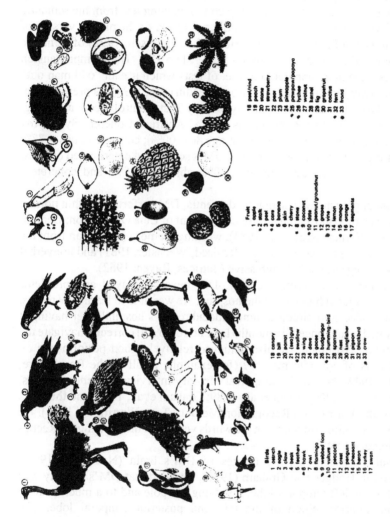

Figure 3. Reproduction of two pages from the *Oxford English Picture Dictionary*. The dots beside the words at the bottom illustrate words that DM was unable to retrieve in April 1997. Reproduced by permission of Oxford University Press. From *Oxford English Picture Dictionary* by E. C. Parnwell © Oxford University Press 1977.

435

published cases of semantic dementia (see for example Hodges, Graham, N., & Patterson, 1995; Hodges, Patterson, & Tyler, 1994), DM's performance on these tests of word production certainly represents a reduction from his premorbid level.

DM was less impaired on tests of word and picture comprehension, scoring within the control range on the word–picture matching test from the semantic battery (DM = 46/48, controls = 47.4, SD = 1.1) and on the picture version of the Pyramids and Palm Trees Test (Howard & Patterson, 1992) of semantic association (DM = 49/52, controls = 51.2, SD = 1.3). His comprehension difficulties were more apparent on a set of tests which use an "odd man out" word synonymy paradigm (adapted from Breedin et al., 1994). At presentation, DM scored as follows: Verb–Noun Synonymy Test (controls score at ceiling; chance = 33%)—verbs = 69%, nouns = 62%; Abstract–Concrete Synonymy Test—abstract nouns = 81% (control range 86–100%); concrete nouns = 77% (control range 90–100%). A year later, DM's scores had deteriorated on most of these tests: verbs = 69%, nouns = 50%, abstract = 65%, and concrete = 65%.

Like other patients with semantic dementia, DM performed within normal limits on tests of visuospatial ability (Judgement of Line Orientation; Benton, de Hamsher, Varney, & Spreen, 1983), working memory (digit span from the Wechsler Adult Intelligence Scale—Revised; Wechsler, 1981) and nonverbal problem-solving (Raven's Progressive Matrices; Raven, 1962).

With respect to episodic memory, DM never displayed any problems when tested either at home or in the hospital. He was able to learn new routes, such as a 10-decision circuit around Addenbrooke's hospital after having it demonstrated to him once. Six months later he could still correctly navigate the route without assistance. He also achieved relatively good performance on standard tests of episodic memory (for example, recall of the Rey Figure; Osterreith, 1944; the Autobiographical Memory Interview; Greene, Hodges, & Baddeley, 1995; Kopelman et al., 1989; Graham et al., 1998; and the faces version of the Warrington Recognition Memory Test; Warrington 1984). He was, however, mildly impaired on the words version of the Warrington Recognition Memory Test.

Coronal T_1 weighted MRI images of DM's brain (November 1995), reproduced in Hodges and Graham (1998), revealed that DM's atrophy was confined to the left temporal lobe, involving the pole and to a much smaller extent the inferior region of the mid and posterior temporal lobe. The hippocampal complex appeared normal. A recent voxel-based morphometry study confirmed the asymmetric pattern of pathology in DM revealing significant atrophy to the left temporal pole with preservation of the hippocampus, the entorhinal cortex and caudal portion of the perirhinal cortex bilaterally (Mummery et al., 2000).

EXPERIMENT 1

An investigation of the effects of home rehearsal
with vocabulary on DM's word production

Given that DM had been recording and practising words he found difficult
to produce since the onset of his anomia, he seemed the ideal case in which to
investigate whether repeated practice with vocabulary would be an effective
strategy for patients with semantic memory impairments. In the following
experiment (reported in Graham et al., 1999c), we found convincing evidence
that rehearsal of the names of concepts combined with pictures and/or real
objects resulted in a significant improvement in DM's word production (as
measured by category fluency). We will briefly review the experiment here;
further details can be found in Graham et al. (1999c).

Methods and procedure

Using the performance of DM and six male, age- and education-matched
control subjects on category fluency for 26 noun categories which DM had
never practised, we created three sets comprising four categories each (Set 1:
"herbs and spices", "chocolate bars", "television shows", and "magazines and
newspapers"; Set 2: "breakfast cereals", "musical groups", "stones and gems",
and "makes of car"; Set 3: "names of companies", "names of charities", "names
of mountains", and "rivers"). These sets were matched for the performance of
the control subjects and also separately for DM, enabling direct comparison of
performance across the three sets during practice and once rehearsal had
ceased. Four additional "red herring" categories were selected for DM to
practise ("drinks", "famous sites", "diseases", and "trees"), so as to provide
distraction from the categories of interest. For some of the categories, DM
rehearsed with real exemplars (e.g., 20 herb and spice bottles; 20 cereal boxes),
while for others the practice was based on items seen in books (e.g., trees;
stones and gems).

For clarity, a complete outline of the experiment is listed below (see Figure 4
for a schematic diagram of the experimental procedure):

April 1997 (Baseline): DM was tested on category fluency for a large
number of nonpractised categories. These provided the data for the category
selection described above and for DM's baseline performance on the 16 categories comprising Sets 1, 2, and 3.

23 June 1997 (Start of Experiment): DM was asked to work on a total of 100
items from six categories regularly over the coming 2 weeks. These categories
were: herbs and spices, chocolate bars, magazines and newspapers, television
shows, famous sites, trees (i.e., Set 1, plus two foil categories). He was told to
practise the items as he had been practising with the *Oxford English Picture*

438

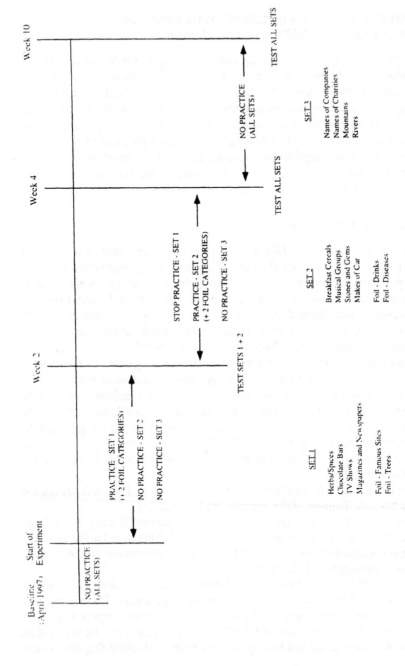

Figure 4. A schematic diagram describing Experiment 1, showing when and what categories DM practised week by week. The categories used in each practised/non-practised set are shown on the figure.

Dictionary (OEPD) and his self-generated material. He was also instructed that he must spend no more than 30 minutes a day practising the new categories and that, during this time, he should also continue to practise as usual with his word notebook and face book. To ensure that DM co-operated with this aspect of the experiment, we asked him to fill in a sheet detailing how often he practised with all the stimuli (see Appendix A).

7 July 1997 (Week 2): DM was given a category fluency test for each of the six categories he had been practising for the past 2 weeks (Set 1 plus foils) and for each of the six new categories he was about to practise (breakfast cereals, musical groups, stones and gems, makes of cars, drinks and diseases (Set 2 plus two new foil categories). He was then requested to start practising the six new categories and to stop rehearsing the previous six categories. As for the prior 2 weeks, he was asked to fill in a sheet detailing how often he practised (limiting his drill on the new categories to 30 minutes per day).

21 July 1997 (Week 4): DM was given all 16 categories in a category fluency test. This included Set 1 and Set 2 (the eight categories he had practised at different times), the four foil categories, and the four categories from the matched Set 3 that he had never practised. He was then asked to stop practising all these categories.

1 September 1997 (Week 10): The category fluency test administered at Week 4 was repeated (with the categories in a different order). DM assured us that he had not been practising the categories, although he admitted that he was finding it difficult to avoid rehearsing television shows and makes of car because he came across them regularly. He also pointed out that he was now practising rivers because they were in the *OEPD*.

10 November 1997 (Week 20): Ten weeks after the end of the experiment (a total of 20 weeks from the start of the study), we retested DM's ability to perform category fluency on the 16 categories. During these additional 10 weeks, DM was free to practise any of the categories he wished as we had told him the experiment was finished.

Results

Appendix A, consisting of one of the sheets used by DM to record his exercises, demonstrates that DM regularly practised with the new items (as well as his word list and face book) during the appropriate learning phase. The times recorded on the sheet, and discussions with DM's wife who had kept an eye on how often he rehearsed the words, confirmed that DM had followed instructions and practised the items for no longer than 30 minutes per day. De-briefing of DM after the experiment verified that he was using similar practice methods to those he used with his own material: object naming—hiding the name of the item and attempting to produce it; and the creation of category-based lists of the test stimuli.

Overall, DM showed striking and statistically significant effects of rehearsal in a comparison of his performance before and after practice on the seven categories given to DM to practice (originally eight, but we excluded makes of car because it turned out that he had been practising this category since April 1997) (Wilcoxon Signed Rank Test, Ws = 2.4, $p < .05$).

A similar analysis was used to assess the impact of DM ceasing his daily drill on his success in category fluency: DM's performance on the seven categories at 10 weeks, after he had stopped the exercises on all categories (excluding makes of car), was significantly lower than his performance after 2 weeks of practice (Ws = 2.4, $p < .05$) but still reliably higher than his scores at the baseline (Ws = 2.2, $p < .05$).

Figure 5 compares DM's performance on the three category sets, excluding makes of cars and rivers because DM had not stopped practising these two semantic categories. We also eliminated magazines and newspapers from Set 1 to produce an equal number of categories in the three sets (purely by luck, magazines and newspapers had been matched to makes of cars and rivers for both DM and the control subjects at the start of the experiment). In terms of improvement on category fluency, it is clear that DM showed a dramatic increase in the number of exemplars produced for the categories in both Sets 1 and 2 after 2 weeks home drill, outperforming the control subjects.

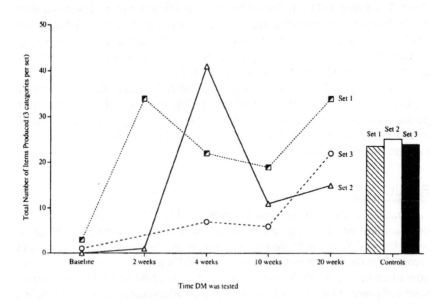

Figure 5. A comparison of DM's performance on Sets 1, 2, and 3 from Experiment 1. To make the comparison between each set meaningful, "magazines and newspapers" was excluded from Set 1, "makes of car" from Set 2, and "rivers" from Set 3. The graph also shows the mean of the controls for each set.

Unfortunately, in Set 1, DM had lost approximately one third of the new items (34 items dropping to 22) 2 weeks after he stopped practising, and by 8 weeks could only produce 19 exemplars in this set. In Set 2, 6 weeks after he had stopped drilling on the items in these categories, DM's category fluency scores had dropped by over two-thirds (41 to 11).

Figure 5 also indicates that, at 20 weeks, DM's performance on all three sets of categories had improved, especially Sets 1 and 3, compared with his scores at 10 weeks. Note that Set 3, which comprised the categories that DM never prac- tised in our experiment, had gradually improved since the baseline until, at 20 weeks, DM's score on these was at a level similar to that of the control subjects. This offers a clear demonstration of how DM notices items or categories on which he is failing and then goes on to practise them, with beneficial conse- quences. For example, DM was initially unable to produce the names of *any* companies (one of the categories in Set 3), yet at 20 weeks, he produced 18 company names.

In DM's case there was an exceedingly high, and in some cases perfect, overlap between his responses on category fluency, including the item order, and either the list of items that he was given by us to learn or the list that he created in his notebook in order to practice a category. Table 1 illustrates this effect for a category from Set 1, magazines and newspapers, and for one of the foil categories, trees. DM's responses to trees reveal another interesting facet of his performance on the category fluency tests: The production of a small number of speech errors (for example, "oat tree" instead of "oak tree", "cider" instead of "cedar", and "earth" instead of "birch").

Out of a total of 254 category fluency responses DM made 27 errors (approximately 11% of his total responses). Although this is a relatively low error rate, the errors are still noteworthy since control subjects essentially never make errors of these types in category fluency. The majority of DM's errors (89%) were phonologically related to the target—blends comprising phonemic segments of within-list items (e.g., "opaz" instead of "opal" and "topaz"; "tives" as a blend of "thyme" and "chives") and other phonemic errors that were not obvious blends of phoneme segments within the list but were clearly phonologically related to a specific list item (e.g., "earth" for "birch").

Discussion

In Experiment 1, DM showed a striking effect of practice. He produced many more items in category fluency after 14 days (approximately 30 minutes rehearsal per day) of exposure to lists of appropriate exemplars than he did prior to practice. By contrast, he showed little change in performance on matched categories which he did not rehearse. These results clearly demonstrate that it is possible for a patient with semantic dementia to relearn previously familiar names that have become difficult to produce. When DM stopped practising the

TABLE 1

Examples documenting the consistency between DM's responses
in Experiment 1 and the order of items in our lists or his notebook
for "magazines and newspapers" and "trees"

List order	DM's response
Magazines and newspapers	
The Times	Times
The Guardian	Guardian
The Independent	Independent
The Daily Telegraph	The Daily Telegraph
Daily Mail	The Daily Mail
The Express	Express
The Sun	The Sun
New Scientist	New Scientist
Time	Time
Reader's Digest	Reader's Digest
	Time
Hello	Hello
OK Magazine	OK Magazine
Tatler	Tatler
Good Housekeeping	Good Housekeeping
Woman	Woman
Vogue	Vogue
Gardener's World	**words, Garden**, [Gardener's World]
Golf World	Punch
Punch	Sainsbury's Magazine
Sainsbury's Magazine	M and S Magazine
Trees	
Oak tree	
Palm	Palm
Fir	**Fire**, fir
Cedar	
Willow	Willow
Beech	Beech
Birch	**Earth**
Chestnut	Chestnut
Pine	**Pin**
Sycamore	
Yew	Yew
	Oat, *oak tree*
	Cider, *no cedar*
	Sycamore

DM's errors (of accuracy) are shown in bold and items where DM deviated
from his list order are in italics.

semantic categories, his performance declined, although not quite to baseline levels, suggesting that it was continual exposure to the vocabulary that was supporting his better word production.

Importantly, DM's responses on the category fluency tests after practice were characterised by striking overlap with his practice lists, both in content and order. He hardly ever produced an exemplar in any of the eight practised semantic categories unless the item was included in his practice list (selected either by us or by him); that is, there was no generalisation to new within-category items that he had presumably known premorbidly. Furthermore, for the majority of categories, DM produced the items on the category fluency tests in an order very similar to the order of occurrence either on our lists or in his notebook. These results reveal that DM's performance on these tests was highly constrained by his practice and suggests that he was producing the exemplars in category fluency *by rote*. *The Concise Oxford Dictionary* (Sykes, 1976 p. 980) defines this term as "by mere habituation, as knowledge got by repetition, from unintelligent memory". Our proposal is that, whereas the category fluency test is usually considered to tap semantic memory, for DM performing category fluency for his practised sets, it was more akin to traditional word-list learning tasks of episodic memory. DM had memorised the items and, in the category fluency tests, attempted to remember them as lists.

DM's most common errors—phonemic blends and other phonological errors—also suggest production via rote episodic memory. Generation of category exemplars exclusively from semantic memory is unlikely to yield errors of these types. Indeed we have essentially never observed such errors in category fluency (or in any other semantically driven word production task, such as naming) by other patients with semantic dementia: they typically give either very few, or sometimes no, correct exemplar names, but also no incorrectly pronounced names.

By contrast with the complete absence of such errors in their category fluency, patients with semantic dementia *have* been observed to make errors of these types, especially phonological exchanges and blends, in a different task—immediate serial recall of strings of three to four previously familiar words of which the patients' comprehension is now degraded (Knott, Patterson, & Hodges, 1997; Patterson, Graham, N., & Hodges, 1994). Patterson et al. argued that, in semantic dementia, the deterioration of conceptual knowledge results in a gradual loss of "binding" between semantic and phonological representations. As a result, under conditions of high phonological load, the patients make phonological transposition errors like those made by normal subjects reproducing short sequences of nonwords. We suggest here that DM's manner of performing category fluency can be considered akin to the data from other patients with semantic dementia when they were recalling strings of three to four familiar words with degraded meaning. DM's phonemic blends reflect two factors: (1) his impoverished understanding of the test stimuli—his errors typically occurred in categories of which he had little knowledge (e.g., stones and gems, herbs and spices); and (2) the stress placed on the phonological system by the requirement to produce a long sequence of items.

EXPERIMENT 2

A two year follow-up of the effects of DM's home drill with "forgotten" vocabulary

Given that DM was able to benefit from practice with vocabulary at home, we predicted that he would not show the usual pattern of profound deterioration on word production tasks shown by other patients with semantic dementia. In general, patients with this syndrome present with a mild to moderate anomia which worsens dramatically over time (Hodges et al., 1995). A similar deterioration has been noted on tests of picture and word comprehension (Hodges et al., 1994). In DM's case, however, we might predict a rather unusual pattern of longitudinal performance on tests of word production: Poor performance initially, followed by an improvement in production of practised words until a point in time when practice is no longer effective (i.e., a bell-shaped pattern).

In terms of performance on tests of semantic memory, however, the pattern should be rather different. In the experiment described previously, there was a strong, although unsubstantiated, suggestion that DM was producing words in category fluency for which he possessed little or no semantic knowledge. For example, on one occasion he produced the name "aubergine", but was unable to explain to the experimenter exactly what an aubergine was. This implies that on tests of semantic knowledge, we might see the usual pattern of decline documented previously in semantic dementia (i.e., a progressive, and seemingly unstoppable, deterioration of semantic memory).

In order to address these hypotheses, we had the opportunity to test DM again approximately 2 years after we started the experiment described above. During this time, DM had continued to practise at home with lists of words and different pictorial encyclopaedias (including the *OEPD*). Although he had given up rehearsing with famous people, he remained equally, if not more, obsessed by his vocabulary practice.

Method

DM was given category fluency from the semantic battery (Hodges et al., 1992, 1995; Hodges & Patterson, 1995) and the word version of the Pyramid and Palm Trees Test (PPT) of associative semantic knowledge (Howard & Patterson, 1992) on seven (six for the words PPT) separate occasions. These data points were April 1995, November 1995, July 1996, April 1997, November 1997, June 1998, and April 1999 (category fluency only).

Results

Figure 6a shows DM's performance on category fluency over the seven testing sessions starting in April 1995 and finishing in April 1999. In April 1995, DM showed a mildly impaired level of performance on category fluency (approximately $-2.0\,z$-scores below the control mean). The striking longitudinal finding by July 1996 was that DM's ability to produce exemplars in category fluency had improved by approximately 50%, to the extent that he now out-performed many control subjects. Further testing revealed that there was little change in DM's ability to perform category fluency for over 2 years. In April 1999, however, DM's score dropped substantially. At this point, his performance was virtually identical to the one he achieved on the first testing session in April 1995.

Other effects that we noted on DM's category fluency performance on the seventh and final testing session are illuminating with regard to our hypothesis about rote learning. For the first time since we had been testing him, DM produced a number of non-category responses (e.g., "cement" as a household item; "beak" as a bird; "canvas" as a vehicle; and "garlic" as an animal). These inappropriate category inclusions are germane to a further, striking effect: When asked to provide semantic information about a number of the items he had successfully produced on the category fluency test, DM was profoundly impaired. For example, for both "punt" and "barge"—items he had provided for the category, "types of boat"—DM responded that he did not know what the word meant. Similarly, when asked to describe a "dalmatian", he said he had no idea what a dalmatian was, despite the fact that he had produced this word correctly in the category, "types of dog". DM's inability to produce detailed, or even sometimes any, semantic information about the words which he generated in category fluency was evident in all the categories tested.

Figure 6b illustrates that DM's improvement on tests used in our longitudinal battery only extended to tasks tapping word production. On the word version of the Pyramid and Palm Trees Test DM showed a consistent decline in performance.

Discussion

The 2 year follow-up of DM's performance on category fluency has provided further support for the hypotheses tested in the previous experiment and discussed in detail in Graham et al. (1999c). DM showed a remarkable improvement, and subsequent preservation, of his performance on category fluency over time. In fact, it was only in April 1999 that we found any evidence of a decline in his ability to produce words when given a category label, and even at this point, DM was still performing as well as he had done when he first presented. This pattern is in direct contrast to that shown by many other patients with semantic dementia and, given the results from the experiment which

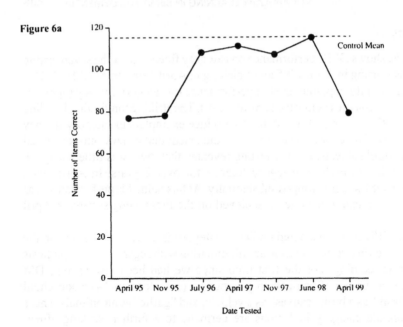

Figure 6a

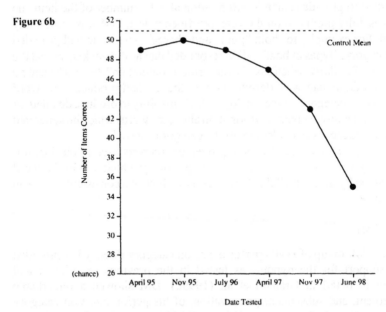

Figure 6b

Figure 6. DM's performance on (a) category fluency from the semantic battery (Hodges et al., 1992, 1995; Hodges & Patterson, 1995) on seven separate occasions (April 1995, November 1995, July 1996, April 1997, November 1997, June 1998, and April 1999); and (b) the word version of the Pyramid and Palm Trees Test on six occasions (April 1995, November 1995, July 1996, April 1997, November 1997, June 1998).

investigated the effects of practice on DM's word production, constitutes further evidence that home drill substantially improved his ability to produce previously "difficult-to-retrieve" words on tests of word production.

One of the most striking results from this final experiment, however, relates not to DM's reduction in the number of words generated in category fluency in April 1999 but rather to his inability to produce semantic information about many of the items that he *did* generate correctly in the fluency task. We suggest that this is additional support for our earlier proposal that DM was using rote memory in order to support his learning (i.e., that he was learning in a mechanical manner without proper reflection or understanding of the materials in question). Furthermore, DM's lack of knowledge about the exemplars he provided illustrates that this type of rote learning, even with pictures and descriptions of the names of concepts, had little impact on his deteriorating semantic system. In support of this hypothesis, DM's performance on the Pyramid and Palm Trees Test declined over time, a pattern that has been documented previously in other cases with semantic dementia (Hodges et al., 1994; 1995).

GENERAL DISCUSSION

The two experiments described in this paper (see also the other experiments described in Graham et al., 1999c), demonstrate that a patient with semantic dementia, DM, could relearn words that were difficult for him to produce in spontaneous speech or on tests of word production such as picture naming and category fluency. Furthermore, analyses of DM's performance when he stopped practising revealed that it was the repeated exposure to test stimuli which was boosting his word production: 10 weeks post-practice in Experiment 1, DM was only able to produce 40% of the exemplars that he had managed to recall at the end of a fortnight's daily practice. Experiment 1 also suggests that DM's learning was tightly constrained by the stimuli that he was practising: He almost never produced exemplars that he had not practised and he appeared to have learned items by rote, typically producing instances in an order that matched the lists that he had been rehearsing. A further result of interest from Experiment 1 was the production of some phonemic blend errors (e.g., "opaz" in place of the contiguous exemplars "opal" and "topaz") which once again suggests that DM was performing category fluency for his practised categories as an episodic recall task. In the assessments of Experiment 2, which occurred 2 years after the start of the other experiments, DM still showed a remarkable ability to produce exemplars on category fluency, although his performance had declined from earlier testing sessions. At this point, for the first time, he produced some inappropriate category exemplars and was consistently unable to provide semantic information about many of the exemplars he had provided in the fluency test. The data from this study strongly point to rote memory as DM's learning method and confirm the hypothesis raised in the Introduction that patients with semantic dementia are capable of new learning, presumably due to the relative preservation of the hippocampal complex early in the disease. It is important to note the specificity of this learning: There was little beneficial impact of DM's home drill on his degraded knowledge base as exemplified by his lack of improvement on semantic tests, such as the Pyramid and Palm Trees Test (Howard & Patterson, 1992), and his poor knowledge of the meaning of the exemplars produced during category fluency.

Why did practice benefit DM?

DM is not the only patient with semantic dementia to have self-initiated word rehearsal as an attempted remedy for anomia (see Funnell, 1995; Graham & Hodges, 1997), but this strategy seems to have been particularly effective in DM's case. Elsewhere, we have argued that several factors may have resulted in the success of DM's practice, in particular: (1) the use of a rich and varied set of stimuli, which included descriptions, drawings and photographs of the concepts corresponding to DM's unretrievable names; and (2) the mild degree of both his anomia and his semantic impairment when he initiated this word drill (see Graham et al., 1999c, for more details). At least one other patient, AM, who practised "forgotten" words but failed to show any beneficial effects of practise was both more anomic and had a greater degree of semantic memory impairment than DM (Graham & Hodges, 1997). It is possible, therefore, that patients with semantic dementia will only show a benefit of practice at a relatively mild stage of word-production and comprehension deficits.

The other, more theoretically interesting, proposal relates to the fact that DM drilled on words and pictures concurrently, thereby co-activating the semantic and phonological representations of a given concept. AM, the patient mentioned previously, rehearsed with alphabetically organised word lists, thus predominantly activating phonological representations. Several studies on the relative effectiveness of different paradigms for the facilitation of word-retrieval in aphasic stroke patients (Cohen, Engel, Kelter, & List, 1979; Howard et al., 1985a, b; Patterson, Purell, & Morton, 1983) have suggested that such phonologically based techniques (e.g., word repetition, Patterson et al., 1983) are significantly less effective than those which also require semantic processing (e.g., word–picture matching, Howard et al., 1985a, b). In fact, the studies by Howard and colleagues strongly suggest that effective facilitation in word production may depend upon concurrent activation of the semantic and phonological representations of the specific concept/name.

This interpretation may also explain why DM was measurably anomic when he first presented (despite his self-initiated year of home drill). DM's initial notebooks were not in fact organised by semantic category: For example, sewing machine, shears, study, shandy, retract, flour, lid, etc. (see Figure 1). Practice with these stimuli would have been purely phonological in nature and may only have produced short-term assistance which would not have accumulated from day to day. By contrast, his later materials, the *OEPD*, and his other lists, used a combination of words and pictures which were arranged by category: Practice with these would result in a more beneficial strategy, whereby he was co-activating semantic and phonological representations of his difficult-to-produce words. The other possibility is that DM may not have been practising the items that were included in our semantic tests (e.g., ostrich, frog, helicopter, sledge, etc.) having not noticed that he was having trouble producing these words in spontaneous speech. When he started using the *OEPD* for practice, he would be more likely to encounter the types of stimuli which comprise the semantic battery and, therefore, we might expect an improvement on his performance on tasks which require him to produce the names of these exemplars.

It is important to note that, despite the potential importance of activating both semantic and phonological representations, the semantic information that DM was acquiring or relearning was probably rather minimal—in many instances, perhaps no more than the fact that a particular name belonged to a particular category or list. This point is illustrated in the final experiment in which DM was unable to produce any information about many of the words he successfully retrieved during category fluency. We emphasise again, therefore, that, for DM, this word learning was more in the nature of rote verbal learning than semantically-based vocabulary learning.

The final experiment in our series raises a further interesting question: Given that DM's home drill has been a highly successful technique for boosting his word production, why did he show a substantial drop in performance on category fluency in 1999? There are a number of factors that could have caused this effect. First, DM may not at this stage have been practising as consistently as he has done over the previous few years. It is unlikely that this is the predominant explanation for DM's drop in performance as his wife has reported no decline in the *amount* of time he spends working on his words at home. In fact, DM has become increasingly obsessed with his vocabulary practice and in April 1999 was spending 7–8 hours a day looking at his books. A more plausible explanation relates to the *quality* of DM's practising: Given DM's drop by 1998 into the seriously impaired range on the Pyramid and Palm Trees Test of word comprehension (Figure 6b), it is clear that his semantic system was becoming significantly degraded. Reduced semantic activation would have a detrimental impact on his ability to retain and retrieve recently learnt or relearnt words. A third, and not mutually exclusive, factor relates to DM's capacity for new learning. While episodic memory is preserved early in semantic dementia, later on in the disease new learning of verbal and nonverbal materials becomes compromised (see Graham et al., 1999b). If DM's relearning of vocabulary is largely episodically, rather than semantically, dependent, it is possible that his poorer performance on word production is directly associated with a decrease in his ability to learn from practice.

Implications for therapy for patients with semantic impairments

While the experiments described here suggest that repeated exposure to vocabulary may be a successful therapeutic strategy, at least as measured by DM's marked improvement on our tests of word production, it is important to note that DM's perpetual homework has had a negative impact on his psychological well-being, which raises questions about the value of this strategy in semantic dementia. DM had full insight into the progressive nature of his anomia and comprehension impairments, and was aware that when he ceased practising he risked losing the items that he had painstakingly learned or regained. As a result, he became increasingly obsessed with practising previous lists and also with adding new names of objects and concepts to his lists as the ranks of inaccessible words swelled. Over time, therefore, the number of words, pictures, faces, and names that he has been forced to practise has become overwhelming, leading to periods of depression and frustration both in DM and other members of his family. Although these "side effects" provide a sobering counterpoint to the success of DM's word practice, this caution may not apply to all patients. The relative benefits and risks will probably vary significantly from case to case depending on both cognitive factors and personality.

There has recently been considerable interest in the relative effectiveness of techniques of learning which allow or even encourage the learner to make and then correct errors, as compared with regimes designed only to permit correct responses that get reinforced. The principle of errorless learning techniques is not that the person will always be able to produce the correct response, but that frank errors—which themselves may get encoded and remembered—are avoided. Baddeley and Wilson (1994) showed that brain injured amnesic patients scored better on a word-completion task using errorless learning compared with the more traditional trial-and-error method. Name learning and picture recognition have also been shown to benefit from this technique (Wilson, Baddeley, Evans, & Shiel, 1994; see Wilson & Evans, 1996 for a review) and a recent paper by Clare, Wilson, Breen, and Hodges (1999) described a successful treatment regime based on errorless learning, in which a patient in the early stages of Alzheimer's disease relearned the names of members of his bowls club.

Although neither we, nor certainly DM, had designed his homework drills to fit an errorless learning principle, in retrospect it seems possible that his learning could be considered consistent with this technique. The majority of patients with semantic dementia (especially those, like DM, with predominantly left-temporal atrophy, Lambon Ralph et al., in press) produce relatively few frankly incorrect responses in their attempts to name. The most common failures are "don't know" responses, plus some circumlocutions, superordinates (e.g., "animal"), and comments (e.g., "Oh, I've got one of them at home"). It is possible, therefore, that DM's homework drill in naming consisted mainly of either producing the correct name or producing nothing and immediately looking up the correct name—i.e., a kind of implicit use of an errorless procedure. Further studies should address this topic and whether other anomic patients, especially those with a nonprogressive semantic disorder, could benefit from learning techniques which facilitate the co-activation of semantic and phonological representations.

REFERENCES

Alvarez, P., & Squire, L.R. (1994). Memory consolidation and the medial temporal lobe: A simple network model. *Proceedings of the National Academy of Science, 91*, 7041–7045.

Baddeley, A.D., & Wilson, B.A. (1994). When implicit learning fails: Amnesia and the problem of error elimination. *Neuropsychologia, 32*, 53–68.

Benton, A.L., de Hamsher, K., Varney, N.R., & Spreen, O. (1983). *Judgement of Line Orientation*. New York: Oxford University Press.

Breedin, S.D., Saffran, E.M., & Coslett, H.B. (1994). Reversal of the concreteness effect in a patient with semantic dementia. *Cognitive Neuropsychology, 11*, 617–660.

Clare, L., Wilson, B.A., Breen, K., & Hodges, J.R. (1999). Errorless learning of face–name associations in early Alzheimer's disease. *Neurocase, 5*, 37–46.

Cohen, R., Engel, D., Kelter, S., & List, G. (1979). Kurz- und Langzeiteffekte von Benennenhilfen bei Aphatikern. In G. Peuser (Ed.), *Studien zur Sprachtherapie*. Munich: Wilhelm Fink.

Diesfeldt, H.F.A. (1992). Impaired and preserved semantic memory functions in dementia. In L. Bäckman (Ed.), *Memory functioning in dementia*. Amsterdam: Elsevier Science.

Funnell, E. (1995). A case of forgotten knowledge. In R. Campbell & M. Conway (Eds.), *Broken memories* (pp. 225–236). Oxford, UK: Blackwell.

Graham, K.S. (1995). *Semantic memory impairment and anomia in progressive fluent aphasia.* Unpublished Ph.D. thesis, University of Cambridge, Cambridge, UK.

Graham, K.S., Becker, J.T., & Hodges, J.R. (1997). On the relationship between knowledge and memory for pictures: Evidence from the study of patients with semantic dementia and Alzheimer's disease. *Journal of the International Neuropsychological Society, 3*, 534–544.

Graham, K.S., & Hodges, J.R. (1997). Differentiating the roles of the hippocampal complex and the neocortex in long-term memory storage: Evidence from the study of semantic dementia and Alzheimer's disease. *Neuropsychology, 11*, 77–89.

Graham, K.S., Murre, J.M.J., & Hodges, J.R. (1999a). Episodic memory in semantic dementia: A computational approach based on the TraceLink model. In J. Reggia, E. Ruppin, & D. Glanzman (Eds.), *Disorders of brain, behaviour and cognition: The neurocomputational perspective (Progress in Brain Research).* (pp 47–65). Amsterdam: Elsevier Science.

Graham, K.S., Patterson, K., & Hodges, J.R. (1999b). Episodic memory: New insights from the study of semantic dementia. *Current Opinion in Neurobiology, 9*, 245–250.

Graham, K.S., Patterson, K., Pratt, K.H., & Hodges J.R. (1999c). Re-learning and subsequent forgetting of semantic category exemplars in a case of semantic dementia. *Neuropsychology, 13*, 359–380.

Graham, K.S., Pratt, K.H., & Hodges, J.R. (1998). A reverse temporal gradient for public events in a single case of semantic dementia. *Neurocase, 4*, 461–470.

Graham, K.S., Simons, J.S., Pratt, K.H., Patterson, K., & Hodges, J.R. (2000). Insights from semantic dementia on the relationship between episodic and semantic memory. *Neuropsychologia, 38*, 313–324.

Greene, J.D.W., Hodges, J.R., & Baddeley, A.D. (1995). Autobiographical memory and executive function in early dementia of Alzheimer type. *Neuropsychologia, 33*, 1647–1670.

Harasty, J.A., Halliday, G.M., Code, C., & Brooks, W.S. (1996). Quantification of cortical atrophy in a case of progressive fluent aphasia. *Brain, 119*, 181–190.

Hodges, J.R., Garrard, P., & Patterson, K. (1998). Semantic dementia. In A. Kertesz & D. Munoz (Eds.), *Pick's disease and Pick's complex*, (pp. 83–104). New York: Wiley-Liss.

Hodges, J.R., & Graham, K.S. (1998). A reversal of the temporal gradient for famous person knowledge: Implications for the neural organisation of long-term memory. *Neuropsychologia, 36*, 803–825.

Hodges, J.R., Graham, N., & Patterson, K. (1995). Charting the progression in semantic dementia: Implications for the organisation of semantic memory. *Memory, 3*, 463–495.

Hodges, J.R., & Patterson, K. (1995). Is semantic memory consistently impaired early in the course of Alzheimer's disease? Neuroanatomical and diagnostic implications. *Neuropsychologia, 33*, 441–459.

Hodges, J.R., & Patterson, K. (1996). Nonfluent progressive aphasia and semantic dementia: A comparative neuropsychological study. *Journal of the International Neuropsychological Society, 2*, 511–524.

Hodges, J.R., Patterson, K., Oxbury, S., & Funnell, E. (1992). Semantic dementia: Progressive fluent aphasia with temporal lobe atrophy. *Brain, 115*, 1783–1806.

Hodges, J.R., Patterson, K., & Tyler, L.K. (1994). Loss of semantic memory: Implications for the modularity of mind. *Cognitive Neuropsychology, 11*, 505–542.

Howard, D., & Patterson, K. (1992). *Pyramids and Palm Trees: A test of semantic access from pictures and words.* Bury St Edmunds, UK: Thames Valley Test Company.

Howard, D., Patterson, K., Franklin, S., Orchard-Lisle, V., & Morton, J. (1985a). The facilitation of picture naming in aphasia. *Cognitive Neuropsychology, 2*, 49–80.

Howard, D., Patterson, K., Franklin, S., Orchard-Lisle, V., & Morton, J. (1985b). Treatment of word retrieval deficits in aphasia: A comparison of two therapy methods. *Brain, 108*, 817–829.

Knott, R., Patterson, K., & Hodges, J.R. (1997). Lexical and semantic binding effects in short term-memory: Evidence from semantic dementia. *Cognitive Neuropsychology, 14*, 1165–1216.

Kopelman, M.D., Wilson, B.A., & Baddeley, A.D. (1989). The autobiographical memory interview: A new assessment of autobiographical and personal semantic memory in amnesic patients. *Journal of Clinical Experimental Neuropsychology, 11*, 724–744.

Lambon Ralph, M.A., Howard, D., Nightingale, G., & Ellis, A.W. (1998). Are living and non-living category-specific deficits causally linked to impaired perceptual knowledge? Evidence from a category-specific double dissociation. *Neurocase, 4*, 311–338.

Lambon Ralph, M.A., McClelland, J.L., Patterson, K., Galton, C., & Hodges J.R. (in press). No right to speak? The relationship between object naming and semantic impairment: Neuropsychological evidence and a computational model. *Journal of Cognitive Neuroscience.*

McClelland, J.L., McNaughton, B.L., & O'Reilly, R. (1995). Why there are complementary learning systems in the hippocampus and neocortex: Insights from the successes and failures of connectionist models of learning and memory. *Psychological Review, 102*, 419–437.

Mesulam, M.M. (1982). Slowly progressive aphasia without generalised dementia. *Annals of Neurology, 11*, 592–598.

Mummery, C.J., Patterson, K. Price, C.J. Ashburner, J. Frackowiak, R.S.J., & Hodges, J.R. (2000) A voxel based morphometry study of semantic dementia: The relationship between temporal lobe atrophy and semantic dementia. *Annals of Neurology, 47*, 36–45.

Murre, J.M.J. (1996). TraceLink: A model of amnesia and consolidation of memory. *Hippocampus, 6*, 675–684.

Osterreith, P.A. (1944). Le test de copie d'une figure complexe. *Arch Psychologie, 30*, 206–256.

Parnwell, E.C. (1977). *Oxford English picture dictionary*. Oxford: Oxford University Press.

Patterson, K., Graham, N., & Hodges, J.R. (1994). The impact of semantic memory loss on phonological representations. *Journal of Cognitive Neuroscience, 6*, 57–69.

Patterson, K., Purell, C., & Morton, J. (1983). Facilitation of word retrieval in aphasia. In C. Code & D.J. Muller (Eds.), *Aphasia therapy*, (pp. 76–87). London: Arnold.

Pick, A. (1892). Uber die Beziehungen der senilen Hirnatrophie zur Aphasie [On the manifestations of aphasia in senile brain atrophy]. *Prager Medizinische Wochenschrift, 17*, 165–167.

Raven, J.C. (1962). *Coloured progressive matrices sets A, AB, B*. London: H.K. Lewis.

Schwartz, M.F., Marin, O.S.M., & Saffran, E.M. (1979). Dissociations of language function in dementia: A case study. *Brain and Language, 7*, 277–306.

Snodgrass, J.G., & Vanderwart, M. (1980). A standardised set of 260 pictures: Norms for name agreement, familiarity and visual complexity. *Journal of Experimental Psychology: General, 6*, 174–215.

Snowden, J.S., Goulding, P.J., & Neary, D. (1989). Semantic dementia: A form of circumscribed cerebral atrophy. *Behavioural Neurology, 2*, 167–182.

Snowden, J.S., Griffiths, H.L., & Neary, D. (1994). Semantic dementia: Autobiographical contribution to preservation of meaning. *Cognitive Neuropsychology, 11*, 265–288.

Snowden, J., Griffiths, H.L., & Neary, D. (1995). Autobiographical experience and word meaning. *Memory, 3*, 225–246.

Snowden, J.S., Griffiths, H.L., & Neary, D. (1996a). Semantic-episodic memory interactions in semantic dementia: Implications for retrograde memory function. *Cognitive Neuropsychology, 13*, 1101–1137.

Snowden, J.S., Neary, D., & Mann, D.M.A. (1996b). *Fronto-temporal lobar degeneration: fronto-temporal dementia, progressive aphasia, semantic dementia*. New York: Churchill Livingstone.

Squire, L.R. (1992). Memory and the hippocampus: A synthesis from findings with rats, monkeys, and humans. *Psychological Review, 99*, 195–231.

Srinivas, K., Breedin, S.D., Coslett, H.B., & Saffran, E.M. (1997). Intact perceptual priming in a patient with damage to the anterior inferior temporal lobes. *Journal of Cognitive Neuroscience, 9*, 490–511.

Sykes, J.B. (1976). *The concise Oxford dictionary of current English (Sixth edition)*. Oxford: Oxford University Press.

Warrington, E.K. (1975). Selective impairment of semantic memory. *Quarterly Journal of Experimental Psychology, 27*, 635–657.

Warrington, E.K. (1984). *Recognition Memory Test*. Windsor, UK: NFER Nelson.

Wechsler, D.A. (1981). *Wechsler Adult Intelligence Scale—Revised. Test manual*. New York: Psychological Corporation.

Wilson, B.A., Baddeley, A.D., Evans, J.J., & Shiel, A. (1994). Errorless learning in the rehabilitation of memory impaired people. *Neuropsychological Rehabilitation, 4*, 307–326.

Wilson, B.A., & Evans, J.J. (1996). Error-free learning in the rehabilitation of people with memory impairments. *Journal of Head Trauma Rehabilitation, 11*, 54–64.

Manuscript received July 1999
Revised manuscript received April 2000

APPENDIX A

DAY	WORDS		FACES		NEW ITEMS	
	START	FINISH	START	FINISH	START	FINISH
EXAMPLE	12.20	1.00	3.05	4.15	7.45	8.15
23rd June	6=00	6·30	/		2=30	3=15.
24th June	5=00	5=40	9=30	10=05	3·4?	4=15
25th June	10=00	10=40 AM.	9=00 PM	9=30 PM	8·30 PM	9=00 PM
26th June	9-30	10=00 AM	/		5=00	5=35 PM
27th June	2:30 PM	3=00	10=00	10=15 PM	5=00	5=25 PM
28th June	10=00	10=30	/		/	
29th June	12=00	12·30	7.15 PM	7=35	8=30 PM	9=00
30th June	10-00	10-30 AM	/		8=45	9=15 PM
1st July	11=30	12=00	6=00 ?	6=20	3=00	5=30
2nd July	3=00	3=30	/		9=30 PM	9=50
3rd July	2=00	2=35	10:30 PM	10=45	9=15	9=40 PM
4th July	3=00	3=30	10=00	10=20 PM	6=00	6=20 ?
5th July	10=30	11=00	/		11=00	11=20
6th July	10=15	10=45	/		7=00	7=30 PM

A copy of one of the sheets used by DM to record the length of time he practised the categories in Experiment 1.

Influence of anosognosia on treatment outcome among dementia patients

Deborah C. Koltai, Kathleen A. Welsh-Bohmer,
and Donald E. Schmechel

*Joseph and Kathleen Bryan Alzheimer's Disease Research Center,
Duke University Medical Center, Durham, USA*

This study was a preliminary investigation of the effects of a Memory and Coping Program among mild to moderate dementia patients. A total of 24 elderly participants were randomly assigned to treatment and waiting-list control conditions. A pre-test, post-test design was used, with group comparisons of change scores on objective cognitive tests and subjective ratings of mood and memory. While encouraging trends emerged suggesting improvement among those who received treatment, group differences did not reach statistical significance. However, when outcomes were compared by treatment subgroups with and without anosognosia, significant differences emerged. Participants with insight made significantly greater gains in perceived memory functioning that those without insight. In contrast, informants perceived greater gains among treatment subjects relative to controls independent of insight status. The need for additional research to further delineate the influences of anosognia, baseline cognition, and affective status, and other potential intervention outcome modifiers is discussed, with attention to instrumentation and methodological considerations.

Correspondence should be sent to Deborah C. Koltai, Bryan ADRC, Duke University Medical Center, 2200 West Main Street, Suite A230, Durham, NC 27705, USA.

This work was supported by NIA Grant AG05128 to the Bryan ADRC. The authors wish to thank Dr Carl Pieper and Dr Laurence Branch of the Center for the Study of Aging and Human Development at Duke University Medical Center for consultation provided during the investigation.

INTRODUCTION

The devastating consequences of Alzheimer's disease (AD) and other dementias can be observed in many ways. While progressive cognitive deterioration is the cardinal sign of neurodegenerative illnesses, depression and other affective reactions are also frequently observed. Functional disability and behavioural problems inevitably follow. These domains are not mutually exclusive: One disability frequently gives rise to others, requiring attention to additive and interactive factors (Diehl, Willis, & Schaie, 1995; Koltai & Branch, 1998; Lawton, 1986). While substantial progress has been made in recent decades with the clarification of neuropathological processes, identification of susceptibility genes, and pharmacological treatments, millions of persons and families continue the struggle of contending with dementia. Until prevention and cure are obtained, efforts to optimise cognitive abilities and adjustment should continue.

Despite the relative absence of systematic research in this area, many clinicians provide memory training programmes or individual cognitive training to patients with dementia. Clinical interventions are typically used in preclinical or early stages when such methods can best be learned and incorporated into behaviour, potentially resulting in improved skills and a slowed rate of decline. Bäckman (1990) points out that the "negative view of memory training in AD may have been premature", and notes that successful studies differ in theoretical rationales, samples, and dependent measures.

Demonstration of a successful nonpharmacological treatment of the behavioural symptoms associated with dementia would represent a major advance. Such work could potentially influence patient functioning, caregiver burden, clinical practice, and health care policy. This preliminary investigation of an integrated intervention programme targeting cognitive abilities and emotional adjustment among early dementia patients represents one such effort to capture the gains frequently observed by clinicians, but rarely tested empirically. The intervention is driven by the need to maximise both functioning, use of residual capacities, and quality of life for patients with dementia. The study of the intervention is driven by the need to make the gains and limits of such services publicly verifiable.

There is some evidence that intervention has merit. Specific techniques targeting distinct goals have proven effective. For example, Camp, Foss, O'Hanlon, and Stevens (1996) used a spaced retrieval technique to train patients with AD to remember to use a calendar, and McKitrick, Camp, and Black (1992) applied this technique to teach AD patients to perform a prospective memory task. Errorless learning and associative techniques have been used with dementia patients to improve learning or retention duration of face–name pairs (Clare, Wilson, Breen, & Hodges, 1999; Hill, Evankovich, Sheikh, & Yesavage, 1987). Camp and colleagues (1996) contend that "it is possible to design effective, pragmatically useful memory interventions" for this population.

Others have used intervention programmes with promising results. A programme involving cognitive stimulation resulted in stable cognitive and behavioural functioning over time among those receiving treatment relative to comparison group deterioration (Quayhagen & Quayhagen, 1989). These investigators later trained both caregivers and AD patients in a home-based cognitive stimulation programme and found improved cognition relative to control and placebo passive activity groups, and the experimental and placebo activity groups had fewer behavioural problems than the control group (Quayhagen et al., 1995).

While some intervention techniques and programmes target cognition, other efforts emphasise affective functioning. The rationale of doing so is clear, given the potential impact of depression on cognition (Alexopoulos et al., 1993; Emery & Oxman, 1992; Lichtenberg, Ross, Millis, & Manning, 1995; Nussbaum, 1994) and the high prevalence of depression among dementia patients. A recent study found that among AD patients, 28% had dysthymia, and another 23% met criteria for major depression (Migliorelli et al., 1995). Even in the absence of marked depression, patient reports of further reduced cognitive efficiency during periods of emotional distress highlight a potential target for improving function. Wagner, Teri, and Orr-Rainey (1995) found that among behaviour problems of special care unit demented patients, those related to emotional distress were second only to problems related to memory impairment. These studies emphasise the need to identify and treat emotional factors that lead to excess disability, or greater than warranted functional incapacity (Brody, Kleba, Lawton, & Silverman, 1971). Successful treatment of depression, even in the context of a progressive neurodegenerative illness, may optimise the use of residual capacities and delay the need for institutionalisation.

Although few in number, efforts of this kind that focus on symptom mitigation and adjustment among depressed dementia patients have been documented. Encouraging preliminary results of a behavioural treatment suggest reduced depression in both patients and caregivers who are initially depressed (Teri, Logsdon, Wagner, & Uomoto, 1994; Teri & McCurry, 1994). Clinical examples illustrate that benefit can be realised from psychotherapy (e.g., Hausman, 1991; Miller, 1989). Others emphasise the benefits of group therapy to address coping and acceptance of emotional reactions, with areas of therapeutic potential outlined (Davies, Robinson, & Bevill, 1995; LaBarge & Trtanj, 1995; Yale, 1989). Guidelines for psychotherapy, behaviour management, and cognitive or environmental strategies have been put forth, as well as the necessary modifications to techniques (e.g., Greene, Ingram, & Johnson, 1993; Hausman, 1991; Jutagir, 1993; Solomon & Swabo, 1992; Teri & Gallagher-Thompson, 1991; Teri et al., 1994; Verwoerdt, 1981; Weiner, 1991; Whitehead, 1991). However, the need for additional controlled study of the treatment of affective and behavioural disorders in this population has also been emphasised (e.g., Labarge, Rosenman, Leavitt, & Cristiani, 1988; Teri et al., 1992; Whitehead, 1991).

The need for interventions targeting memory and coping skills is well established, given the known relationships between cognition and affect, and their impact on functional and health status and health care utilisation (e.g., Branch & Jette, 1982; Branch et al., 1988; Diehl et al., 1995; Fitz & Teri, 1994; Galanos, Fillenbaum, Cohen, & Burchett, 1994; Greiner, Snowdon, & Schmitt, 1996; Reuben, Rubenstein, Hirsch, & Hays, 1992; Rockwood, Stolee, & McDowell, 1996). What is lacking are systematic studies empirically demonstrating short-term and long-term intervention efficacy on cognition, affect, and functional outcomes, and an understanding of the effects of potential modifying variables for individual patients. Preliminary evidence of the effects of general mental status on treatment offers some guidelines for intervention selection (Hill, Yesavage, Sheikh, Friedman, 1989; Yesavage, Sheikh, Friedman, & Tanke, 1990). A classification system of memory interventions based on methodologies, types of mental processing involved, and memory systems engaged also has been described (Camp et al., 1993). Factors potentially modifying outcome have been outlined (Koltai & Branch, 1999). However, these represent only preliminary efforts to understand what modifies intervention outcome. Given this, decisive statements regarding intervention efficacy appear to be premature. The present study thus evolved to evaluate empirically the effects of intervention.

This study was a preliminary investigation of the effects of a Memory and Coping Program (MCP) among patients with mild to moderate dementia who were experiencing difficulty adjusting to their cognitive losses. MCP is an integrated intervention programme targeting cognitive abilities and emotional adjustment among early dementia patients. Secondary aims of examining the influence of potential modifying variables emerged as their effects became evident during the course of intervention.

METHOD

Subjects

Eligible participants were referred to the intervention programme from within the Bryan ADRC Neurological Disorders Clinic. After screening and acquisition of informed consent, 24 elderly subjects aged 60–84 with mild to moderate dementia were enrolled. Only one eligible potential participant declined to participate, stating that he would be uncomfortable in a group setting. Inclusion criteria for this study were: (1) age 60 or older; (2) mild to moderate dementia as determined by ratings of 0.5–1.0 on the Clinical

TABLE 1
Selected sample characteristics

	Treatment (n = 14) Mean (SD)	Control (n = 8) Mean (SD)
Age	72.9 (6.7)	73.9 (7.2)
Education	15.0 (4.0)	15.0 (3.0)
Baseline MMSE	22.9 (3.6)	26.6 (2.5)*
Baseline GDS	7.0 (5.2)	6.5 (2.9)
Baseline informant rated GDS	14.7 (6.3)	8.3 (5.1)*
Test–retest interval (days)	47.3 (12.0)	41.0 (3.3)

*$p < .05$

Dementia Rating (CDR) Scale (Hughes et al., 1982) and evidence of cognitive compromise on neurological mental status examination; and (3) adequate language skills to participate in treatment as indicated by ability to give informed consent/assent.

Table 1 illustrates selected sample characteristics. Mann-Whitney U comparisons showed that treatment and control groups did not differ in age, education, or baseline depression as measured by the Geriatric Depression Scale (GDS; Yesavage et al., 1983). However, despite random assignment, the control group had a significantly higher mean Mini-Mental Status Exam (MMSE; Folstein, Folstein, & McHugh, 1975) score than the treatment group, and less mean depressive symptomatology as rated by informants on a parallel form of the GDS. These differences warrant attention when reviewing the results.

Design

A randomised pre-test, post-test design was used. Subjects were randomly assigned to one of three groups: individual MCP (n = 8), group MCP (n = 8), or waiting-list control (n = 8). The test battery was administered within two weeks of beginning treatment and within two weeks post-treatment. Waiting-list control subjects were evaluated with the same time interval; there were no significant differences in test–retest interval between the three conditions.

Subjects randomised to the group MCP condition were divided (by order of enrolment) into two groups of four, each of which participated in five one-hour weekly intervention sessions addressing cognitive and affective functioning. Subjects randomised to the individual MCP condition completed one-on-one sessions (mean sessions = 6). When available, caregivers joined the sessions during the last 10–15 minutes for a general review. Subjects randomised to the waiting-list control condition received small group MCP after all testing had been completed. The first author conducted all MCP sessions.

After 8% attrition, data were available for 14 treatment and 8 control subjects. Specifically, two subjects in the group MCP condition did not complete the post-test due to serious illness. In addition, one subject in the individual MCP condition was unable to have an informant complete pre-test questionnaires. Subjects in the individual and group MCP conditions were pooled for statistical comparisons because of the small sample size and similar outcomes.

Intervention

MCP is an integrated intervention programme that utilises multiple cognitive, compensatory, and coping strategies to address abilities and adjustment. Each technique used in MCP is published or used in clinical practice. Some of the interventions have been modified for the specific needs of this population. Details of each training component can be found in Appendix 1. MCP involves training and practice in the following techniques:

1. Spaced retrieval (Camp et al., 1996).
2. Face–name recall strategy (Bäckman et al., 1991; Hill et al., 1987; Wilson, 1987; Yesavage et al., 1990).
3. Verbal elaboration (Wilson, 1987).
4. Concentration/Overt repetition.
5. External aids (Sohlberg & Mateer, 1989).
6. Coping strategies.

Measures

Outcome measures were selected to address general adjustment, depressive symptomatology, perceived cognitive status, and cognitive performance. Measures relevant to these analyses included:

Geriatric Depression Scale (GDS; Yesavage et al., 1983). This is a commonly used questionnaire made up of simple, straightforward questions that were selected specifically to screen for depressive symptomatology in elderly populations (Brink et al., 1982). Construct validity, sensitivity, and specificity have been demonstrated (e.g., Koenig, Meador, Cohen, & Blazer, 1988; Yesavage et al., 1983).

Relative GDS. This is a parallel form of the GDS. Relatives of the subjects completed this questionnaire to provide a measure of their perception of the subjects' affective status.

Everyday Memory Questionnaire (EMQ; Sunderland, Harris, & Baddeley, 1983).   The EMQ is a self-rated measure of memory functioning that was developed to reflect both the occurrence and frequency of memory failures in everyday life (Sunderland et al., 1983).

Relative EMQ.   This parallel form of the EMQ was included to establish the occurrence and frequency of the subjects' memory failures from the informants' perspective.

Consortium to Establish a Registry for Alzheimer's Disease test battery (CERAD: Morris et al., 1989).   This cognitive screening battery includes the MMSE, a list-learning and memory task, abbreviated Boston Naming Test, categorical fluency, and Rosen figures of constructional praxis.

Anosognosia ratings.   The therapist rated each treatment subject on a dichotomised variable of insight versus no insight, while blind to their total dataset. Formal measures of insight were not employed, as examination of this variable was not initially anticipated. However, when the potential impact of anosognosia became apparent, therapist ratings, which are an accepted rating practice (see discussion section), were employed. Subjects were rated as having insight if they demonstrated a basic understanding of the presence of cognitive deficits that extended beyond normal age-related memory difficulties and their impact on functioning.

RESULTS

Treatment efficacy was examined using change scores between baseline and post-test, to adjust for baseline individual differences. Because the data can be considered ordinal, the Mann-Whitney *U* statistic was used for data analyses. The use of nonparametric analyses represents a conservative approach that may have resulted in an underestimate of the effects of intervention. However, in order to avoid violating assumptions regarding normal distribution, it was the most appropriate approach to employ for comparisons between the treatment and control groups.

As expected, group differences were not found on selected comparisons involving objective cognitive measures. Change scores on the MMSE were compared by group, as well as total words learned across three trials and recall after a brief intervening task on the CERAD list-learning task. These measures do not allow for the application of MCP techniques (e.g., face–name recall), and lack of change on traditional cognitive tests is a common finding in such studies despite improvement on performance-based tasks designed to measure treatment outcome. In contrast, change was expected on rating scales measuring perceived functioning. Encouraging trends were revealed on both subject and informant ratings of memory functioning, with greater gains among the treatment group as compared to controls. These trends occurred despite the observed baseline group differences (lower MMSE and higher RGDS scores among the treatment group). However, despite the trends, the differences in change scores were not statistically significant. Table 2 illustrates these findings.

During the course of the intervention, variables that were potentially influencing treatment outcome became apparent. One of the variables was anosognosia, or the lack awareness of deficits. While systematic examination of such variables was outside the scope of the study given the sample size and lack of planned measures to assess them, the therapist rated subjects on insight status, without knowledge of their dataset. Eight treatment group subjects were rated as having insight, whereas the remaining six were rated as not having insight.

Particularly relevant findings emerged regarding perceived changes in memory functioning as reported on the Everyday Memory Questionnaire (EMQ; Sunderland et al., 1983), and the parallel form completed by relatives (REMQ). These perceived changes are illustrated in Figure 1.

Figure 1A illustrates EMQ change scores for each subject, by treatment and control groups. Note that the frequencies reveal a trend towards more improvement among the treatment group. Treatment subjects showed an advantage over control subjects on the decline in EMQ scores (indicating

TABLE 2
Comparisons between treatment and control groups on selected outcomes

	Treatment (n = 14) Mean (SD)	Control (n = 8) Mean (SD)
Change in objective measures†		
MMSE	−0.21 (? 9)	0.75 (2.4)
WLM—Total	0.64 (1.7)	1.63 (2.8)
WLM—Recall	0.64 (1.3)	−0.25 (1.8)
Change in subjective ratings††		
GDS	−1.21 (2.5)	0.13 (3.0)
RGDS	−1.62 (4.4)	−1.38 (4.1)
EMQ	−6.43 (14.3)	−1.00 (14.1)
REMQ	−3.54 (14.7)	5.75 (10.4)

WLM—Total: Total words recalled over three learning trials; WLM—Recall: Delayed recall after a brief intervening task; † An increase in scores indicates improvement for all objective measures; †† A reduction in scores indicates improvement for all subjective measures.

A

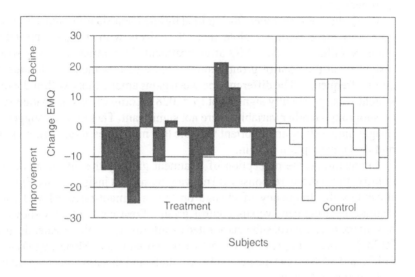

B

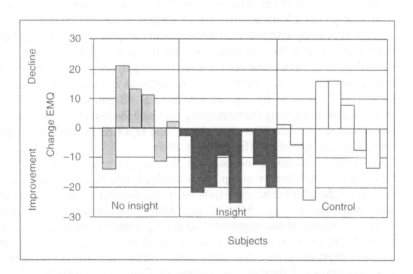

Figure 1. 1A = individual subject EMQ scores by group. 1B = individual subject EMQ change scores by insight subgroup.

463

improvement), between assessments, Mean Δ(SD) = –6.4 (14.3) and –1 (14.1), respectively, $p < .375$. However, note the variability in response within the treatment group.

EMQ change scores were then tallied by anosognosia groupings: Figure 1B illustrates these findings. Note that all subjects with insight reported less memory failures on the EMQ after treatment. In contrast, subjects without insight or in the control group reported more or less memory failures with similar frequency. The difference between gains among those with and without insight was statistically significant ($p = .028$). Comparisons of change scores by subgroup on other variables were not significant. These results suggest that insight may well be an important variable that moderates actual treatment gain and/or the perception of gain.

Interestingly, the perception of treatment gain by the informants did not confirm this pattern; responses did not vary by subject insight status. Figure 2A illustrates the frequency of change on the informant-rated REMQ for the sample, by treatment versus control group. Treatment subjects showed an advantage over control subjects as rated by informants, with a greater decline in REMQ scores (improvement) between assessments, Mean Δ(SD) = –3.5 (14.7) and +5.8 (10.4), respectively, $p < .065$, and this advantage approached statistical significance.

As was done with the EMQ change scores, REMQ change scores were then tallied by anosognosia subgroups: Figure 2B illustrates these findings. While perceived improvement occurred more frequently than decline among treatment group informants relative to control group informants, the mean change reported by informants of the treatment group with insight did not differ from that reported by informants of the treatment group without insight ($p = .886$). In contrast to the results noted by insight subgroup among subjects, informants' perceptions did not seem to differ as a function of whether the subject was rated as having, or not having, insight. Instead, informants perceived benefit among the treatment group independent of insight status, and this advantage in gain relative to the change reported for the control group approached statistical significance ($p = .065$).

Exploratory comparisons between the insight and no insight groups revealed that the former group acknowledged significantly more memory failures on the EMQ at baseline ($p = .045$), and showed a trend towards being less impaired on the MMSE ($p = .067$). Exploratory nonparametric Spearman's correlations suggested that among treatment subjects, the change in GDS was inversely related to baseline GDS ($r = –.527, p = .05$), so more baseline depression was associated with a greater reduction of depressive symptomatology. Likewise, the change in EMQ was inversely related to baseline EMQ ($r = –.648, p = .01$), so more perceived memory failures at baseline was related to more reduction of complaints. Finally, baseline GDS and EMQ were significantly related ($r = .591, p = .03$).

A

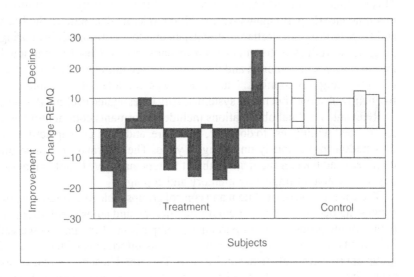

B

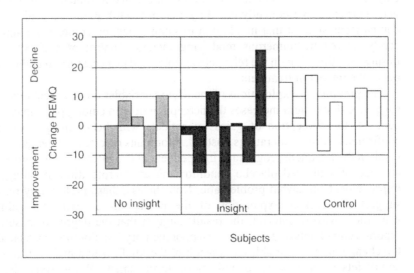

Figure 2. 2A = individual REMQ change scores by group. 2B = individual REMQ change scores by insight subgroup.

CONCLUSIONS

This preliminary investigation demonstrated the feasibility of recruiting and retaining elderly participants with mild to moderate dementia in the Memory and Coping Program. Reliable attendance and low attrition (2/24) during the programme reflected the enthusiasm of participants. Clearly, individuals in the early stages of dementia and their relatives are motivated to learn methods of optimising functioning. This study was an attempt to capture gains frequently observed but rarely systematically investigated in clinical practice.

Relevant anecdotal observations included informants commenting on their loved ones' willingness to do more, talk more, and even give up activities that they had been previously unwilling to yield. The information gained during treatment and the communication that it fosters may have benefits that extend beyond the goal of impacting memory and coping.

The comparison of treatment and control groups yielded encouraging trends suggesting better perceived memory functioning and adjustment after participation in the programme. In particular, comparison of the gain perceived by informants of treatment group subjects versus informants of the comparison group approached statistical significance. This trend in such a small sample is promising, and consistent with therapist observations and subject and informant reports of improvement. The lack of statistical significance is unlikely to be accounted for by lack of efficacy, or the inherent problems in empirical investigations of therapies addressing concerns rooted in the individuals' existence so eloquently noted by Yalom (1980). Rather, the additional comparisons suggest that in addition to sample size, outcomes were significantly altered by numerous modifying factors. Control of such variance through stratification on the relevant variables will be necessary to understand better the impact of treatment.

The preliminary explorations of modifying variables on treatment outcome suggested that insight increases the perception of gain among participants. In contrast, the perception of gains by patients with better insight was not confirmed by informant ratings. Instead, informants reported greater gains as a result of the treatment programme independent of insight status. Of course, the absence of a blinded placebo condition makes interpretation of ratings of improvement somewhat problematic. Nonetheless, these preliminary results suggest that further exploration of the perception of treatment gain is warranted. Also of interest, the results suggest that the degree of baseline-reported complaints of depression and poor memory functioning was related to the change in these variables as a result of the MCP, with a higher degree of complaints being associated with more improvement. While some degree of association between these variables could be anticipated given that the change scores considered baseline status, the results suggest variance in gain as a function of baseline status, and further exploration of this relationship would be useful in future studies. As expected, baseline memory complaints and depression were also related. Finally, although based on a very small sample, the results were consistent with the literature on anosognosia, with the subgroup rated as having insight reporting more memory problems and showing a trend towards having less impaired mental status. This latter finding is consistent with studies demonstrating the association between anosognosia and disease severity (McDaniel, Edland, Heyman, & CERAD Clinical Investigators, 1995; Starkstein et al., 1997). Further study is necessary to clarify whether insight accounts for variance in treatment outcome independent of disease severity.

Clinical reports have associated frontal dysfunction with lack of insight into diminished abilities or appropriate behaviour (e.g., McGlynn & Schacter, 1989; Neary, 1990). Indeed, executive functions, which are those cognitive abilities typically associated with frontal lobe integrity, are thought to be responsible for complex behaviour planning, initiation, monitoring, and execution (Lezak, 1995). It is reasonable to hypothesise that the benefit of intervention among anosognostic patients may be hindered due to decreased motivation resulting from a lack of appreciation for the need for effortful processing. There may also be a decreased ability to acquire intervention techniques due to the executive dysfunction frequently associated with this condition. Further study would be beneficial to refine intervention approaches by such subgroups.

Limitations of the current study include the fact that some findings may be an artifact of the small sample size; further study in larger, well-defined groups is warranted. In addition, due to the lower reliability of change scores and regression to the mean, some of these findings could be attributed to error. The variance within Alzheimer's disease and other dementias is considerable and stratification on relevant variables would be useful. The use of a blinded placebo condition would reduce the potential for bias related to the Hawthorne effect on ratings. The use of therapist ratings alone to define insight is also less than optimal. In addition to the need for further investigation with a large sample size and a blinded placebo condition, these results suggest a number of factors warranting attention in future study.

First among these, the measurement of anosognosia deserves further exploration. McGlynn and Schacter (1989) also highlight the need for more attention to how anosognosia is defined operationally. Some investigators operationally define anosognosia in AD by comparing the patient's ratings to those obtained from their caregiver (Kotler-Cope & Camp, 1995; McGlynn & Kaszniak, 1991; Migliorelli et al., 1995; Seltzer, Vasterling, Hale, & Khurana, 1995; Starkstein et al., 1995, 1997), or by comparing subject ratings to objective performance-based scores (Anderson & Tranel, 1989). Others have compared patient and relative performance estimations to actual performance (McGlynn & Kaszniak, 1991). Still others use physician or psychologist ratings of insight

(McDaniel et al., 1995; Sevush & Leve, 1993; Reed, Jagust, & Coulter, 1993; Verhey, Ponds, Rozendaal, & Jolles, 1995). Methods using informant ratings as the comparison standard have significant problems, namely the validity of caregiver ratings (Prigatano, 1996). Numerous studies have shown the limited shared variance between subjective ratings and objective test performance, even when used with normal elders or informants (Herzog & Rodgers, 1989; Koss et al., 1993; Jonker, Launer, Hooijer, & Lindeboom, 1996; LaRue et al., 1996; Scogin & Rohling, 1989). Indeed, examination of the data presented by McGlynn and Kaszniak (1991) indicates that while informants are more accurate than subjects at estimating performance, they also make considerable over- and under-estimation errors. Because subjective ratings share little variance with objective performance, it seems imprudent to operationally define another variable by them. At present, a combination of methods to operationally define anosognosia may be the most prudent approach given the limits of each individual method, and within-subject longitudinal monitoring of insight seems important given the possible impact of intervention directly on this variable.

Second, more attention to outcome measures is indicated. Clarification of actual versus perceived gain, and how this varies as a function of insight, would advance our understanding of how best to measure treatment efficacy and may provide information about differential benefits of intervention for different target populations. For some, gain may be related to a reduction in affective distress. Others may improve in cognitive efficiency or functional capacities. Because excess health care utilisation and its associated costs has been demonstrated in the context of affective disorders, cognitive impairment, or functional disability, intervention that impacts any of these spheres may prove worth while. However, growth in our understanding of likely outcomes for various target treatment groups would require further attention to instrumentation. In this study, improvement was not expected or found on objective cognitive measures. Clearly, expansion of outcome measures to include training-related instruments that would allow for application of the interventions is needed. A meta-analytic study of the effects of mnemonic training showed that larger gains are found on tasks that specifically allow for use of the newly acquired skills (Verhaeghen, Marcoen, & Goossens, 1992). The majority of published, standardised face–name recall tasks preclude effective use of the strategies taught in the intervention due to very short stimulus presentation times. The majority of published verbal list learning tasks require rapid, sequential presentation of words, which also precludes effective use of the strategies taught during the intervention. Modification of existing tasks to allow for application of the techniques could be accomplished by piloting tasks using simultaneous presentation of words and longer presentation times of face–name pairs or words, all of which would assist the process of association. Including such tasks would also clarify the discrepancies between subject and informant perceptions of gain.

Again, study with training-related performance tasks is needed to determine whether anosognosia modifies actual gain, or whether differential response is limited to perception of gain among treatment subjects, and to delineate the influences of anosognosia versus disease severity. Also, measures of participant practice and caregiver assistance may also be influenced by insight and other factors, and could clarify the effects of motivation on outcome.

Further clarification of the impact of treatment on perceived versus actual gain using such instruments could have profound effects on selection of potential candidates for treatment. If anosognosia truly hinders treatment gain as suggested by the perception of participants in this study, such services may be inappropriate for this subgroup. However, the greater gain perceived by treatment subject informants relative to control group informants suggests that perhaps participants do actually benefit from treatment, although those with anosognosia may not be able to appreciate such gain, just as they do not appreciate the magnitude of deficits prior to treatment. If this is indeed the case, ethical practice would require a clear delineation of expected gains, and perception of gains, within this context.

Third, retention of subjective rating scales of mood and cognition is essential to detect perceived training gains. Despite the limited ability of subjective measures to predict object performance, these ratings are not without merit as perceived gain may be just as important as objective gain for some. Indeed, if such a gain results in a reduction of excess disability, health care utilisation and costs may also be reduced, and overall quality of life may improve.

Finally, investigation of other potential modifying variables, such as diagnosis or the frequency or length of intervention sessions, would be useful. It is reasonable to hypothesise that diagnosis may influence outcome in addition to disease severity, motivation, and insight, as different illnesses have various neuroanatomical substrates that could differentially affect an individual's potential to benefit from various types of intervention. Likewise, the utility of intervention is in part contingent on the ability of each subject to learn the techniques. Therefore, performance during training should be monitored to account for variance attributable to the degree of strategy acquisition. In addition, the timing and duration of instruction, particularly the effect of booster or maintenance sessions, may affect short-term and long-term outcomes.

This preliminary investigation demonstrates that significant positive treatment gain as a result of a nonpharmacological memory and coping intervention programme is possible among early stage dementia patients. Further study with a larger sample size allowing for the use of multivariate statistical analyses is clearly indicated. Ideally, such an investigation would better define anosognosia operationally, include a blinded placebo condition, and use self-report measures, training-related tasks, and objective cognitive measures. Doing so would clarify whether gain is true or perceived, and would provide the necessary means to disentangle the effect of modifying variables, such as anosognosia, and baseline cognitive and affective status. Clarification of how *actual* and *perceived* gain varies as a function of such variables would advance our understanding of how best to measure treatment efficacy and may provide information about the differential benefits of intervention for various target populations.

REFERENCES

Alexopoulos, G., Meyers, B., Young, R., Mattis, S., & Kakuma, T. (1993). The course of geriatric depression with reversible dementia: A controlled study. *American Journal of Psychiatry, 150,* 1693–1699.

Anderson, S., & Tranel, D. (1989). Awareness of disease states following cerebral infarction, dementia, and head trauma: Standardized assessment. *Clinical Neuropsychologist, 3,* 327–339.

Bäckman, L., (1990). Plasticity of memory functioning in normal aging and Alzheimer's disease. *Acta Neurologica Scandinavica, 82,* 32–36.

Bäckman, L. (1992). Memory training and memory improvement in Alzheimer's disease: Rules and exceptions. *Acta Neurologica Scandinavica, 85,* 84–89.

Bäckman, L. (1996). Utilizing compensatory task conditions for episodic memory in Alzheimer's disease. *Acta Neurologica Scandinavica, 165,* 109–113.

Bäckman, L., Josephsson, S., Herlitz, A., Stigsdotter, A., & Viitanen, M. (1991). The generalizability of training gains in dementia: Effects of an imagery-based mnemonic on face–name retention duration. *Psychology and Aging, 6,* 498–492.

Bird, M., & Luszcz, M. (1991). Encoding specificity, depth of processing, and cued recall in Alzheimer's disease. *Journal of Clinical and Experimental Neuropsychology, 13,* 508–520.

Branch, L., & Jette, A. (1982). A prospective study of long-term care institutionalization among the aged. *American Journal of Public Health, 72,* 1373–1379.

Branch, L., Wetle, T., Scherr, P., Cook, N., Evans, D., Hebert, L., Masland, E., Keough, M., & Taylor, J. (1988). A prospective study of incident comprehensive medical home care use among the elderly. *American Journal of Public Health, 78,* 255–259.

Brink, T., Yesavage, J., Lum, O., Heersema, P., Adey, V., & Rose, T. (1982). Screening tests for geriatric depression. *Clinical Gerontologist, 1,* 37–44.

Brody, E., Kleban, M., Lawton, M.P., & Silverman, H., (1971). Excess disabilities of mentally impaired aged: Impact of individualized treatment. *Gerontologist, Summer Part I,* 124–133.

Camp, C., Foss, J., O'Hanlon, A., & Stevens, A. (1996). Memory interventions for persons with dementia. *Applied Cognitive Psychology, 10,* 193–210.

Camp, C., Foss, J., Stevens, A., Reichard, C., McKitrick, L., & O'Hanlon, A. (1993). Memory training in normal and demented elderly populations: The E-I-E-I-O model. *Experimental Aging Research, 19,* 277–290.

Clare, L., Wilson, B., Breen, K., & Hodges, J. (1999). Errorless learning of face–name association in early Alzheimer's disease. *Neurocase, 5,* 37–46.

Davies, H., Robinson, D., & Bevill, L. (1995). Supportive group experience for patients with early-stage Alzheimer's disease. *Journal of the American Geriatric Society, 43,* 1068–1069.

Diehl, M., Willis, S., & Schaie, K. (1995). Everyday problem solving in older adults: Observational assessment and cognitive correlates. *Psychology and Aging, 10,* 478–491.

Emery, V., & Oxman, T. (1992). Update on the dementia spectrum of depression. *American Journal of Psychiatry, 149,* 305–317.

Fitz, A., & Teri, L. (1994). Depression, cognition, and functional ability in patients with Alzheimer's disease. *Journal of the American Geriatrics Society, 42*, 186–191.

Folstein, M., Folstein, S., & McHugh, P. (1975). Mini-Mental State: A practical method for grading the cognitive state of patients for the clinician. *Journal of Psychiatric Research, 12*, 189–198.

Galanos, A., Fillenbaum, G., Cohen, H., & Burchett, B. (1994). The comprehensive assessment of community-dwelling elderly: Why functional status is not enough. *Aging: Clinical and Experimental Research, 6*, 343–352.

Greene, J., Ingram, T., & Johnson, W. (1993). Group psychotherapy for patients with dementia. *Southern Medical Journal, 86*, 1033–1035.

Greiner, P., Snowdon, D., & Schmitt, F. (1996). The loss of independence in activities of daily living: The role of low normal cognitive function in elderly nuns. *American Journal of Public Health, 86*, 62–66.

Hausman, C. (1991). Dynamic psychotherapy with elderly demented patients. In G. Jones & B. Miesen (Eds.), *Caregiving in dementia* (pp. 181–198). Amsterdam: Routledge.

Herlitz, A., Adolfsson, R., Bäckman, L., & Hilsson, L-G. (1991). Cue utilization following different forms of encoding in mildly, moderately, and severely demented patients with Alzheimer's disease. *Brain and Cognition, 15*, 119–130.

Herlitz, A., & Viitanen, M. (1991). Semantic organization and verbal episodic memory in patients with mild and moderate Alzheimer's disease. *Journal of Clinical and Experimental Neuropsychology, 13*, 559–574.

Herzog, A., & Rodgers, W. (1989). Age differences in memory performance and memory ratings as measured in a sample survey. *Psychology and Aging, 4*, 173–182.

Hill, R. Evankovich, K., Sheikh, J., & Yesavage, J. (1987). Imagery mnemonic training in a patient with primary degenerative dementia. *Psychology and Aging, 2*, 204–205.

Hill, R., Yesavage, J., Sheikh, J., & Friedman, L. (1989). Mental status as a predictor of response to memory training in older adults. *Educational Gerontology, 15*, 633–639.

Hughes, C., Berg, L., Danziger, W., Cohen, L., & Martin, R. (1982). A new clinical scales for the staging of dementia. *British Journal of Psychiatry, 140*, 566–572.

Jonker, C., Launer, L., Hooijer, C., & Lindeboom, J. (1996). Memory complaints and memory impairment in older individuals. *Journal of the American Geriatrics Society, 44*, 44–49.

Jutagir, R. (1993). Geropsychology and neuropsychological testing: Role in evaluation and treatment of patients with dementia. *Mount Sinai Journal of Medicine, 60*, 528–531.

Koenig, H., Meador, K., Cohen, H., & Blazer, D. (1988). Self-rated depression scales and screening for major depression in the older hospitalized patient with medical illness. *Journal of the American Geriatrics Society, 36*, 699–706.

Koltai, D., & Branch, L. (1998). Consideration of intervention alternatives to optimize independent functioning in the elderly. *Journal of Clinical Geropsychology, 4*, 333–349.

Koltai, D., & Branch, L.G. (1999). Cognitive and affective interventions to maximize abilities and adjustment in dementia. *Annals of Psychiatry: Basic and Clinical Neurosciences, 7*, 241–255.

Koss, E., Patterson, M., Ownby, R., Stuckey, J., & Whitehouse, P. (1993). Memory evaluation in Alzheimer's disease: Caregivers' appraisals and objective testing. *Archives of Neurology, 50*, 92–97.

Kotler-Cope, S., & Camp, C. (1995). Anosognosia in Alzheimer disease. *Alzheimer Disease and Associated Disorders, 9*, 52–56.

LaBarge, E., Rosenman, L., Leavitt, K., & Cristiani, T. (1988). Counseling clients with mild senile dementia of the Alzheimer's type: A pilot study. *Journal of Neurologic Rehabilitation, 2*, 167–173.

LaBarge, E., & Trtanj, F. (1995). A support group for people in the early stages of dementia of the Alzheimer type. *Journal of Applied Gerontology, 14*, 289–301.

LaRue, A., Small, G., McPherson, S., Komo, S., Matsuyama, S., & Jarvik, L. (1996). Subjective memory loss in age-associated memory impairment: Family history and neuropsychological correlates. *Aging, Neuropsychology, and Cognition, 3*, 132–140.

Lawton, M.P. (1986). Contextual perspectives: Psychosocial influences. In L. Poon, T. Crook, K. Davis, C. Eisdorfer, B. Gurland, A. Kaszniak, & L. Thompson (Eds.), *Handbook for clinical memory assessment of older adults* (pp. 32–42). Washington, DC: American Psychological Association.

Lezak, M. (1995). *Neuropsychological assessment.* New York: Oxford University Press.

Lichtenberg, P., Ross, T., Millis, S., & Manning C. (1995). The relationship between depression and cognition in older adults: A cross-validation study. *Journal of Gerontology, 50*, P25–P32.

McDaniel, K., Edland, S., Heyman, A., & CERAD Clinical Investigators (1995). Relationship between level of insight and severity of dementia in Alzheimer disease. *Alzheimer Disease and Associated Disorders, 9*, 101–104.

McGlynn, S., & Kaszniak, A. (1991). When metacognition fails: Impaired awareness of deficit in Alzheimer's disease. *Journal of Cognitive Neuroscience, 3*, 183–189.

McGlynn, S., & Schacter, D. (1989). Unawareness of deficits in neuropsychological syndromes. *Journal of Clinical and Experimental Neuropsychology, 11*, 143–205.

McKitrick, L., Camp, C., & Black, F.W. (1992). Prospective memory intervention in Alzheimer's disease. *Journal of Gerontology, 47*, P337–P343.

Miller, M. (1989). Opportunities for psychotherapy in the management of dementia. *Journal of Geriatric Psychiatry & Neurology, 2*, 11–17.

Migliorelli, R., Teson, A., Sabe, L., Petracca, G., Petracchi, M., Leiguarda, R., & Starkstein, S. (1995). Anosognosia in Alzheimer's disease: A study of associated factors. *Journal of Neuropsychiatry, 7*, 338–344.

Migliorelli, R., Teson, A., Sabe, L., Petracchi, M., Leiguarda, R., & Starkstein, S. (1995). Prevalence and correlates of dysthymia and major depression among patients with Alzheimer's disease. *American Journal of Psychiatry, 152*, 37–44.

Morris, J., Heyman, A., Mohs, R., Hughes, P., Van Belle, G., Fillenbaum, G., Mellits, E., & Clark, C. (1989). The Consortium to Establish a Registry of Alzheimer's Disease (CERAD), I: Clinical and neuropshycological assessment of Alzheimer's disease. *Neurology, 39*, 1159–1165.

Neary, D. (1990). Dementia of frontal lobe type. *Journal of the American Geriatrics Society, 38*, 71–72.

Nussbaum, P. (1994). Pseudodementia: A slow death. *Neuropsychology Review, 4*, 71–90.

Prigatano, G. (1996). Behavioural limitations TBI patients tend to underestimate: A replication and extension to patients with lateralized cerebral dysfunction. *Clinical Neuropsychologist, 10*, 191–201.

Quayhagen, M., & Quayhagen, M. (1989). Differential effects of family-based strategies on Alzheimer's disease. *Gerontologist, 29*, 150–155.

Quayhagen, M., Quayhagen, M., Corbeil, R., Roth, P., & Rodgers, J. (1995). A dyadic remediation program for care recipients with dementia. *Nursing Research, 44*, 153–159.

Reed, B., Jagust, W., & Coulter, L. (1993). Anosognosia in Alzheimer's disease: Relationships to depression, cognitive function, and cerebral perfusion. *Journal of Clinical and Experimental Neuropsychology, 15*, 231–244.

Reuben, D., Rubenstein, L., Hirsch, S., & Hays, R. (1992). Value of functional status as a predictor of mortality: Results of a prospective study. *American Journal of Medicine, 93*, 633–669.

Rockwood, K., Stolee, P., & McDowell, I. (1996). Factors associated with institutionalization of older people in Canada: Testaing a multi-factorial definition of frailty. *Journal of the American Geriatrics Society, 44*, 578–582.

Scogin, F., & Rohling, M. (1989). Cognitive processes, self-reports of memory functioning, and mental health status in older adults. *Journal of Aging and Health, 1*, 507–520.

Seltzer, B., Vasterling, J., Hale, M., & Khurana, R. (1995). Unawareness of memory deficit in Alzheimer's disease: Relation to mood and other disease variables. *Neuropsychiatry, Neuropsychology, and Behavioural Neurology, 8*, 176–181.

Sevush, S., & Leve, N. (1993). Denial of memory deficit in Alzheimer's disease. *American Journal of Psychiatry, 150*, 748–751.

Sohlberg, M., & Mateer, C. (1989). *Introduction to cognitive rehabilitation: Theory and practice.* New York: Guilford Press.

Solomon, K., & Szwabo, P. (1992). Psychotherapy for patients with dementia. In J. Morley, R. Coe, R. Strong, & G. Grossberg (Eds.), *Memory function and aging-related disorders* (pp. 295–319). New York: Springer.

Starkstein, S., Chemerinski, E., Sabe, L., Kuzis, G., Petracca, G., Teson, A., & Leiguarda, R. (1997). Prospective longitudinal study of depression and anosognosia in Alzheimer's disease. *British Journal of Psychiatry, 171*, 47–52.

Starkstein, S., Vazquez, S., Migliorelli, R., Teson, A, Sabe, L., & Leiguarda, R. (1995). A single-photon emission computed tomographic study of anosognosia in Alzheimer's disease. *Archives of Neurology, 52*, 415–420.

Sunderland, A., Harris, J., & Baddeley, A. (1983). Do laboratory tests predict everyday memory? A neuropsychological study. *Journal of Verbal Learning and Verbal Behavior, 22*, 341–357.

Teri, L., & Gallagher-Thompson, D. (1991). Cognitive-behavioural interventions for treatment of depression in Alzheimer's patients. *Gerontologist, 31*, 413–416.

Teri, L., Logsdon, R., Wagner, A., & Uomoto, J. (1994). The caregiver role in behavioral treatment of depression in dementia patients. In E. Light, G. Niederehe, & B. Lebowitz (Eds.), *Stress effects on family caregivers of Alzheimer's patients: Research and interventions* (pp. 185–204). New York: Springer.

Teri, L., & McCurry, S. (1994). Psychosocial therapies. In C. Coffey, J. Cummings, M. Lovell, & G. Pearlson (Eds.), *The American Psychiatric Press textbook of geriatric neuropsychiatry* (pp. 662–682). Washington, DC: American Psychiatric Press.

Teri, L., Rabins, P., Whitehouse, P., Berg, L., Reisberg, B., Sunderland, T., Eichelman, B., & Phelps, C. (1992). Management of behavior disturbance in Alzheimer disease: Current knowledge and future directions. *Alzheimer Disease and Assocaited Disorders, 6*, 77–88.

Verhaeghen, P., Marcoen, A., & Goossens, L. (1992). Improving memory performance in the aged through mnemonic training: A meta-analytic study. *Psychology and Aging, 7*, 242–251.

Verhey, F., Ponds, R., Rozendaal, N., & Jolles, J. (1995). Depression, insight, and personality changes in Alzheimer's disease and vascular dementia. *Journal of Geriatric Psychiatry and Neurology, 8*, 23–27.

Verwoerdt, A. (1981). Individual psychotherapy in senile dementia. In N. Miller & G. Cohen (Eds.), *Clinical aspects of Alzheimer's disease and senile dementia* (pp. 187–208). New York: Raven Press.

Wagner, A., Teri, L., & Orr-Rainey, N. (1995). Behavior problems of residents with dementia in special care units. *Alzheimer Disease and Associated Disorders, 9*, 121–127.

Weiner, M. (1991). Psychological and behavioral management. In M. Weiner (Ed.), *The dementias: Diagnosis and management* (pp. 107–133). Washington, DC: American Psychiatric Press.

Whitehead, A. (1991). Twenty years a-growing: Some current issues in behavioural psychotherapy with elderly people. *Behavioural Psychotherapy, 19*, 92–99.

Wilson, B. (1987). *Rehabilitation of memory.* New York: Guilford Press.

Yale, R. (1989). Support groups for newly diagnosed Alzheimer's clients. *Clinical Gerontologist, 8*, 86–89.

Yalom, I. (1980). *Existential psychotherapy.* New York: Basic Books.

Yesavage, J., Brink, T., Rose, T., Lum, O., Huan, V., Adey, M., & Leirer, V. (1983). Development and validation of a geriatric depression screening scale: A preliminary report. *Journal of Psychiatric Research, 17*, 37–44.

Yesavage, J., Sheikh, J., Friedman, L., & Tanke, E. (1990). Learning mnemonics: Roles of aging and subtle cognitive impairment. *Psychology and Aging, 5*, 133–137.

Manuscript received August 1999
Revised manuscript received March 2000

APPENDIX 1
INTERVENTION: MEMORY AND COPING
PROGRAM (MCP)

MCP is an integrated intervention programme that targets memory functioning and adjustment. The techniques utilised in MCP are applied in clinical practice and have received attention in the literature. Strategies are introduced, modelled, and practised, and the material is reviewed at the end of the session with available caregivers. Practice assignments are given. Subjects are given notebooks to promote their taking notes, and a written summary of the content of sessions is given to each subject.

The use of multiple training procedures is justified in a number of ways. First, studies have found that AD patients show clear improvements in episodic memory when "support", such as encoding instructions and cues, has been provided at both acquisition and retrieval (Bäckman 1992, 1996; Bird & Luszcz, 1991), suggesting that the *quantity* of support affects outcome. Second, there is evidence for differential gains in response to the various *types* of support provided and mnemonic strategies taught by level of dementia severity (e.g., Herlitz, Adolfsson, Bäckman, & Nilsson, 1991; Herlitz & Viitanen, 1991; Hill et al., 1989; Yesavage et al., 1990). Finally, in clinical practice, inter-subject variability is often observed in strategy preference and abiltiy, supporting the utility of multiple approaches to maximise chances of benefit. MCP covers the following content:

Introduction.   Participants briefly discuss what they hope to gain from MCP. The remainder of the session is devoted to instruction about memory. Changes associated with normal aging and various neurological disorders are discussed. This allows for a general, non-threatening introduction to MCP during which information is provided in a supportive setting.

Face–name recall.   Name recall is one of the most frequent complaints among memory impaired persons. A face–name technique is taught that has been used successfully in numerous training studies with normal elders, dementia patients, and traumatic brain injury patients to improve the number of face–name pairs learned or the length of retention duration (e.g., Bäckman et al., 1991; Hill et al., 1987; Wilson, 1987; Yesavage et al., 1990). The strategy typically involves: (1) identifying a distinctive facial feature, (2) creating a visual association with the name (e.g., "Turtle" for the last name "Tuttle"), and (3) connecting the visual association with the prominent feature. Studies have found, however, that dementia patients have difficulty learning and executing the third step of this strategy (Bäckman et al., 1991; Hill et al., 1987). Therefore, the strategy was modified and included the following simpler steps: (1) repeat the name several times, (2) create a visual association with the name (e.g., "Turtle" for the last name "Tuttle"), and (3) include the person in the visual association image (e.g., Mr. Tuttle should be visualised interacting with the turtle).

External aids.   This session addresses environmental support. (1) Subjects are instructed in the use of calendars/appointment books to assist recalling what they will do and what they have done. Organisational benefits are highlighted. Subjects are taught to check these aids regularly by associating them with a regularly performed activity (e.g., reviewing it at meals) to facilitate the development of this activity as a routine. (2) Subjects are instructed to use notes or index cards as retrieval cues and to help organise information they wish to convey. (3) Environmental adaptations that decrease the frequency of memory failures are encouraged, such as placing a phone pad next to the telephone to serve as a cue to take messages.

Verbal elaboration.   This session focuses on using verbal elaboration and association to increase attention and the chances of storage. While many strategies are based on verbal elaboration, studies suggest that individuals with central nervous system compromise show more recall gains with the story technique than with others (Wilson, 1987). This technique involves associating the information to be learned by creating a story with the target information being the key elements.

Concentration/overt repetition.   This session focuses on increasing concentration through simple repetition. Subjects are encouraged to use overt or covert verbal repetition to reduce the likelihood of intrusions from internal or external distractions, and to facilitate concentration. For instance, subjects are encouraged to state out loud the goal of their activity while pursuing it to decrease the likelihood of becoming distracted.

Spaced retrieval.   The technique of spaced retrieval is taught to facilitate learning and recall. This strategy requires subjects to retrieve the information to be learned at successively longer intervals, while shortening the interval length when there is a retrieval failure. There is evidence that this technique involves relatively effortless learning and may rely upon implicit, rather than explicit, memory systems (Camp et al., 1996). While Camp and colleagues (1996) suggest that mild AD patients may be able to use the strategy alone, caregivers typically play a role by requesting information retrieval. Caregivers typically enjoy learning this strategy when they join subjects at the end of the session, as it can be used to reduce repetitious questions in addition to facilitating storage.

Coping strategies.   The need to address emotional distress stems not only from quality of life concerns, but also from reports of further reduced cognitive efficiency during periods of emotional distress. This session involves discussions of how mood and memory influence one another, and the importance of monitoring mood and seeking assistance if needed. Adaptive coping strategies (e.g., exercise, relaxation techniques, communication) are reviewed. Identification and participation in rewarding activities is supported. Communication is emphasised as a valuable tool for gaining insight, expressing concerns, and establishing appropriate levels of independence.

Long-term maintenance of treatment gains following a cognitive rehabilitation intervention in early dementia of Alzheimer type: A single case study

Linda Clare[1], Barbara A. Wilson[2], Gina Carter[3],
John R. Hodges[2], and Malcolm Adams[4]

[1]*Sub-department of Clinical Health Psychology,
University College London, UK,*
[2]*MRC Cognition and Brain Sciences Unit, Cambridge, UK,*
[3]*Training Course in Clinical Psychology, University of Southampton, UK,*
[4]*School of Health Policy and Practice, University of East Anglia, UK*

It has been suggested that "memory retraining" has no lasting effect beyond the end of the treatment session (Rabins, 1996). Although this is contradicted by cognitive rehabilitation studies showing that gains can be demonstrated and maintained, few researchers have presented long-term follow-up data. Recent studies (Clare, Wilson, Breen, & Hodges, 1999; Clare et al., 2000) have provided post-intervention follow-up data for one participant that was collected over a 9 month period, during which performance on trained face–name associations remained at ceiling levels. This paper reports a further, naturalistic follow-up of this participant over an additional period of two years, during which his recall of 10 trained face–name associations was evaluated and compared to performance on three untrained, previously-known items retained as part of the full set of stimulus materials throughout the whole study. Recall remained relatively stable over year 1 and showed a modest decline for both trained and previously-known items during year 2. Differences between year 1 and year 2 were significant only for untrained items. At the end of year 2, performance on trained items remained well above initial baseline levels. These results are discussed in the

---

Correspondence should be sent to Linda Clare, Sub-department of Clinical Health Psychology, University College London, Gower Street, London WC1E 6BT, UK. Telephone: 020 7679 1844, Fax: 020 7916 1989, Email: l.clare@ucl.ac.uk.

The authors would like to thank VJ and his sister for making this study possible and for their continued support and enthusiasm.

context of information derived from neuropsychological assessment, scans and self-report measures. It is argued, on the basis of the results presented here, that long-term maintenance of gains resulting from targeted cognitive rehabilitation interventions is possible, and that in view of this it will be important to evaluate the broader impact of cognitive rehabilitation interventions on quality of life and on the progression of dementia.

Cognitive rehabilitation interventions targeting memory functioning in dementia remain somewhat controversial. Some commentators have argued that such interventions are not beneficial. Rabins (1996) has suggested that "memory retraining" may result in adverse outcomes in terms of increased frustration for patients and depression for caregivers, and has commented that: "Although cognitive retraining appears to achieve modest, short-term improvement in cognitive function, this improvement does not persist beyond the training session" (p. 38). This view subsequently found its way into a US consensus statement on interventions for people with dementia of Alzheimer type (DAT) (Small et al., 1997), which supported the usefulness of drug treatments but perceived little benefit in psychological approaches. It has been noted, however, that the psychological needs of people with dementia are commonly ignored within the framework of a largely medical approach (British Psychological Society, 1994). A recent review of empirically validated treatments for older people identified memory therapy as a "probably efficacious" method of slowing decline in dementia (Gatz et al., 1998), suggesting that it may offer some benefits to people with dementia and their families.

Clearly, there is a need to resolve the controversy about cognitive rehabilitation in order to establish what kinds of interventions are likely to be helpful to people with dementia and their families, and to ensure that they are protected where possible from potential adverse effects of intervention. Key questions which remain to be answered about cognitive rehabilitation include the extent to which gains can be maintained over time, the impact of interventions on well-being and quality of life, and what contribution, if any, this approach can make to slowing the progression of DAT. This paper focuses primarily on the first of these questions.

The application of cognitive rehabilitation in early dementia is based on a strong theoretical rationale derived from evidence regarding the neuropsychology and neuroanatomy of memory impairments in DAT and the capacity of the person with DAT for new learning (Clare, 1999). It is also compatible with models which emphasise the psychosocial needs of the person with dementia (Kitwood, 1997), since it aims to contribute to the promotion of adjustment and coping (Cottrell & Schulz, 1993; Droes, 1997; Hagberg, 1997; Woods & Britton, 1985) and the reduction of excess disability (Reifler & Larson, 1990).

On theoretical grounds, it can be predicted that maintenance of gains over a substantial period of time should be possible, at least to some extent. This argument derives from consideration of both memory processes and memory structures. Investigation of memory in terms of the processes of encoding, storage and retrieval permits an evaluation of the stages of processing most affected in DAT. While short-term forgetting, within the first 30 s of exposure to a stimulus, is impaired (Kopelman, 1985), long-term forgetting appears to be relatively spared (Christensen et al., 1998; Kopelman, 1992). Thus, although there may be some subtle difficulties in maintaining information in long-term memory (Christensen et al., 1998), the memory problem in DAT does not appear to be primarily one of impaired storage. This explanation cannot, of course, account for the presence of retrograde memory deficits (Glisky, 1998), but in relation to new learning, the major deficit is thought to lie in encoding and acquisition of new memories (Christensen et al., 1998; Greene, Baddeley, & Hodges, 1996; Kapur, 1994; Kopelman, 1992) rather than in storage.

This view is underpinned by a developing understanding of the contributions of different brain areas to the processes of encoding, storing and retrieving memories. The anatomical areas most affected in the early stages of DAT are the medial temporal lobe structures, notably the transentorhinal region and the hippocampal complex; these are critical in the establishment and consolidation of new episodic memories, but are thought by most researchers not to be required for long-term storage (Glisky, 1998; Graham & Hodges, 1997; Squire & Knowlton, 1995; for a contrasting view see Nadel & Moscovitch, 1997). Establishment and consolidation of semantic memories is thought to be less dependent on the hippocampus than is the case for episodic memories (Glisky, 1998; Kitchener, Hodges, & McCarthy, 1998; Vargha-Khadem et al., 1997). While medial temporal lobe pathology is linked to the failure to rapidly encode new semantic information in an adequate manner, Glisky (1998) and Kitchener et al. (1998) suggest that other brain areas may be able slowly to integrate new semantic information with existing knowledge if given repeated structured training trials. Thus, it is hard for people with DAT to establish links to prior semantic knowledge at encoding. However, if strategies are provided that enhance this linking function, or if the stimuli themselves drive appropriate semantic processing, then adequate learning can be achieved (Thoene & Glisky, 1995), and storage and retrieval may then proceed adequately.

This argument suggests that interventions which place a strong emphasis on effective encoding, and which provide a demonstration of successful learning, should have the capacity to permit long-term maintenance, and that this is most likely to occur for semantic knowledge. From a clinical perspective, it is important to consider how interventions can be structured in such a way as to facilitate maintenance. Among the possible factors that may influence maintenance of treatment gains, continued input in the form of 'top up' sessions may be important (Woods, 1996b; Bäckman, 1992). It can also be hypothesised that maintenance is most likely where intervention targets are of direct relevance to the person's daily life, and where the participant is aware of his or her memory difficulties and motivated to put new learning into practice (Clare et al., 2000). Finally, the evaluation of performance needs to be balanced against an assessment of the progression of the disorder and concurrent decline in cognitive functioning (Little, Volans, Hemsley, & Levy, 1986).

A wide range of evidence is available suggesting that appropriately-designed interventions may have positive effects on memory functioning and providing little support for the view that these interventions produce significant levels of frustration or depression (for reviews, see Bäckman, 1992, 1996; Clare, 1999; Clare et al., 1999, 2000; Woods, 1996a, 1996b). The evidence base does, however, have some important limitations. In particular, presentation of follow-up data is limited. Some studies reporting positive results of intervention present no follow-up-data (e.g., McEvoy & Patterson, 1986). More typically, studies present follow-up data that indicate gains are maintained beyond the immediate treatment session, but report only relatively short follow-up periods (e.g., Abrahams & Camp, 1993; Camp, 1989; Hill, Evankovich, Sheikh, & Yesavage, 1987). Although these studies clearly show that gains can be maintained for reasonable time periods, the use of longer follow-up periods would provide more convincing evidence of genuine lasting benefit. A small number of studies have begun to present longer-term follow-up data. For example, Clare et al. (1999, 2000) report 6 month and 9 month follow-up data, while Bourgeois (1990, 1992) reports maintenance of gains from training in using a memory wallet 30 months after the end of intervention.

In order to be able to demonstrate that cognitive rehabilitation interventions have the potential to impact on quality of life, and perhaps on the course of DAT, it will be important to show that the theoretical arguments supporting the likelihood of long-term maintenance, outlined above, are borne out in practice and that gains can be maintained over considerable time periods. The present study is a naturalistic follow-up of one participant who completed a cognitive rehabilitation intervention which had direct relevance to his daily life, reported in detail in Clare et al. (1999). The participant performed at ceiling when followed up 1, 3, 6, and 9 months after the end of his intervention; during this time, his performance was not only put into practice in the real-life setting, but was supported by daily practice. It was hypothesised that his knowledge of the face–name associations was sufficiently well-consolidated to be maintained over a substantial period without specific additional practice, and that forgetting would occur only very slowly. The present study follows his performance over the next 2 years, during which time the learning was put to use in the real-life setting but no additional daily practice was carried out.

METHOD

Participant

VJ[1] was 74 years old at the start of the present follow-up study. He was a single man, living with his sister, who formerly worked in the construction industry. He first attended the memory clinic in 1993 and was given a diagnosis of early-stage DAT. VJ, supported by his sister, joined the memory therapy study in 1996.

Background: The initial intervention

VJ's original intervention consisted of training in the names of 11 members of his social club. Photographs of club members were used to teach the face–name associations, which was done using an errorless method incorporating visual imagery, vanishing cues, and expanding rehearsal. An additional three known (and therefore untrained) items were retained in the set to provide encouragement, since performance on these items was at ceiling during baseline assessment. Generalisation sessions were conducted at the club. Mean recall scores for the 11 trained items increased from 20% at initial baseline to 98% following intervention and 100% at 1, 3, 6, and 9 month follow-up. Following training, VJ practised the items daily using the photographs as well as during his weekly visit to his club.

Procedure

After the 9 month follow-up visit, the following arrangement was agreed with VJ. He would stop his daily practice with the photographs and return these to the researcher, so that practice of the face–name associations was confined to club meetings. He would be assessed regularly on the set of face–name associations by means of a free recall test trial of all items, both trained and untrained, but given no feedback on his answers.

The test trials were given during weekly visits to VJ's home during year 1 (1997–1998) and monthly visits during year 2 (1998–1999). One recall trial was given during each visit. The photographs were presented one at a time in random order, and VJ was asked to say the first name of the person shown in the photograph. Responses were recorded verbatim and no feedback was given about whether or not the responses were correct.

At the end of year 1 and year 2, VJ was given a neuropsychological assessment using measures reported in the initial and post-intervention assessments in the original study, so that his results on the recall task could be viewed in the context of any observed changes in his cognitive functioning. VJ and his sister completed self-report measures used in the earlier study, to allow an evaluation

---

[1] VJ is designated "Participant A" in Clare et al. (2000).

of mood and carer strain. Neuroimaging data from 3-D magnetic resonance imaging (MRI) scans carried out at the end of year 1 and year 2 were also available.

At the end of year 2, VJ expressed a desire to resume practice of the face–name associations. He was therefore given an album containing all the photographs and names so that he could refer to it whenever he wished.

Materials

The materials used in the study were 13 Polaroid photographs of members of VJ's club. One photograph, of a club member who had died, was removed from the original set of 14 at the request of VJ's sister, leaving a total of 10 trained and 3 untrained items.

Design and analysis

This naturalistic follow-up study yielded 44 recall scores obtained at weekly intervals in year 1, and 12 scores obtained at monthly intervals in year 2. There were eight occasions during year 1 where visits were not possible due to holidays or illness. The scores on the free recall trials were out of a maximum of 10 for trained and 3 for untrained items. Neuropsychological test scores and self-report scores on a range of measures were collected to allow an evaluation of concurrent changes in cognitive functioning and well-being.

Analysis of the data for both trained and untrained items began with visual inspection of the graphs of year 1 and year 2 scores. Linear trend lines based on regression equations derived from a least-squares model were included in the graphs to assist with the visual inspection. Kendall's tau was used as a non-parametric measure of trend for each category of items in each year. A matched set of 12 scores for year 1 and year 2 was selected by calculating the mean score for trials within each calendar month of year 1, thus yielding 12 monthly mean scores for year 1 corresponding to those for the year 2 monthly trials. The matched set of scores for year 1 and year 2 were then analysed using the ITSACORR interrupted time-series analysis method described by Crosbie (1993). A summary of the matched set of scores is shown in Appendix A.

Standardised measures

The neuropsychological assessment covered general cognitive functioning, visuospatial perception, and memory, using the following measures.

General cognitive functioning:

- Mini-Mental State Examination (MMSE; Folstein, Folstein, & McHugh, 1975).
- National Adult Reading Test (NART; Nelson & Willison, 1991).

- Standard Progressive Matrices (SPM; Raven, 1976).
- Speed and Capacity of Language Processing (SCOLP; Baddeley, Emslie, & Nimmo-Smith, 1992).

Visuospatial perception:

- Visual Object and Space Perception Battery (VOSP; Warrington & James, 1991).
- Unfamiliar Face Matching (Benton, Hamsher, Varney, & Spreen, 1983).

Working memory:

- Digit span, forwards and backwards.

Episodic memory:
- Rivermead Behavioural Memory Test (RBMT; Wilson, Cockburn, & Baddeley, 1985).
- Doors and People (Baddeley, Emslie, & Nimmo-Smith, 1994).

Semantic memory:

- Famous Faces (Greene & Hodges, 1996).
- Famous Names (Greene & Hodges, 1996).

The self-report measures were chosen in order to assess perceptions of memory problems, behaviour, affect and caregiver strain. The following measures were used:

- Memory Symptoms Questionnaire (Kapur & Pearson, 1983) – VJ and his sister each independently rated VJ's memory functioning on this scale.
- Hospital Anxiety and Depression Scale (HADS; Snaith & Zigmond, 1994)—VJ and his sister each completed this scale on their own behalf.
- Caregiver Strain Index (CSI; Robinson, 1983)—VJ's sister rated her own level of strain on this scale.

RESULTS

The results of the neuropsychological assessment, self-report measures, and neuroimaging will be presented first, followed by the results for the recall trials.

Neuropsychological and questionnaire measures

Details of the neuropsychological assessments are summarised in Table 1. The initial and post-intervention neuropsychological assessments carried out in 1996 and 1997 suggested that VJ's general cognitive abilities before the onset of DAT were likely to have been in the high average range, and showed that his current functioning remained above average, although speed of information

TABLE 1
VJ: Results of neuropsychological assessments

Test	(max. possible score)	Initial June 1996 Raw	SS	Post-intervention March 1997 Raw	SS	Interim October 1998 Raw	SS	Final October 1999 Raw	SS
MMSE	(30)	25		26		23		22	
NART errors[1]	(50)	15	112			17	108	20	106
Ravens SPM[1]	(60)	37	118	30	107	32	110	30	107
SCOLP									
Spot the word	(60)	51		52		52		53	
Speed of information processing	(No. in 120 s)	37		31		23		22	
VOSP									
Shape detection	(20)					20		20	
Object decision	(20)					20		19	
Position discrimination	(20)					20		20	
Benton unfamiliar face matching	(54)			44				43	
Digit span (No. of digits)									
Forward		7						5	
Backward		5						4	
RBMT									
Standardised profile score	(24)	2	6				1		0
Story immediate	(21)	0				0		0	
Story delayed	(21)	0				0		0	

Test	(max. possible score)	Initial June 1996		Post-intervention March 1997		Interim October 1998		Final October 1999	
		Raw	SS	Raw	SS	Raw	SS	Raw	SS
Doors and People[2]									
Visual			5		5		4		5
Verbal			4		4		<4		<3
Recall			4		3		<3		<3
Recognition			6		5		4		3
Famous faces									
Identification	(50)	12.5						6.5	
Naming	(50)	5.5						0	
Famous names									
Recognition	(60)	49						53	
Identification	(60)	39.5						19	

[1]Standard Score equivalents for these tasks: M = 100 and SD = 15.
[2]Standard Scores for subtests of this task: M = 10 and SD = 3.
See text for abbreviations.

processing was mildly impaired. Perceptual skills, including processing of unfamiliar faces, were within the normal range. Memory was severely impaired and VJ had particular difficulty in identifying and naming famous people from photographs. There was little change between initial and post-intervention assessments apart from a mild decline in scores for abstract reasoning and speed of information processing.

When reassessed at the end of year 1 of the present study (1998), the most evident change was a further decline in scores for speed of information processing and episodic memory. General cognitive functioning remained stable, and perceptual skills remained within the normal range. At the end of year 2 (1999), VJ's scores were very similar to those achieved at the end of year 1. His digit span was lower than at the initial assessment in 1996, indicating a decline in auditory–verbal working memory. Ability to name and identify famous people from photographs had also declined further. While the ability to recognise famous names remained at the same level as in 1996, ability to give identifying information about the individuals concerned had also declined.

To summarise, while some aspects of cognitive functioning remained intact, especially lexical knowledge and perceptual skills, there was a gradual decline in abstract reasoning, speed of information processing, working memory, episodic memory, and semantic memory over the study period. MMSE scores, too, showed a mild decline.

The ratings made by VJ and his sister on the questionnaire measures are summarised in Table 2. At initial assessment, VJ rated his memory problems as more severe than did his sister. There was no report of anxiety, depression or caregiver strain. Over the study period VJ's own rating of the severity of his memory difficulties showed a mild decrease, while his sister's ratings remained fairly stable, so that at the end of the study period they each gave equivalent ratings of severity. Levels of anxiety and depression for both VJ and his sister remained within normal limits. VJ's sister did not report any significant increase in caregiver strain.

Informally, VJ and his sister reported some changes; for example, VJ now tended to accompany his sister to her various activities rather than remaining at home alone. Such changes did not seem to be viewed as a problem by either VJ or his sister, but were accepted as a useful adaptation to the situation. VJ continued to manage well at home, to drive in familiar locations, and to use the various strategies he had developed to assist his memory.

Neuroimaging findings

On first attending the memory clinic in 1993 VJ underwent CT and HMPAO-SPECT scanning. The CT scan was normal, in keeping with very early dementia of Alzheimer type, and the SPECT scan showed mild hypoperfusion

TABLE 2
Ratings made by VJ and his sister on the self-report measures

Measure	(Max. possible score)	Initial June 1996	Post-intervention March 1997	Interim October 1998	Final October 1999
MSQ					
VJ's self-rating	(20)	11	9	9	5
Carer's rating of VJ	(20)	6	4	3	5
HADS VJ's self-rating					
Anxiety	(21)	1	4	8	5
Depression	(21)	0	3	2	6
HADS carer's self-rating					
Anxiety	(21)	1	3	5	4
Depression	(21)	3	1	4	5
CSI					
Carer's self-rating	(13)	0	0	1	1

See text for abbreviations.

in the left temporal lobe. In November 1998 and September 1999 VJ underwent 3-D MRI scans as part of a study of structural brain imaging in the dementias. Assessment of coronal T_1 images revealed mild, but definite, bilateral hippocampal atrophy as indicated by enlargement of the temporal horn of the lateral ventricle and reduction in height of the hippocampal formation.

Recall trials

Scores on the weekly recall trials in year 1 are shown in Figure 1. For the 10 trained items, the number correct varied between 5 and 10, with a mean of 8. There was a barely perceptible trend towards slightly lower performance over the course of the year (Kendall's tau = −.066, NS). For the three untrained items, scores remained consistently at ceiling until the final three sessions, when on two occasions one name was not recalled (Kendall's tau = −.291, $p < .05$). Thus, there was little change in performance over the year, although a degree of variability in recall was evident for the trained items, but at the end of the year problems with the untrained items began to emerge.

The pattern observed in year 2 was somewhat different to that seen in year 1. Scores on the monthly recall trials in year 2 are shown in Figure 2. Scores for the 10 trained items ranged from 5–9, with a mean of 7.08. Again, a degree of variability was evident, with a phase of low scoring in the middle of the year, followed by a peak and another trough. However, a moderate trend towards lower scores was evident over the course of the year (Kendall's tau = −.461,

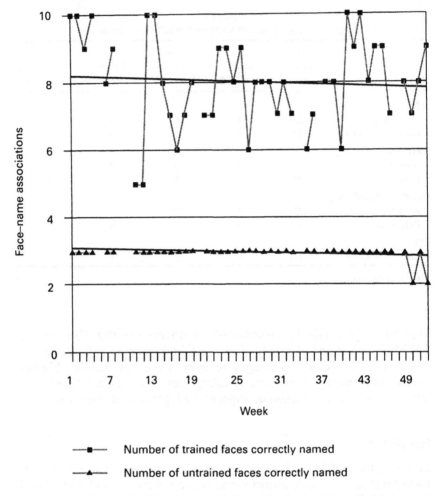

Number of trained faces correctly named

Number of untrained faces correctly named

Figure 1. Scores for recall of face–name associations achieved on weekly recall trials in year 1. Regression equations for the linear trend lines are as follows: trained items, $y = -0.0074x + 8.1962$, $R^2 = 0.0064$; untrained items, $y = -0.005x + 3.087$, $R^2 = 0.1231$.

$p < .05$). Scores for the three untrained items ranged from 1–3, with a mean of 2. Here, too, a trend towards lower scores was evident over the course of the year (Kendall's tau $= -.569$, $p < .05$).

Comparison of year 2 scores with the matched set of year 1 scores using ITSACORR showed a significant change in recall performance for untrained items [overall change: $F(2, 19) = 4.05$, $p < .05$; change in slope: $t_{19} = -2.837$, $p < 0.02$], but no significant change for trained items [overall change: $F(2, 19) = 1.52$, n.s.; change in slope: $t_{19} = -1.72$, n.s.].

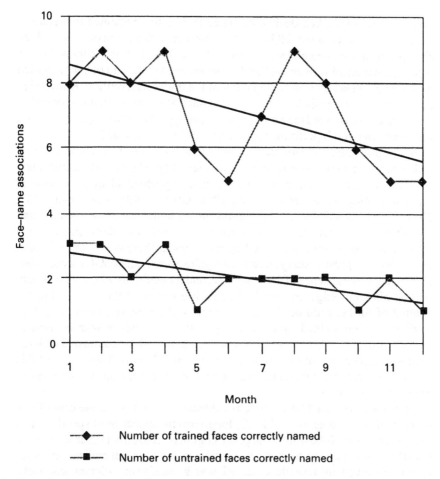

Figure 2. Scores for recall of face–name associations achieved on monthly recall trials in year 2. Regression equations for the linear trend lines are as follows: trained items, $y = -0.2692x + 8.8333$, $R^2 = 0.3585$; untrained items, $y = -0.1399x + 2.9091$, $R^2 = 0.4662$.

DISCUSSION

This naturalistic follow-up study evaluated the long-term maintenance of the effects of a cognitive rehabilitation intervention. In the initial intervention, VJ had learned the names of 11 members of his club, increasing his recall from 20% at baseline to 100% at 1, 3, 6, and 9 month follow-up. This success was supported by daily practice. The present study assessed what happened to his knowledge once daily practice was stopped, and showed that his learning was maintained to a considerable extent. During year 1 there was minimal decline, with a mean score of 80% correct. Scores for year 2 provided evidence of a somewhat more marked decline but nevertheless this remained moderate in nature, since scores never fell below 50% correct, with a mean of 71%, and the change was not statistically significant. VJ's performance on the trained items therefore remained well above baseline levels even at the end of year 2, which was nearly 3 years after the completion of the initial intervention. Knowledge of untrained, previously known items remained at ceiling until the very end of year 1, and then showed moderate decline during year 2, reflecting a significant difference in overall performance and rate of decline in year 2.

It was predicted on theoretical grounds that once information was successfully encoded and stored in memory, as achieved by VJ during the initial intervention, storage and retrieval should be able to proceed adequately, without rapid forgetting (Christensen et al., 1998; Glisky, 1998; Kopelman, 1985, 1992; Thoene & Glisky, 1995). The follow-up to the initial intervention had already demonstrated that maintenance was possible with daily practice, and VJ's performance remained at ceiling levels under these conditions (Clare et al., 1999). The present study showed that gains were maintained to a considerable extent in the absence of daily practice, under conditions where VJ was only putting his knowledge into use in the real-life setting of the club, and in the context of further mild decline in some areas of cognitive functioning. This decline was highlighted by the development of difficulties with previously known names included in the set as untrained items, which contrasted with the relative maintenance of performance on the trained items. The results of this study, therefore, are consistent with predictions derived from the findings of experimental studies.

The study described here provides evidence that, at least in the case of one individual with a diagnosis of DAT, long-term maintenance of specific gains can be observed following a targeted cognitive rehabilitation intervention. Clearly it is necessary to exercise caution in drawing generalisations from results observed in a single case. VJ was a consistent, tolerant and well-organised man who acknowledged and accepted his memory problems and actively attempted to devise coping strategies to minimise their impact. Thus he may have been particularly amenable to an intervention of this type, and he was certainly highly motivated to participate. Nevertheless, similar levels of success have been demonstrated in initial interventions with other individuals (e.g., Clare et al., 2000), and the study indicates that long-term maintenance is possible. Future research on cognitive rehabilitation in DAT needs to incorporate long-term follow-up of participants to provide more evidence about maintenance of gains.

Future research will also need to address the question of the interaction between repeated testing and maintenance of gains. In the present study, no feedback on performance was provided during test trials. It is possible, however, that the test trials in themselves had a positive effect on performance (Landauer & Bjork, 1978). The differing frequencies of test trials may have contributed to the differential rates of decline in performance in year 1 and year 2, although the pattern of performance on untrained items indicates that this is not the whole story. This issue could be addressed, for example, by dividing the trained items into matched groups and varying the frequency of testing across the groups.

The possible interaction between frequency of testing and rates of decline also has a positive aspect. This relates to the clinical observation that continued input may be necessary after the end of a cognitive rehabilitation intervention to facilitate maintenance (Woods, 1996b; Bäckman, 1992). If a recall trial without feedback does indeed have the potential to improve performance, it is likely that a regular recall trial which incorporates feedback on performance would be a more effective way of maintaining performance. This does not necessarily require professional input; in many cases the procedure could be facilitated by a partner, friend, volunteer, care worker or other supporter, as appropriate, with professional back up available at intervals and when needed. For some people with early stage DAT, self-help methods may be sufficient.

It has been claimed that cognitive rehabilitation interventions result in depression and frustration. As the present study demonstrates, this is not necessarily so. The ratings made by VJ and his sister on the self-report measures provide no evidence of negative effects resulting either from the initial intervention or from the subsequent follow-up. On the contrary, VJ remained motivated to resume his regular practice of the face–name associations at the end of the follow-up study. He commented that he found it helpful to know the names because this enabled him to take an active role in club sessions. The intervention therefore met its target of being directly relevant to VJ's daily life, and this relevance remained important at the end of the present study. At the initial assessment in 1996 it had been noted that there might be a danger of withdrawal from participation in the club because of problems with remembering names. Clearly, this had not occurred, although it is not possible to determine the role played by the intervention in ensuring VJ's continued attendance. Future research needs to identify more precisely both the factors that may influence outcome and the broader impact of specific interventions.

The application of cognitive rehabilitation approaches in dementia has been criticised on the grounds that gains are not maintained beyond the immediate treatment session. The present study clearly refutes this suggestion. This finding is supported by the results of the small number of earlier studies reporting long-term follow-up data (e.g., Bourgeois, 1992; Clare et al., 2000). Evidence of this kind suggests that there is a rationale for evaluating the impact of well-designed and appropriately targeted cognitive rehabilitation interventions, which result in demonstrable changes in performance or behaviour, on quality of life and on the course of DAT.

The evidence presented here suggests that cognitive rehabilitation for people in the early stages of DAT should not be dismissed as ineffective or unhelpful. Cognitive rehabilitation may offer distinct benefits for some individuals and their families, and may contribute to ensuring that their psychological needs are met.

REFERENCES

Abrahams, J.P., & Camp, C.J. (1993). Maintenance and generalisation of object naming training in anomia associated with degenerative dementia. *Clinical Gerontologist, 12*, 57–72.

Bäckman, L. (1992). Memory training and memory improvement in Alzheimer's disease: Rules and exceptions. *Acta Neurologica Scandinavica, Supplement 139*, 84–89.

Bäckman, L. (1996). Utilizing compensatory task conditions for episodic memory in Alzheimer's disease. *Acta Neurologica Scandinavica, Supplement 165*, 109–113.

Baddeley, A.D., Emslie, H., & Nimmo-Smith, I. (1992). *Speed and capacity of language processing.* Bury St Edmunds, UK: Thames Valley Test Company.

Baddeley, A.D., Emslie, H., & Nimmo-Smith, I. (1994). *Doors and people: A test of visual and verbal recall and recognition.* Bury St Edmunds: Thames Valley Test Company.

Benton, A.L., Hamsher, K.D., Varney, N.R., & Spreen, O. (1983). *Contributions to neuropsychological assessment.* Oxford: Oxford University Press.

Bourgeois, M.S. (1990). Enhancing conversation skills in patients with Alzheimer's disease using a prosthetic memory aid. *Journal of Applied Behavior Analysis, 23*, 29–42.

Bourgeois, M.S. (1992). Evaluating memory wallets in conversations with persons with dementia. *Journal of Speech and Hearing Research, 35*, 1344–1357.

British Psychological Society, Professional Affairs Board (1994). *Psychological well-being for users of dementia services* (Division of Clinical Psychology Briefing Paper No. 2). Leicester, UK: British Psychological Society.

Camp, C.J. (1989). Facilitation of new learning in Alzheimer's disease. In G. Gilmore, P. Whitehouse, & M. Wykle (Eds.), *Memory and aging: Theory, research and practice* (pp. 212–225). New York: Springer.

Christensen, H., Kopelman, M.D., Stanhope, N., Lorentz, L., & Owen, P. (1998). Rates of forgetting in Alzheimer dementia. *Neuropsychologia, 36*, 547–557.

Clare, L. (1999). Memory rehabilitation in early Alzheimer's disease. *Journal of Dementia Care, 7*, 33–38.

Clare, L., Wilson, B.A., Breen, K., & Hodges, J.R. (1999). Errorless learning of face–name associations in early Alzheimer's disease. *Neurocase, 5*, 37–46.

Clare, L., Wilson, B.A., Carter, G., Gosses, A., Breen, K., & Hodges, J.R. (2000). Intervening with everyday memory problems in early Alzheimer's disease: An errorless learning approach. *Journal of Clinical and Experimental Neuropsychology, 22*, 132–146.

Cottrell, V., & Schulz, R. (1993). The perspective of the patient with Alzheimer's disease: A neglected dimension of dementia research. *The Gerontologist, 33*, 205–211.

Crosbie, J. (1993). Interrupted time-series analysis with brief single-subject data. *Journal of Consulting and Clinical Psychology, 61*, 966–974.

Droes, R.M. (1997). Psychomotor group therapy for demented patients in the nursing home. In B.M.L. Miesen & G.M.M. Jones (Eds.), *Care-giving in dementia: Research and applications* (Vol. 2). London: Routledge.

Folstein, M.F., Folstein, S.E., & McHugh, P.R. (1975). "Mini-mental state": A practical method for grading the cognitive state of patients for the clinician. *Journal of Psychiatric Research, 12*, 189–198.

Gatz, M., Fiske, A., Fox, L., Kaskie, B., Kasl-Godley, J.E., McCallum, T.J., & Wetherell, J.L. (1998). Empirically validated psychological treatments for older adults. *Journal of Mental Health and Aging, 4*, 9–45.

Glisky, E.L. (1998). Differential contribution of frontal and medial temporal lobes to memory: Evidence from focal lesions and normal aging. In N. Raz (Ed.), *The other side of the error term*. Amsterdam: Elsevier Science.

Graham, K.S., & Hodges, J.R. (1997). Differentiating the roles of the hippocampal complex and the neocortex in long-term memory storage: Evidence from the study of semantic dementia and Alzheimer's disease. *Neuropsychology, 11*, 77–89.

Greene, J., Baddeley, A., & Hodges, J. (1996). Analysis of the episodic memory deficit in early Alzheimer's disease: Evidence from the Doors and People test. *Neuropsychologia, 34*, 537–551.

Greene, J.D.W., & Hodges, J.R. (1996). Identification of famous names and famous faces in early Alzheimer's disease: Relationship to anterograde episodic and general semantic memory. *Brain, 119*, 111–128.

Hagberg, B. (1997). The dementias in a psychodynamic perspective. In B.M.L. Miesen & G.M.M. Jones (Eds.), *Care-giving in dementia: Research and applications*, (Vol. 2). London: Routledge.

Hill, R.D., Evankovich, K.D., Sheikh, J.I., & Yesavage, J.A. (1987). Imagery mnemonic training in a patient with primary degenerative dementia. *Psychology and Aging, 2*, 204–205.

Kapur, N. (1994). *Memory disorders in clinical practice*. Hove, UK: Lawrence Erlbaum Associates Ltd.

Kapur, N., & Pearson, D. (1983). Memory symptoms and memory performance of neurological patients. *British Journal of Psychology, 74*, 409–415.

Kitchener, E.G., Hodges, J.R., & McCarthy, R. (1998). Acquisition of post-morbid vocabulary and semantic facts in the absence of episodic memory. *Brain, 121*, 1313–1327.

Kitwood, T. (1997). *Dementia reconsidered: The person comes first*. Buckingham, UK: Open University Press.

Kopelman, M.D. (1985). Rates of forgetting in Alzheimer-type dementia and Korsakoff's syndrome. *Neuropsychologia, 23*, 623–638.

Kopelman, M.D. (1992). Storage, forgetting and retrieval in the anterograde and retrograde amnesia of Alzheimer dementia. In L. Bäckman (Ed.), *Memory functioning in dementia*. Amsterdam: Elsevier Science.

Landauer, T.K., & Bjork, R.A. (1978). Optimum rehearsal patterns and name learning. In K.M. Gruneberg, P.E. Morris, & R.N. Sykes (Eds.), *Practical aspects of memory* (pp. 625–632). New York: Academic Press.

Little, A.G., Volans, P.J., Hemsley, D.R., & Levy, R. (1986). The retention of new information in senile dementia. *British Journal of Clinical Psychology, 25*, 71–72.

McEvoy, C.L., & Patterson, R.L. (1986). Behavioral treatment of deficit skills in dementia patients. *Gerontologist, 26*, 475–478.

Nadel, L., & Moscovitch, M. (1997). Memory consolidation, retrograde amnesia and the hippocampal complex. *Current Opinion in Neurobiology, 7*, 217–227.

Nelson, H.E., & Willison, J.R. (1991). *National Adult Reading Test (NART)* (2nd ed.). Windsor, UK: NFER-Nelson.

Rabins, P.V. (1996). Developing treatment guidelines for Alzheimer's disease and other dementias. *Journal of Clinical Psychiatry, 57*, 37–38.

Raven, J.C. (1976). *Standard progressive matrices*. Oxford: Oxford Psychologists Press.

Reifler, B.V., & Larson, E. (1990). Excess disability in dementia of the Alzheimer's type. In E. Light & B.D. Lebowitz (Eds.), *Alzheimer's disease treatment and family stress*. New York: Hemisphere.

Robinson, B.C. (1983). Validation of a caregiver strain index. *Journal of Gerontology, 38*, 344–348.

Small, G.W., Rabins, P.V., Barry, P.P., Buckholtz, N.S., DeKosky, S.T., Ferris, S.H., Finkel, S.I., Gwyther, L.P., Khachaturian, Z.S., Lebowitz, B.D., McRae, T.D., Morris, J.C., Oakley, F., Schneider, L.S., Streim, J.E., Sunderland, T., Teri, L.A., & Tune, L.E. (1997). Diagnosis and treatment of Alzheimer disease and related disorders: Consensus statement of the American Association for Geriatric Psychiatry, the Alzheimer's Association and the American Geriatric Society. *Journal of the American Medical Association, 278*, 1363–1371.

Snaith, R.P., & Zigmond, A.S. (1994). *The Hospital Anxiety and Depression Scale*. Windsor, UK: NFER-Nelson.

Squire, L.R., & Knowlton, B.J. (1995). Memory, hippocampus, and brain systems. In M. Gazzaniga (Ed.), *The cognitive neurosciences*. Boston, MA: MIT Press.

Thoene, A.I.T., & Glisky, E.L. (1995). Learning of face–name associations in memory impaired patients: A comparison of different training procedures. *Journal of the International Neuropsychological Society, 1*, 29–38.

Vargha-Khadem, F., Gadian, D.G., Watkins, K.E., Connelly, A., Paesschen, W.V., & Mishkin, M. (1997). Differential effects of early hippocampal pathology on episodic and semantic memory. *Science, 277*, 376–380.

Warrington, E., & James, M. (1991). *Visual object and space perception battery*. Bury St Edmunds, UK: Thames Valley Test Company.

Wilson, B.A., Cockburn, J., & Baddeley, A.D. (1985). *The Rivermead Behavioural Memory Test*. Bury St Edmunds, UK: Thames Valley Test Company.

Woods, R.T. (1996a). Cognitive approaches to the management of dementia. In R.G. Morris (Ed.), *The cognitive neuropsychology of alzheimer-type dementia*. Oxford: Oxford University Press.

Woods, R.T. (1996b). Psychological "therapies" in dementia. In R.T. Woods (Ed.), *Handbook of the clinical psychology of ageing* (pp. 575–600). Chichester, UK: John Wiley.

Woods, R.T., & Britton, P.G. (1985). *Clinical psychology with the elderly*. London: Croom Helm.

Manuscript received December 1999
Revised manuscript received October 2000

APPENDIX A

Matched set of year 1 and year 2 scores used in the time-series analysis

	Year 1			Year 2	
Month	Trained items mean (max 10)	Untrained items mean (max 3)	Month	Trained items score (max 10)	Untrained items score (max 3)
1	9.75	3	1	8	3
2	8.5	3	2	9	3
3	7.5	3	3	8	2
4	7	3	4	9	3
5	7.33	3	5	6	1
6	8.2	3	6	5	2
7	7.75	3	7	7	2
8	7	3	8	9	2
9	7.25	3	9	8	2
10	9.25	3	10	6	1
11	8.25	3	11	5	2
12	7	2.33	12	5	1

From efficacy to effectiveness to diffusion: Making the transitions in dementia intervention research

Cameron J. Camp

Myers Research Institute of the Menorah Park Center for Senior Living, Beachwood, Ohio, USA

Translating research outcomes into clinical application in neuropsychological rehabilitation is seen as requiring two critical transitions. The first is a transition in research outcome emphasis from efficacy (demonstrating that an intervention works under controlled conditions) to effectiveness (demonstrating that an intervention works as implemented in real-world contexts). The second is a transition in which effective interventions are required to be diffused within caregiving systems to enable them to be implemented on a large scale. Examples of these transitions are provided within the context of designing interventions for persons with dementia.

INTRODUCTION

Ideally, a new technology, directed at a societal problem, would first be developed and shown to be effective in an applied research setting; the generality of that effective technology would then be demonstrated; finally, the technology would be applied on a larger scale, with continued measurement of its generality and effectiveness. ... (behavioural) technologies mostly lie unnoticed in our ever-proliferating professional journals.   (Stolz, 1981, p. 491–492)

Correspondence should be addressed to Cameron J. Camp, Myers Research Institute, 27100 Cedar Road, Beachwood, OH 44122 (216) 831-5452 x 133; fax: (216) 595-7331; e-mail: Ccamp@Myersri.com.

Support for preparation of this manuscript was provided by Grant TRGC-95-016 from the Alzheimer's Association, Grants 1R21 MH57851-01 and 1R25 MH57418-01 from the National Institutes of Mental Health, and Grant 1R01 AG1790-01 from the National Institute on Aging to the author.

The focus of this paper is on making transitions. Researchers in neuro-psychological rehabilitation are well-trained to design interventions and assess their efficacy in persons with neurological disorders. A premise of this paper is that this is a necessary but far from sufficient condition for interventions to impact the lives of large numbers of neurologically impaired individuals in positive and meaningful ways. To achieve such impact, intervention research must make two critical transitions. First, interventions that may have proven successful in tightly controlled studies must demonstrate that they can work in uncontrolled, real-world settings. This is the transition from efficacy to effec-tiveness. The distinction between efficacy and effectiveness, as well as criteria for designing effective interventions, will be examined. Second, once proven effective, interventions must be diffused within caregiving systems. The process of diffusion of interventions will be discussed as well. This is the transi-tion from demonstrating effectiveness to making effective interventions acces-sible to large numbers of persons with neurological disorders. It is a second premise of this paper that interventions are not truly effective unless they are disseminated.

In order to help clarify these discussions, they will be framed within the context of designing interventions for persons with dementia. Additionally, examples of interventions for persons with dementia illustrating the process of making transitions from efficacy to effectiveness to diffusion will be provided. However, the issues involved in making such transitions should be relevant to all researchers interested in rehabilitation of neurological disorders.

EFFICACY VERSUS EFFECTIVENESS

A useful way to distinguish basic and applied research is to examine the distinc-tion between efficacy—which might be considered a paramount value for basic research, and effectiveness—a critical feature of applied research. Phillips and Knopman (1999), working from a health services research perspective, define these concepts thus (p. 228):

> Analyses of efficacy are probably best defined as inquiries into the likelihood that individuals in a defined population will benefit from a treatment when it is provided under ideal, or tightly controlled, conditions. Inquiries into effectiveness, in its broadest and most meaningful sense, investigate the distribution and impact of a treat-ment as it is employed in the everyday operation of the health care system.

It is noteworthy that this distinction between efficacy research and effective-ness research has been echoed in a recent description of research priorities formulated at the National Institute of Mental Health's Adult and Geriatric Treatment and Preventive Interventions Research Branch (Liebowitz & Rudorfer, 1998). These authors, working from a psychopharmacological research perspective, describe efficacy studies as research done under a "regulatory model", i.e., research tied to requirements of drug approval and registration. Studies conducted within this model, analogous to "basic" research in Cook and Campbell's (1979) scheme, place such a high premium on internal validity that (p. 1) ". . . the inclusions and exclusions are so limiting, the conditions of treatment delivery are so optimized, and the outcomes so narrowly defined, that generalization is virtually impossible". Thus, as with Cook and Campbell's description of basic research, external validity is given low priority in "intervention" research involving drugs when a regulatory model is used and efficacy is paramount. Further evidence for the premium placed on efficacy in this model is the use of specially trained clinicians to deliver the treatment to samples of "pure" disease cases.

On the other hand, Liebowitz and Rudorfer (1998) describe effectiveness research under a public health research model, such as that described by Phillips and Knopman (1999). Within this model, exclusion criteria are minimal, disorders are complex and include comorbidities, samples are designed to ensure generalisability and are usually large, and outcomes of treatment in real-world settings are the primary focus. This model parallels the applied research perspective described by Cook and Campbell (1979).

Liebowitz and Rudorfer (1998) went further to describe the charge of their new branch at the National Institute of Mental Health. They proposed that research should be supported that uses a public health model to accelerate the development and widespread application of treatments for mental disorders. They noted that small, well-controlled studies with high internal validity should be seen as a beginning, not an end. Treatment should be broadly defined to include pharmacotherapy, other somatic interventions, and psychosocial treatments that would include both rehabilitation and preventive interventions (including prevention of relapse and recurrence).

DESIGNING EFFECTIVE NEUROPSYCHOLOGICAL INTERVENTIONS FOR DEMENTIA

Assuming that a *Zeitgeist* is appearing that emphasises the need to demonstrate effectiveness in intervention research, how can persons in the field of neuropsychological rehabilitation take steps to ensure that their interventions will be effective? Consider the case of medication used to treat symptoms of dementia. Gifford et al. (1999) examined the use of tacrine, a cholinesterase inhibitor, to treat symptoms of Alzheimer's disease (AD) in nursing home settings. Using a database that included the entire population of nursing home residents in four states of the USA over a four-year period, they found that physicians often prescribed the drug for persons who did not fit the profile of those for whom the drug had been efficacious. The drug was often not administered at appropriate dosage levels, and was delivered intermittently rather than at the prescribed times (four times a day). Such a pattern is not necessarily surprising in what Phillips and Knopman (1999) describe as a "'neurologist-free' environment". Given that neuropsychologists may not often have regular access to environments serving persons with dementia, especially in the USA with its currently structured managed care environment, how can interventions be developed that will be effective within "neuropsychologist-free" environments?

The following is a set of parameters those hardy souls venturing into this domain should carefully consider. Effective interventions for dementia:

- *Must be robust enough to be effective when applied in a variety of settings, including long-term care, assisted living, and private homes.* Caregivers in a number of different settings have to deal with behavioural problems associated with dementia, such as repetitive vocalisations, aggressive behaviours, or apathy. Ideally, interventions should not be setting-specific, especially when the progression of dementia can cause individuals to be placed in different settings at different stages of dementia.
- *Usually must work with mixed dementias and other comorbidities.* Individuals in early stages of AD who fit inclusion criteria for regulatory model/clinical trials research are nonexistent in long-term care settings where dementia care commonly is being delivered. Comorbidity is the norm, while mixed dementias or dementias of relatively unknown aetiology are commonplace. Interventions for dementia, to be effective, must accommodate heterogeneous populations, and often must work across a range of levels and types of dementia.
- *Must be able to be delivered effectively by existing caregivers and professionals.* Psychologists and neuropsychologists will not be called upon to deliver interventions on a large scale. This will be done, instead, by rehabilitation and recreational/activities therapists, social workers, nursing staff, volunteers and family members. Interventions that cannot be successfully implemented with existing staffing will not be effective.
- *Must fit within existing health care system parameters.* Nursing staff, therapists, etc., sometimes work within severely constricted parameters. Demands of time, record-keeping, and day-to-day job responsibilities restrict their ability to implement new interventions. This is especially true if interventions require additional time or must be conducted outside of regular job routines. In addition, if supervisory staff do not value an intervention or see it as outside the normal duties of a staff member, the intervention will not be implemented, no matter how efficacious it might be.
- *Usually must be tied to reimbursement.* Either indirectly, as in the case where providing the intervention is seen as part of a staff member's

regular job routine, or directly, as when an intervention can be applied and then billed to a third party, interventions must be tied to reimbursement. To expect that interventions will be implemented with persons with dementia over and above regular job routines or free of charge by professionals under severe pressure to meet quotas for billable hours is naïve.

The above conditions may be thought of as necessary for interventions developed by applied research to be effective, but they are not sufficient. In order to have a widespread impact, researchers must deal with the issue of diffusion of interventions into caregiving systems.

DIFFUSION OF INTERVENTIONS

Charness (1998) discussed the issue of the diffusion of knowledge as it relates to applied gerontological research, and many of his points are germane to the current discussion. He concluded that successful diffusion of knowledge, in general, depends on four critical features:

- *Science/engineering*: Does the intervention work as intended? Note that the original design of the telephone was substantially revamped by Thomas Edison before it could be made commercially viable (e.g., Edison separated transmission and reception functions within the device).
- *Infrastructure:* Does an infrastructure exist that would allow widespread access to new information or technology?
- *Price*: Will the price allow widespread access to and adoption of the new knowledge? A variety of forces, including competition in the marketplace, marketing and perhaps advertising strategies, manufacturing techniques, etc., influence this feature.
- *Standards*: Will standards be required and/or adopted in order for the knowledge to be widely diffused? Examples of this issue include adoption of standards for computer software and floppy disk formatting, Betamax vs. VHS for videotape recorders, etc.

Charness, using examples from diffusion of knowledge about aging and performance derived from ongoing research efforts, estimated that the likely impact of conference presentations and academic publications on older adults in general was slight. Diffusing knowledge thorough popular media and trade journals was likely to have moderate to high impact, with legislation having the highest impact on the everyday lives of older adults (see Stolz, 1981 for examples of legislation being influenced—or not—by applied psychological research). With regard to patents and products, effects on older adults were estimated to be slight unless these were carefully marketed.

There is a clear lesson to be learned from Charness' observations, reinforced by our experience in designing interventions for dementia. It is this: simply demonstrating its efficacy under ideal conditions, or even its effectiveness in a real-world setting, is not sufficient for an intervention to be successfully diffused within existing systems providing care to persons with dementia. Camp (1999b) made a similar point (p. 180):

> The lab-based, treatment efficacy approach to intervention research can identify interventions that are potentially useful. However, unless interventions can be utilized by target populations . . . such interventions may not be effective. External validity becomes paramount if memory interventions are to have any sort of meaningful impact on the lives of older adults. It is possible to create effective memory interventions, but the transition from efficacious to effective treatment can only take place in real-world settings, and must produce sufficient return for the time and effort expended in their implementation.

Family members, nursing staff, social workers, rehabilitation professionals, etc., who deliver care to persons with dementia almost universally will not translate research findings published in journals or presented at conferences into dementia care practice. In real-world contexts, interventions can be viewed as products that must be marketed, and that are expected to work "right out of the box". Even if a successful intervention/product exists, it must be made accessible to its target population/market. And as is the case with many products, there must also be a support system and training available for those who use the intervention. In order to illustrate these points, two examples describing attempts to transform findings from research into widely disseminated interventions will be described.

MODELS FOR MAKING TRANSITIONS

Case study 1: Spaced-retrieval, a memory intervention

One approach for transforming research findings is to use basic research findings to develop a treatment efficacy study, followed by treatment effectiveness studies. An example of this is the case of spaced-retrieval (SR). SR is a memory intervention in which information is successfully recalled at expanding intervals (e.g., immediate recall, recall after a 10-s interval, followed by recall after a 20-s interval, followed by a recall after intervals of 30 s, 1 min, 2 min, 4 min, etc.) If a respondent fails at a recall attempt, the person is provided the correct response and asked to recall it immediately. Then, the next interval is shortened to that of the last successful recall interval. SR has been called a shaping technology applied to memory (Bjork, 1988). (For an extensive review of the development of SR as a memory intervention, as well as discussion of the theoretical basis of SR, the reader is referred to Camp, Bird, & Cherry, 2000).

First developed as an efficacy study using college students as participants (Landauer & Bjork, 1978), SR was later adapted for use with cognitively impaired populations (Camp, 1989; Moffat, 1989; Schacter, Rich, & Stampp, 1985). Camp and his colleagues (Camp, Foss, O'Hanlon, & Stevens, 1996a; Camp, Foss, Stevens, & O'Hanlon, 1996b), in a larger study using persons meeting clinical criteria for diagnosis of probable AD (McKhann et al., 1984), demonstrated the efficacy of the intervention. In that study, persons with AD were trained to remember to "redeem" coupons for money across intervals lasting seven days and to use a calendar to perform daily activities such as chores or keeping appointments. Other efficacy studies on a smaller scale have also been conducted (e.g., Cherry & Simmons-D'Gerolamo, 1999; Cherry, Simmons, & Camp, 1999; McKitrick, Camp, & Black, 1992; Riley, 1992).

In an attempt to make the transition from efficacy to effectiveness in the implementation of SR, Brush and Camp studied the effects of applying SR to specific clinical goals of speech/language pathologists (Brush & Camp, 1998a, 1998b, 1999). In their studies, long-term care residents with dementia were successfully trained by speech/language pathologists to meet goals ranging from remembering a room number to using a daily routine list to remembering to take a swallow of liquid after eating a bite of solid food (a treatment for dysphagia).

We are currently engaged in a large-scale, multi-site study to develop SR as a "standard practice" intervention that can be implemented as a billable procedure by speech/language pathologists within the context of their usual therapy sessions (National Institute of Aging Grant 1R01 AG1790-01). If successful, the study will demonstrate that SR is an effective intervention, and dissemination of the intervention will begin. In anticipation of the dissemination process, a manual describing how SR can be used to meet rehabilitation goals across a number of therapeutic disciplines has been developed (Brush & Camp, 1998c).

Initial results of studies examining the effects of SR in meeting therapeutic goals have been very encouraging. It appears that the SR intervention has the characteristic of Charness' (1998) four critical features. If ongoing research helps refine the SR technique as an effective therapeutic procedure, the criterion for the first critical feature—science/engineering—will be met. Second, an infrastructure exists to disseminate SR in the form of the discipline of speech/language pathology. In addition, our research has shown how SR can be utilised by other rehabilitation disciplines such as physical therapy, occupational therapy, music therapy, and art therapy (Brush & Camp, 1998c). We have also demonstrated that caregivers in home settings can implement SR successfully (McKitrick, 1993; McKitrick & Camp, 1993). Third, the price of the intervention should be nominal—that of reading a training manual, attending a training seminar, or acquiring a videotape. Finally, standards for rehabilitative treatment exist. Often, these standards are strongly influenced by reimbursement agencies, which require evidence of improvement in clients as a requisite for payment. SR can be implemented within the context of standard therapy sessions as a means of enhancing the effectiveness of sessions. For example, SR can be superimposed upon normal therapeutic procedures. Once an expanding retrieval schedule has been implemented, the intervals between recall trials for SR can be filled with other therapeutic activities to reach additional therapeutic goals. Thus, SR can augment current standard practices without significantly increasing time spent within a session.

Case study 2: Activities as interventions for dementia

In the case of SR, efficacy studies led in turn to effectiveness studies designed to lead to dissemination. An alternative scenario, implied in the opening quote by Stolz (1981), provides a variation on this model for making transitions towards an ultimate dissemination of research findings. In this scenario, findings from basic research are culled and incorporated into an intervention that is tested in an applied research setting, i.e., without the stringent controls of a laboratory and/or clinical trials format. External validity, in this second model, has a high value and research is conducted with generalisation of results in mind. In this case, while an intervention has its roots in basic research findings, it is created to meet an immediate need. The thinking behind this approach is that if an intervention cannot prove effective, whether or not it has demonstrated efficacy, it has little value in applied settings. This may be especially true in environments that are highly resistant to change. An example of this line of research is presented next, along with a discussion of its relationship to dissemination of research findings.

A strong argument has been made that interventions for dementia often should take the form of activities designed to accommodate deficits commonly associated with the disorder, in our laboratory (Camp, 2000; 1999a, b; Camp, Koss, & Judge, 1999; Camp & Mattern, 1999; Plautz & Camp, in press; Sterns & Camp, 1998; Vance, Camp, Kabacoff, & Greenwalt, 1996) and elsewhere (e.g., Bowlby, 1993; Buckbee, 1999; Burgio, et al., 1994; Dreher, 1997; Engleman, Altus, & Mathews, 1999; Rancourt, 1991; Weaverdyck, 1991). There are several reasons to recommend this approach. First, research has demonstrated that activities that effectively engage older adults with dementia can also reduce problematic behaviours associated with dementia, increase engagement with the physical and/or social environment, and/or produce more positive affect, in our laboratory (Camp et al., 1997; Judge, Camp, & Orsulic-Jeras, 2000; Orsulic-Jeras, Judge, & Camp, 2000a; Stevens, Camp, King, Bailey, & Hsu, 1998; Stevens, King, & Camp, 1993) and elsewhere (e.g., Aronstein, Olsen, & Schulman, 1996; Barinaga, 1998; Bocksnick & Hall,

1994; Bourgeois, 1992a; 1992b; 1993; Bourgeois, Burgio et al., 1997; Bowlby, 1993; Buettner, 1999; Buettner et al. 1996; Cohen-Mansfield & Werner, 1995; Engelman et al., 1999; Fazio, Chavin, & Clair, 1999; Martichuski, Bell, & Bradshaw, 1996; Volicer & Bloom-Charette, 1999; Ward, Los Kamp, & Newman, 1996; Zgola, 1987). The logic underlying these studies is that if an individual is constructively engaged in an activity that he or she deems interesting and meaningful, the person cannot simultaneously be engaging in "problematic" behaviours associated with dementia such as apathy, agitation, etc.

In addition, there exists an infrastructure to help disseminate this type of intervention. Much dementia care takes place in long-term care settings and adult day care centres. Most such facilities have staff whose primary job responsibility is provision of activities for persons with dementia. In many instances, employment of such personnel is required through licensing regulations. Thus, there is a ready conduit for effective interventions for dementia in the form of activities if this target population of caregivers can be reached. In addition, home health care workers and/or family members caring for individuals with dementia in home settings are a target market for activity-based interventions, and caregivers in these settings may show a preference for implementing activities compared to other psychosocial interventions.

An example of this type of intervention is seen in the evolution of an activity developed for persons with dementia in an adult day care centre who were unable to participate in traditional group activities such as bingo games because of their levels of cognitive impairment. An alternative small group activity was designed for these clients called "memory bingo". As described in detail elsewhere (Camp, 1999a, 1999b), this game was designed to fulfil several functions. The activity had to:

- Appeal to individuals across a large range of impairment, so that heterogeneous groups could take part. This would ensure that as clientele changed, the intervention could continue to be used.
- Be flexible enough that it could be used repeatedly without becoming "stale" to either clients or staff.
- Work with groups of various sizes, and potentially be expandable to very large groups. This would ensure that it could be used in situations where staffing was light and many clients were to be taking part in an activity.
- Be engaging to persons with dementia at the functional level of each individual. While group activities are commonplace in dementia care, the challenge is finding an activity that will not result in a number of participants sleeping, losing track of the activity, wandering away from the activity, or becoming disruptive.
- Provide both cognitive stimulation and social interaction. The development of the sense of community that is so important to good dementia

care in adult day care and long-term care settings depends on the formation of social groups and support systems.

• Accommodate the physical and cognitive changes associated with both aging and dementia.

Wilson (1997) notes that cognitive rehabilitation refers primarily to a process by which professionals work together with a client to optimise a client's level of functioning by alleviating, remediating, or circumventing deficits. In the case of dementia, we have argued for the use of such a cognitive rehabilitation perspective when designing interventions (Camp & Mattern, 1999; Sterns & Camp, 1998).

Creating the activity. The first version of the game was designed to be a highly simplified version of bingo. At the start of the game, four 4-inch × 6-inch index cards, called "answer cards", were placed in front of each participant. On each card were typed words belonging to a particular category, i.e., the "theme" of the particular game being played at that time. For example, the theme of a game might be old television shows. In this case, participants would have four answer cards, placed on the table in front of them in a 2 × 2 array, and each card would have the name of one television show from the past printed on it (e.g., "Have Gun, Will Travel" on the first card, "Father Knows Best" on the second, "I Love Lucy" on the third, and "The Honeymooners" on the fourth). The reverse side of each answer card was left blank. The person leading the game had a stack of "calling cards" that were to be read aloud, one at a time. For example, the game leader might read aloud a calling card containing the item "Gunsmoke". If any of the players had "Gunsmoke" on one of their four answer cards, they turned the matching answer card over so it was showing its blank side. This continued until someone had all blank cards, at which time a "bingo" was declared and a prize awarded. Cards were then taken up, and a new set of answer cards representing a different category was distributed.

The same procedures would be used for games involving other categories such as household items, song titles, famous people, national capitals, etc. Generally, two to three games were played within an hour's time, occupying up to eight persons with moderately advanced dementia. We also found that clients could utilise varying levels of complexity in the content of calling cards. Examples include: Matching the word on the calling card to a word on an answer card (e.g., calling card item "moon"—corresponding answer card item "moon"), completing a sentence or phrase (calling card item "Shine on harvest"—corresponding answer card item "moon"); or answering a question (calling card item "Neil Armstrong was the first person to walk here"—corresponding answer card item "moon"). Thus, the content of the games could be matched to the level of dementia seen in players, with easier stimuli used for more advanced dementia. We also found that participants could take turns reading items from the calling cards aloud to increase their participation and interest in the games.

Several components of the intervention are noteworthy. The clients quickly learned the game's procedures, which should be expected given that procedural or implicit memory is relatively spared far into the course of dementia (see Camp & Foss, 1997). For example, after playing a few sessions of the game, participants would turn over answer cards that matched the calling cards without having to be prompted, even if they stated that they could not remember having played the game before. Thus, a routine was quickly established and clients' attention was focused primarily on the cards and their content. The use of these materials and procedures also takes advantage of external prompts and aids provided by the cards and their spatial arrangement in front of the clients. Clients at any given time could see how many cards were blank and how many still had words. Thus, the intervention was designed to ameliorate disabilities associated with impairments in working memory and executive function. In addition, game participants spontaneously reminisced about item contents that access semantic memory, encouraged by fellow participants and staff.

Finally, attention was given to the construction of the written materials themselves. Following recommendations of Morrell and Echt (1997), as well as utilising feedback from previous studies involving creating activities for persons with dementia (Camp et al., 1997; Camp & Mattern, 1999), we utilised a sans serif typeface for all lettering. Answer cards were in 100 point type size, all in capital letters, while calling cards were printed in 48 point type size, using both upper case and lower case letters where grammatically appropriate. In addition, since persons with dementia have substantially worse spatial contrast sensitivity compared to healthy older adults (Gilmore, Turner, & Mendez, 1991; Gilmore & Whitehouse, 1995), and increasing stimulus contrast is necessary to reduce difficulties in visual stimulus identification in persons with dementia (e.g., Turner, 1990), we ensured that there was a high contrast between letters and background. Further, calling cards and answer cards were laminated using a non-glare material. The materials were therefore constructed to accommodate changes in the visual and perceptual systems associated with both aging and dementia.

In our initial pilot work, we observed that persons normally exhibiting inappropriate vocalisations and other problem behaviours stopped these once their attention focused on the game. Behaviours such as reading items from calling cards, scanning the answer cards, and helping each other if someone forgot to turn over an answer card replaced the disruptive behaviours. In one case, a woman living in an advanced dementia unit who constantly sought attention and made requests for assistance showed none of these behaviours while playing the game, although the behaviours immediately returned once the game was over and put away.

Initial studies using the activity. Once the initial form and procedures of the game had been created, memory bingo became integrated into a larger study of the effects of Montessori-based activities for persons at varying stages of dementia (Judge et al., 2000; Orsulic-Jeras et al., 2000a; Orsulic-Jeras, Schneider, & Camp, 2000b). Maria Montessori was an Italian physician and educator who applied principles of rehabilitation to the education of young children, a technique known as the Montessori Method. For example, the Montessori Method focuses on abilities that are available to the individual and the use of assistive devices/modifications to the environment to accommodate current levels of physical and cognitive functioning. Activities emphasise use of real-world materials, task analysis and task breakdown, practice with activities of daily living, sensory stimulation, working at one's own pace, and developmentally based programming, i.e., activities and materials link to one another progressing from concrete to abstract, simple to complex, etc. Activities are designed to be meaningful, to generate useful products, and to provide social roles for participants: individuals, small groups, or large groups. The use of the Montessori method as an effective approach to providing interventions for dementia has been discussed in our laboratory (e.g., Camp, 1999a; 1999b; Camp et al., 1997, 1999; Vance et al., 1996) and elsewhere (Buckbee, 1999; Dreher, 1997). Thus, memory bingo was part of a larger project involving Montessori-based activities for both individuals and groups of residents at varying stages of dementia. In this study, the game was used as a small group activity presented to persons with dementia in a number of settings, including adult day care and various long-term care units.

In the first setting, adult day care, 19 participants completed a nine-month study. Observational data were gathered when residents were taking part in Montessori-based activities, including memory bingo, and in regular unit programming over a nine-month period. Ten-minute (600-s) observation windows were used. (Details of our observational data recording system are presented in Judge et al., 2000; Orsulic-Jeras et al., 2000a, b; or can be obtained directly from the author.) Our primary focus for this initial study was to determine whether the intervention was better than standard long-term care programming (e.g., group exercise, group sing-along, reality orientation, etc.) at eliciting engagement with the physical and social environments of activities.

We operationally defined different forms of engagement, with a focus on constructive and passive engagement. Constructive engagement (CE) was defined as speaking or commenting and manipulating objects or gesturing that was appropriate to the activity. We contrasted constructive engagement with another form of engagement that we named passive engagement (PE), which was defined as passively observing any aspect of an ongoing activity without vocalising or exhibiting motor responses. Thus, we were interested in the total amount of time residents were engaged (constructive + passive engagement = total engagement) in activities, as well as assessing the different styles of engagement elicited by different activities. As reported elsewhere (Judge et al., 2000), Montessori-based activities elicited significantly more constructive engagement and less passive engagement than regular activities programming. With regard to memory bingo, four participants in adult day care took part in this Montessori-based activity and in regular unit programming. Data regarding their overall levels of observed engagement types are shown in Table 1.

For these four participants, Mini-Mental State Exam scores (MMSE; Folstein, Folstein, & McHugh, 1975) ranged from 12 to 23 (M = 19). All were diagnosed by a neuropsychologist using NINCDS-ADRDA criteria (McKhann et al., 1984) as having dementia: two as having possible AD, and two with mixed dementias.

Although more constructive engagement and less passive engagement were elicited by memory bingo compared to regular programming in this sample, a statistically significant effect was only found for total engagement (TE), t (3) = 2.3, $p < .05$ (one tailed). Although the sample was small, it was interesting to note that participants were either actively or passively engaged in memory bingo for almost the entire amount of observation time. In contrast, in regular programming, participants often engaged in off-task activities such as self-grooming, attempting to talk to passers-by, etc. Given that the adult day care setting where data were gathered placed a heavy emphasis on activities programming, and all participants are community-dwelling, we were interesting in examining the effects of memory bingo in long-term care settings,

TABLE 1

Means (and standard deviations) of observed time spent (in seconds) exhibiting Constructive Engagement (CE), Passive Engagement (PE), Total Engagement (TE), and Non-engagement (NE) by activity type by site

		Site		
Measure	Activity Type	ADC	SCU	LTC-A
CE	Memory Bingo	198[1] (137)	342 (113)	261 (58)
	Regular Programme	72 (74)	82 (37)	32 (24)
PE	Memory Bingo	402 (136)	258 (113)	316 (61
	Regular Programme	368 (115)	276 (138)	88 (74)
TE	Memory Bingo	600 (0.2)	600 (0)	578 (25)
	Regular Programme	440 (139)	358 (175)	120 (94)
NE	Memory Bingo	N/A	0 (0)	12 (27)
	Regular Programme	N/A	74 (74)	148 (63)

[1] 600 total seconds were possible (10-minute observations).

ADC, adult day care; SCU, special care unit for dementia residents; LTC-A, long-term care unit for advanced dementia.

where cognitive and physical functioning are generally lower than in adult day care populations.

The second setting was a special care unit (SCU) designed for persons with early to moderate stages of dementia. Here, 25 residents took part in the programme over a period of nine months. As reported in Orsulic-Jeras, Schneider, and Camp (2000b), and as was the case with the first study, residents on the SCU exhibited significantly more constructive and passive engagement in Montessori-based programming than in regular activities programming.

Four residents on the SCU took part in this activity. MMSE scores for these persons ranged from 5 to 20 (M = 12). All were diagnosed by a neuro-psychologist using NINCDS-ADRDA criteria as having dementia: two as having probable AD, one with possible AD, and one with possible vascular dementia.

In this setting, in addition to constructive and passive engagement, we also measured non-engagement (NE), defined as sleeping or staring blankly into space (i.e., not visually examining any part of the environment) for a period of longer than 10 seconds. This construct can be viewed as one of the behavioural manifestations of apathy, a common behavioural problem in persons with AD and related forms of dementia (Mega, Cummings, Fiorello, & Gornbein, 1996). A previous study using Montessori-based intergenerational programming had shown that non-engagement seen in residents of an SCU could be significantly reduced through effective activity programming (Camp et al., 1997). For the overall (N = 25) sample, relatively little non-engagement was seen on the unit during activities, but when it occurred it did so exclusively during regular programming.

Overall results for memory bingo participants are shown in Table 1. Memory bingo was exceptionally good at eliciting engagement, with all participants engaging in the activity in some form in all memory bingo sessions (M = 600 s across all observation windows). Within regular SCU programming, less total engagement was seen (M = 357 s across all observation windows), a difference that was statistically significant, t (3) = 2.8, $p < .05$. This effect was primarily the result of a significant difference in levels of constructive engagement in the memory bingo activity (M = 342 s) compared to regular SCU activity programming (M = 82 s), t (3) = 4.0, $p < .01$. The difference for passive engagement did not reach significance.

With regard to non-engagement, only three of the four residents displayed this behaviour during regular SCU programming, and its occurrence was of low frequency (M = 20, 128, and 147 s, respectively). However, non-engagement was never observed during memory bingo.

In the third setting, a long-term care unit for persons with advanced dementia, 16 residents took part in a nine-month study. As reported in Orsulic-Jeras et al. (2000a), significantly more constructive engagement and less passive engagement was associated with taking part in Montessori-based programming compared to regular programming, replicating previous findings.

Five older residents took part in memory bingo on this unit. MMSE scores for these persons ranged from 8 to 15 (M = 12). All were diagnosed by a neuropsychologist as having dementia: one as having probable AD, two with possible AD, one with probable vascular dementia, and one with possible vascular dementia. In addition, in this setting we trained activities staff to implement the game, and all observations were made while activities staff were conducting memory bingo as part of a regularly scheduled activity event for the unit. We did this to determine if the intervention had the potential to be effective as well as efficacious. Again, observations were taken over a nine-month period and memory bingo was part of a larger project involving Montessori-based activities for both individuals and groups of residents at varying stages of dementia. Results are shown in Table 1.

As before, memory bingo elicited an extremely high (M = 578 s) level of total engagement, and was significantly greater than during regular unit programming (M = 120 s), t (4) = 11.7, $p < .001$. Compared to the SCU residents, persons on this advanced dementia unit were substantially less likely to be engaged during regular activities programming. All of these residents demonstrated non-engagement during regular programming as well, ranging from an average of 68 s to 242 s per 600-min window, while only one of these residents showed non-engagement during memory bingo (M = 61 s). Memory bingo was associated with significantly more CE and PE, and less NE, than regular programming on this unit.

Staff were extremely positive in their assessment of the intervention, its utility, and its ability to "work". They also noted that problem behaviours such as disruptive vocalisations did not occur when residents were taking part in memory bingo. (It is extremely difficult for a person to be effectively engaged in an activity and simultaneously exhibiting problem behaviours.) As a result, it appeared that memory bingo had the potential to be an effective intervention for persons with dementia. At this point, we were interested in attempting to make the transition to diffusion of the intervention.

Commercialising the intervention

These small studies provided evidence that the intervention was quite success-ful at engaging persons with dementia of varying aetiology who were not engaged to the same extent or quality during regular activities programming in diverse settings. The original version of the game/intervention has since become a staple of programming by regular activities staff within our long-term care and adult day care facilities. Staff find the activity easy to learn and implement, while older adults with dementia learn the procedures after only a few sessions and enjoy both the content of the games as well as the social interactions during games. The original version of the game was not commercialised, and needed modifications in order to be marketed successfully.

We are currently exploring the commercial feasibility and potential of the game and working with a business enterprise to develop an improved prototype of the activity. Instructional materials will be developed so that activities and caregiving staff can implement the game quickly and with minimal training. In addition, instructions will be provided on how to include descriptions of the intervention in plans of care and documentation related to reimbursement. Of course, we will assess the effectiveness of this form of the intervention through research efforts before we begin the process of its diffusion.

With regard to Charness' (1998) critical features for diffusion, we have attempted to ensure that the intervention will work as intended by attempting to use a human factors approach to the design of the intervention, including accommodations for physical and cognitive declines seen in populations with dementia. As mentioned previously, an infrastructure exists for disseminating the intervention through activities staff in long-term care, assisted living, and adult day care settings, as well as through caregivers of persons with dementia living in home settings. Use of inexpensive materials that can be easily mass-produced will help keep the price of the game accessible. While no standards within the industry exist formally, there is an assumption within long-term care, assisted living facilities, and adult day care settings that activities staff must be able to work with large groups of residents or clients. When these persons also have dementia, it is often challenging to keep such persons engaged in group activities. Thus, the "industry standard" of working with large groups of older adults, many of whom have dementia, often coupled with a lack of activities designed to enable such persons to engage constructively in group activities, bodes well for our ability to disseminate the intervention. However, as we attempt to diffuse the intervention in a way that is similar to marketing of a product, we are finding that other skills are needed to ensure that large numbers of persons with dementia might benefit from our work.

Skills/expertise needed for diffusion of interventions

If the model for dissemination of interventions for persons with dementia depicted here has merit, it could also serve as a model for dissemination of neuropsychological rehabilitation interventions in general. Nor does commercialisation of products initially developed through scientific research, e.g., the Rivermead Behavioural Memory Test (Wilson, Cockburn, & Baddeley, 1985), preclude their continued use by basic and applied scientists. As was the case with Thomas Edison, who saw his inventions through the patent and marketing processes with great finesse, those who adopt this model must be more than just good scientist-practitioners. Expertise in a number areas currently absent from the formal training of neuropsychologists must be acquired, formally or informally, or purchased through consultants. A brief list of such areas could include:

- Intellectual property law.
- Marketing.
- Manufacturing processes.
- Cost-effectiveness analysis. This is needed to demonstrate that psycho-social interventions can be as or more effective, and as or less costly than pharmacological interventions, especially over long time frames and for large-scale interventions. (See Lombard, Haddock, Talcott, & Reynes, 1998, for a discussion of the role of cost-effectiveness analyses in psychological practice; see Vogt, 1994, for an interesting discussion of cost-effectiveness perspectives on preventative interventions.)
- Contracts.
- Patent/copyright procedures.
- Influencing public policy/legislation.
- Interacting with media and popular/trade publications. It is possible, of course, simply to publish or otherwise distribute research findings in the hopes that other enterprising individuals will find ways to distribute interventions effectively. Such a course runs several risks, including watching discoveries have no impact or be mismanaged/misused by persons not involved in their creation.

It is also important to remember that if staff do not implement an intervention appropriately (or at all), a problem arises that is an integral part of the intervention process. It is easy to publish an article, or give staff in-service training, and then blame caregivers when the intervention fails. Assigning blame may salve the conscience of researchers who develop an intervention, but it does nothing to enhance the quality of life of persons with dementia. If an intervention is not being used properly, it is our problem. Finding truly effective interventions involves:

- Working with and listening to caregivers.
- Developing training materials and methods necessary to make an intervention effective.
- Creating and becoming part of interdisciplinary teams and understanding their job constraints (Lichtenberg, 1994, 1998).
- Ultimately, working to influence the legislative and managerial systems that will enable interventions to be supported, accepted, and reimbursed on a large scale.

SUMMARY

Individuals providing care for persons with dementia and other neurological disorders, such as rehabilitation staff, recreational therapists, nursing staff, social workers, family members, and volunteers, require effective interventions. Such caregivers are faced with a host of problems when dealing with persons with dementia, their needs are often quite pressing, and they need positive results that can be discerned without resorting to statistical analyses. They deserve to be informed and assisted by researchers.

Persons conducting research involving dementia and other neurological disorders do so on many levels. Basic researchers develop a knowledge base that has the potential for application. Some applied researchers initially attempt to demonstrate the efficacy of interventions under conditions that are controlled as rigidly as possible. Their logic is that if an intervention does not prove efficacious under such conditions, it is not worth exporting to less controlled settings. Other applied researchers make external validity a high priority and attempt to demonstrate that interventions can be successfully applied (usually by research staff) in real-world settings, sometimes skipping the first step of demonstrating treatment efficacy.

Finding ways for researchers to provide assistance to caregivers has been the ultimate focus of this paper. This will require researchers to guide their work through a number of transitions. The outlines of a model for making these transitions was provided. Included in the outline were a number of recommendations for skills, including knowledge and/or expertise, which should be acquired by researchers but generally are not part of their formal training. Before researchers attempt to acquire such skills or provide it to students, however, a final transition must take place—a change of attitudes.

The first attitude that must be changed, as pointed out by an anonymous reviewer, is that of therapeutic nihilism. There is a widespread assumption that persons with dementia cannot learn new behaviours or skills, and therefore any treatment attempting to bring about change in such persons: (1) is doomed to failure; and (2) will provide only frustration for all concerned. This attitude can be seen in some family caregivers as well as paid caregivers, who assume that palliative care for dementia is the best that can be provided. It is also seen in rehabilitation professionals. In the USA, for example, speech and language pathologists as well as occupational and physical therapists often receive little training regarding methods to accommodate memory deficits seen in persons with dementia. This leads to self-fulfilling prophecies—the results of treatments given to persons with dementia are not maintained (due to no efforts or ineffective efforts to provide for memory deficits in this client population). Therefore, it appears obvious that efforts to provide treatment are futile. Similarly, recreational activity therapists are not trained to remediate memory deficits in persons with dementia (and can be placed in positions in long-term care facilities after receiving little or no training about dementia in general). These therapists often are required to document that large numbers of persons with dementia are exposed to activities programming, regardless of the level of participation or engagement exhibited by residents. Under such circumstances, these professionals can understandably adopt the attitude that most persons in their care will not exhibit high levels of engagement, and that this situation cannot be changed.

In addition, at least in the USA, staff of agencies controlling reimbursements for therapy often assume that persons with dementia have little or no capacity for improvement, especially if memory is involved in therapy. Therefore, it is possible for an effective treatment to be provided and yet have reimbursement for it denied solely on the grounds that the client had AD or some other dementing condition. Other barriers to provision of services exist as well. For example, in the USA, speech and language pathologists cannot bill for treatments aimed at improving memory. Memory improvement is solely the domain of occupational therapists. Goals for speech and language pathologists must involve improved communication, although overcoming memory deficits is generally a necessary precursor for improved communication to take place. Defences against providing effective rehabilitation for dementia are multi-layered and formidable.

A final change in attitude must occur in researchers. It will require that researchers be willing to follow their work beyond demonstration into dissemination. It will require that researchers think of intervention as a large-scale enterprise. It will require that researchers be willing to let their interventions be applied by non-researchers in settings without good experimental controls. Without this final transition, researchers will have to accept the strong possibility that their interventions may have no meaningful impact, or that they may lose control over their work. It is the contention of this paper that researchers owe it to patients and to themselves to make this final transition.

REFERENCES

Aronstein, Z., Olsen, R., & Schulman, E. (1996). The nursing assistants use of recreational interventions for behavioral management of residents with Alzheimer's disease. *American Journal of Alzheimer's Disease, May/June,* 26–31.

Barinaga, M. (1998). Alzheimer's treatment that works now. *Science, 282,* 1030.

Bjork, R.A. (1988). Retrieval practice and the maintenance of knowledge. In M. M. Gruneberg, P. Morris, & R. Sykes (Eds.), *Practical aspects of memory* (Vol. 2, pp. 396–401). London: Academic Press.

Bocksnick, J.G., & Hall, B.L. (1994). Recreation activity programming for the institutionalized older adult. *Activities, Adaptation, & Aging, 19,* 1–25.

Bourgeois, M. (1992a). *Conversing with memory impaired individuals using memory aids.* Gaylord, Michigan: Northern Speech Services.

Bourgeois, M. (1992b). Evaluating memory wallets in conversations with persons with dementia. *Journal of Speech and Hearing Research, 35,* 1344–1357.

Bourgeois, M. (1993). Effects of memory aids on the dyadic conversations of individuals with dementia. *Journal of Applied Behavior Analysis, 26,* 77–87.

Bourgeois, M., Burgio, L., Schulz, R., Beach, S., & Palmer, B. (1997). Modifying repetitive verbalizations of community-dwelling patients with AD. *The Gerontologist, 37,* 30–39.

Bowlby, C. (1993). *Therapeutic activities with persons disabled by Alzheimer's Disease and related disorders.* Gaithersburg, MD: Aspen.

Brook, R.H., & Lohr, K.N. (1985). Efficacy, effectiveness, variations, and quality: Boundary-crossing research. *Medical Care, 23,* 710–722.

Brush, J.A., & Camp, C.J. (1998a). Using spaced retrieval as an intervention during speech-language therapy. *Clinical Gerontologist, 19,* 51–64.

Brush, J.A., & Camp, C.J. (1998b). Using spaced retrieval to treat dysphagia in a long-term care resident with dementia. *Clinical Gerontologist, 19,* 96–99.

Brush, J.A., & Camp, C.J. (1998c). *A therapy technique for improving memory: Spaced retrieval.* Beachwood, OH: Menorah Park Center for Senior Living.

Brush, J.A., & Camp, C.J. (1999). Effective interventions for persons with dementia: Using spaced retrieval and Montessori techniques. *Neurophysiology and Neurogenic Speech and Language Disorders, 9,* 27–32.

Buckbee, C. (1999). Montessori methods enhance function. *Provider, 25,* 63–67.

Buettner, L.L. (1999). Simple pleasures: A multilevel sensorimotor intervention for nursing home residents with dementia. *American Journal of Alzheimer's Disease, 14,* 41–52.

Buettner, L.L., Lundegren, H., Lago, D., Farrell, P., & Smith, R. (1996). Therapeutic recreation as an intervention for persons with dementia and agitation: An efficacy study. *American Journal of Alzheimer's Disease, September/October,* 4–12.

Burgio, L.S., Scilley, K., Hardin, M., Janosky, J., Bonino, P., Slater, S.C., & Engberg, R. (1994). Studying disruptive vocalization and contextual factors in the nursing home using computer-assisted real-time observation. *Journals of Gerontology: Psychological Sciences, 49,* P230–P239.

Camp, C.J. (1989). Facilitation of new learning in Alzheimer's disease. In G.C. Gilmore, P.J. Whitehouse, & M.L. Wykle (Eds.), *Memory, aging, and dementia* (pp. 212–225). New York: Springer.

Camp, C.J. (Ed.) (1999a). *Montessori-based activities for persons with dementia: Volume 1.* Beachwood, OH: Menorah Park Center for Senior Living.

Camp, C.J. (1999b). Memory interventions for normal and pathological older adults. In R. Schulz, M.P. Lawton, & G. Maddox, (Eds.), *Annual review of gerontology and geriatrics* (Vol. 18, pp. 155–189). New York: Springer.

Camp, C.J. (2000). Clinical research in long-term care settings: What the future holds. In V. Molinari (Ed.), *Professional issues in long-term care.* New York: Hatherleigh.

Camp, C.J., Bird, M.J., & Cherry, K.E. (2000). Retrieval strategies as a rehabilitation aid for cognitive loss in pathological aging. In R.D. Hill, L. Bäckman, & A.S. Neely (Eds.), *Cognitive rehabilitation in old age* (pp. 224–248). New York: Oxford University Press.

Camp, C.J., & Foss, J.W. (1997). Designing ecologically valid memory interventions for persons with dementia. In D.G. Payne & F.G. Conrad (Eds.), *Intersections in basic and applied memory research* (pp. 311–325). Mahwah, NJ: Lawrence Erlbaum Associates Inc.

Camp, C.J., Foss, J.W., O'Hanlon, A.M., & Stevens, A.B. (1996a). Memory interventions for persons with dementia. *Applied Cognitive Psychology, 10,* 193–210.

Camp, C.J., Foss, J.W., Stevens, A.B., & O'Hanlon, A.M. (1996b). Improving prospective memory task performance in Alzheimer's disease. In M.A. Brandimonte, G.O. Einstein, & M.A. McDaniel (Eds.), *Prospective memory: Theory and applications* (pp. 351–367). Mahwah, NJ: Lawrence Erlbaum Associates Inc.

Camp, C.J., Judge, K.S., Bye, C.A., Fox, K.M., Bowden, J., Bell, M., Valencic, K., & Mattern, J.M. (1997). An intergenerational program for persons with dementia using Montessori methods. *Gerontologist, 37,* 688–692.

Camp, C. J., Koss, E., & Judge, K. S. (1999). Cognitive assessment in late stage dementia. In P. A. Lichtenberg (Ed.), *Handbook of clinical gerontology assessment* (pp. 442–467). New York: John Wiley.

Camp, C.J., & Mattern, J.M. (1999). Innovations in managing Alzheimer's disease. In D.E. Biegel & A. Blum (Eds.), *Innovations in practice and service delivery across the lifespan* (pp. 276–294). New York: Oxford University Press.

Charness, N. (1998). *How do we know if Roybals Centers are working?* Paper presented at the annual convention of the American Psychological Association, San Franciso, August, 1998.

Cherry, K.E., & Simmons-D'Gerolamo, S.S. (1999). Effects of a target object orientation task on recall in older adults with probable Alzheimer's disease. *Clinical Gerontologist, 20,* 39–62.

Cherry, K.E., Simmons, S.S., & Camp, C.J. (1999). Spaced-retrieval enhances memory in older adults with probable Alzheimer's disease. *Journal of Clinical Geropsychology, 5,* 159–175.

Cohen-Mansfield, J., & Warner, P. (1995). Environmental influences on agitation: An integrative summary of an observational study. *American Journal of Alzheimer's Care and Related Disorders and Research, 10,* 32–39.

Cook, T.D., & Campbell, D.T. (1979). *Quasi-experimentation: Design and analysis issues for field settings.* Chicago: Rand-McNally.

Dreher, B.B. (1997). Montessori and Alzheimer's: A partnership that works. *American Journal of Alzheimer's Disease, 12,* 138–140.

Engelman, K.K., Altus, D.D., & Mathews, R.M. (1999). Increasing engagement in daily activities by older adults with dementia. *Journal of Applied Behavioral Analysis, 32,* 107–110.

Fazio, S., Chavin, M., & Clair, A.A. (1999). Activity based Alzheimer care: A national training program. *American Journal of Alzheimer's Disease, 14,* 149–156.

Folstein, M.F., Folstein, S.E., & McHugh, P.R. (1975). Mini-mental state: A practical method of grading the cognitive state of patients for the clinician. *Journal of Psychiatry Research, 12,* 189–198.

Gifford, D.R., Lapane, K.L., Gambassi, G., Landi, F., & Mor, V. (1999). Tacrine use in nursing homes: Implications for prescribing new cholinesterase inhibitors. *Neurology, 50,* 238–244.

Gilmore, G.C., Turner, J.B., & Mendez, M. (1991). Contrast sensitivity and Alzheimer's disease: A comparison of two methods. *Optometry and Vision Science, 68,* 790–794.

Gilmore, G.C., & Whitehouse, P. (1995). Contrast sensitivity in Alzheimer's disease: A one-year longitudinal analysis. *Optometry and Vision Science, 72,* 83–91.

Judge, K.S., Camp, C.J., & Orsulic-Jeras, S. (2000). Use of Montessori-based activities for clients with dementia in adult day care: Effects on engagement. *American Journal of Alzheimer's Disease, 15,* 42–46.

Kaufman, M.M. (1994) Activity-based intervention in nursing home settings. In B.R. Bonder & M.B. Wagner, (Eds.), *Functional performance in older adults* (1st Ed., pp. 306–321). Philadelphia: F.A. Davis.

Landauer, T.K., & Bjork, R.A. (1978). Optimal rehearsal patterns and name learning. In M.M. Gruneberg, P.E. Harris, & R.N. Sykes (Eds.), *Practical aspects of memory* (pp. 625–632). New York: Academic Press.

Lichtenberg, P.A. (1994). *A guide to psychological practice in long-term care.* Binghamton, NY: The Haworth Press.

Lichtenberg, P.A. (1998). *Mental health practice in geriatric health care settings.* New York: The Haworth Press.

Liebowitz, B.D., & Rudorfer, M.D. (1998). Treatment research at the millennium: From efficacy to effectiveness. *Journal of Clinical Psychopharmacology, 18,* 1.

Lombard, D., Haddock, C.K., Talcott, G.W., & Reynes, R. (1998). Cost-effectiveness analysis: A primer for psychologists. *Applied and Preventive Psychology, 7,* 101–108.

Martichuski, D.K. Bell, P.A., & Bradshaw, B. (1996). Including small group activities in large special care units. *Journal of Applied Gerontology, 15,* 224–237.

McKhann, G., Drachman, D., Folstein, M., Katzman, R., Price, D., & Stadlan, E.M. (1984). Clinical diagnosis of Alzheimer's disease: Report of the NINCDS-ADRA Work Group under the auspices of the Department of Health and Human Services Task Force on Alzheimer's Disease. *Neurology, 34,* 939–944.

McKitrick, L.A. (1993). *Caregiver participation in word-retrieval training with anomic Alzheimer's disease patients.* Unpublished doctoral dissertation, University of New Orleans, Department of Psychology, New Orleans, LA, USA.

McKitrick, L.A., & Camp, C.J. (1993). Relearning the names of things: The spaced-retrieval intervention implemented by a caregiver. *Clinical Gerontologist, 14,* 60–62.

McKitrick, L.A., Camp, C.J., & Black, F.W. (1992). Prospective memory intervention in Alzheimer's Disease. *Journal of Gerontology: Psychological Sciences, 47,* 337–343.

Mega, M.S., Cummings, J.L., Fiorello, T., & Gornbein, J. (1996). The spectrum of behavioral changes in Alzheimer's disease. *Neurology, 46,* 130–135.

Moffat, N.J. (1989). Home-based cognitive rehabilitation with the elderly. In L.W. Poon, D.C. Rubin, & B.A. Wilson (Eds.), *Everyday cognition in adulthood and late life* (pp. 659–680). New York: Cambridge University Press.

Morrell, R.W., & Echt, K.V. (1997). Designing written instructions for older adults: Learning to use computers. In A.D. Fisk & W.A. Rogers (Eds.), *Handbook of human factors and the older adult* (pp. 335–362). San Diego: Academic Press.

Orsulic-Jeras, S., Judge, K.S., & Camp, C.J. (2000a). Montessori-based activities for long-term care residents with advanced dementia: Effects on engagement and affect. *The Gerontologist, 40,* 107–111.

Orsulic-Jeras, S., Schneider, N.M., & Camp, C.J. (2000b). Montessori-based activities for long-term care residents with dementia: Outcomes and implications for geriatric rehabilitation. *Topics in Geriatric Rehabilitation, 16,* 78–91.

Phillips, C.D., & Knopman, D.S. (1999). Neurology "with the bark off": Tacrine, nursing home residents, and health services research. *Neurology, 52,* 227–230.

Plautz, R.E., & Camp, C.J. (in press). Activities as agents for intervention and rehabilitation in long-term care. In B.R. Bonder & M.B. Wagner (Eds.), *Functional performance in older adults* (2nd edition). Philadelphia: F.A. Davis.

Rancourt, A.M. (1991). Programming quality services for older adults in long-term care facilities. *Activities, Adaptation, and Aging, 15,* 1–11.

Riley, K.P. (1992). Bridging the gap between researchers and clinicians: Methodological perspectives and choices. In R.L. West & J.D. Sinnott (Eds.), *Everyday memory and aging: Current research and methodology* (pp. 182–189). New York: Springer-Verlag.

Schacter, D.L., Rich, S.A., & Stampp, M.S. (1985). Remediation of memory disorders: Experimental evaluation of the spaced-retrieval technique. *Journal of Clinical and Experimental Neuropsychology, 7,* 70–96.

Sterns, H.L., & Camp, C.J. (1998). Applied gerontology. *Applied Psychology: An International Review, 47,* 175–198.

Stevens, A.B., Camp, C.J., King, C.A., Bailey, E.H., & Hsu, C. (1998). Effects of a staff implemented therapeutic group activity for adult day care clients. *Aging and Mental Health, 2,* 333–342.

Stevens, A.B., King, C.A., & Camp, C.J. (1993). Improving prose memory and social interaction using question asking reading with adult day care clients. *Educational Gerontology, 19,* 651–662.

Stolz, S.B. (1981). Adoption of innovations from applied behavioral research: Does anybody care? *Journal of Applied Behavior Analysis, 14,* 491–505.

Turner, J. (1990). *Visual perception in normal aging and Alzheimer's disease: Influences on picture naming and recognition.* Unpublished doctoral dissertation. Case Western Reserve University, Cleveland, Ohio, USA.

Vance, D., Camp, C., Kabacoff, M., & Greenwalt, L. (1996). Montessori methods: Innovative interventions for adults with Alzheimer's disease. *Montessori Life, 8,* 10–11.

Vogt, T.M. (1994). Cost-effectiveness of prevention programs for older people. *Generations, 18,* 63–68.

Volicer, L. & Bloom-Charette, L. (1999). *Enhancing the quality of life in advanced dementia.* Boston: University School of Medicine.

Ward, C.R., Los Kamp, L., & Newman, S. (1996). The effects of participation in an intergenerational program on the behavior of residents with dementia. *Activities, Adaptation, & Aging, 20,* 61–76.

Weaverdyck, S.E. (1991). Intervention to address dementia as a cognitive disorder. In D.H. Coons (Ed.), *Specialized dementia care units.* (pp. 224–244). Baltimore: Johns Hopkins University Press.

Wilson, B.A. (1997). Cognitive rehabilitation: How it is and how it might be. *Journal of the International Neuropsychological Society, 3,* 487–496.

Wilson, B.A., Cockburn, J., & Baddeley, A. D. (1985). *The Rivermead Behavioral Memory Test.* Bury St. Edmunds, UK: Thames Valley Test Company.

Zgola, J.M. (1987). *Doing things: A guide to programming activities for persons with Alzheimer's Disease and related disorders.* Baltimore: Johns Hopkins University Press.

Manuscript received August 1999
Revised manuscript received February 2000

Subject Index

For Product Safety Concerns and Information please contact our
EU representative GPSR@taylorandfrancis.com Taylor & Francis
Verlag GmbH, Kaufingerstraße 24, 80331 München, Germany